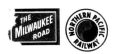

iewoehner

ιota 58367

Chasing
Dirt

Chasing

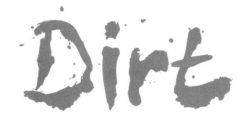

The American Pursuit
of Cleanliness

Suellen Hoy

New York   Oxford
OXFORD UNIVERSITY PRESS
1995

Oxford University Press

Oxford   New York
Athens   Aukland   Bangkok   Bombay
Calcutta   Cape Town   Dar es Salaam   Delhi
Florence   Hong Kong   Istanbul   Karachi
Kuala Lumpur   Madras   Madrid   Melbourne
Mexico City   Nairobi   Paris   Singapore
Taipei   Tokyo   Toronto

and associated companies in
Berlin   Ibadan

Published by Oxford University Press, Inc.,
200 Madison Avenue, New York, New York 10016

Oxford is a registered trademark of Oxford University Press

Library of Congress Cataloging-in-Publication Data
Hoy, Suellen
Chasing Dirt : the American pursuit of cleanliness / Suellen Hoy.
p. cm.   Includes bibliographical references and index.
ISBN 0-19-509420-4
1. Hygiene—United States—History.
2. Sanitation—United States—History.   I. Title.
RA780.H69   1995
614′.4′0973—dc20   94-27129

1 3 5 7 9 8 6 4 2

Printed in the United States of America
on acid-free paper

For Walter

Acknowledgments

Since 1986, when I began this book, many institutions and individuals have shown interest in it. I now have the welcome privilege of publicly thanking them. Although none of them is responsible for any of the book's shortcomings, all of them can rejoice with me in its completion.

I owe a very large debt of gratitude to the National Endowment for the Humanities and the Henry E. Huntington Library. Because of the generosity of both institutions, I was able to take a six-month leave of absence from the North Carolina Division of Archives and History in 1987 to do research on this book. Two years later, I was awarded a British Academy–Huntington Library Exchange Fellowship for a month's research at the British Library. In 1992-93 the National Endowment for the Humanities honored me with a year-long research fellowship; it enabled me to complete a draft. During 1989 I also benefited from a Newberry Library summer grant.

I am especially grateful for the services of so many librarians, archivists, and curators. Some I got to know, and I want to thank them personally: Linda Gregory, Marilyn Witulski, and Marcie Rarick, Interlibrary Loan Division, Hesburgh Library, University of Notre Dame; Archie Motley, Chicago Historical Society; Daniel B. May, Metropolitan Life Insurance Company Archives; Anne Remien, Fitzpatrick Brothers Archives; Darwin H. Stapleton and Thomas Rosenbaum, Rockefeller Archives Center; Mildred Gallik, Soap & Detergent Association Archives; Joel Wurl, Immigration History Research Center at the University of Minnesota; Edward M. Rider, Procter & Gamble Archives; Peter J. Fetterer, Kohler Company Archives; and Jeffrey K. Stine, Lu Ann Jones, and Pete Daniel, National Museum of American History, Smithsonian Institution. Many others, whom I do not know, also served me well—at the National Archives, Library of Congress, State Historical Society of Wisconsin, Schlesinger Library at Radcliffe College, Joseph Regenstein Library at the University of Chicago, Yale University Archives, Massachusetts Historical Society, New York Public Library, and New-York Historical Society. I must also thank my friends at the Little Professor Bookstore in South Bend, Indiana, from whom I purchased many books and received—along with the books—friendly inquiries about my progress and large helpings of good cheer.

For sharing their own experiences and cleanliness stories, for sending newspaper clippings and copies of journal articles, for giving me tips on archival collections and books to read, as well as their kind encouragement, I thank: Andrew Albanese, Barbara Allen, Charlene Avallone, Daniel E. Burnstein, Kathleen Biddick, JoAnne Brown, Robert D. Bugher, Drew Buscareno, Jane C. Busch, E. Wayne Carp, Peg Corwin and Bob Smith, John D'Emilio, Candace Falk, Paula Fass, Maureen Flanagan, Deborah Gardner, Brent D. Glass, Ruth Hardin, Sandra and Thomas C. Hoy, Barbara and Kenneth T. Jackson, Richard Jackson and John Nickerson, Alice Kessler-Harris, Alan M. Kraut, Gail and Jim Leonard, Karen Lystra, Michael P. McCarthy, John F. McClymer, Margaret Mac Curtain, O.P., John McClymer, Jeanne and James H. Madison, Barbara Mellon and Justin Kolb, Martin V. Melosi, Robert Middlekauff, Patricia Mooney-Melvin, Anna K. Nelson, Ronald L. Numbers, Gail O'Brien, Harold L. Platt, William S. Price, Jr., Carmine Prioli, Judith Raftery, Michael C. Robinson, Howard Rosen, Charles E. Rosenberg, Michal Rozbicki, Thomas Schlereth, Bruce Smith, Joel A. Tarr, Martha Vicinus, Louise Wade, Janet Welsh, O.P., Jacqueline S. Wilkie, and Bradley Young. I also thank the Dial Corp., Phoenix, for permitting use of the Dutch Cleanser trademark.

A smaller number of people, historians all, wrote letters of recommendation (not only to the institutions that supported me but also to several that did not) and, in many instances, read and commented on draft chapters of this book. I appreciate very much their continued support and thoughtful criticisms: James H. Cassedy, Ruth Schwartz Cowan, Jeffrey J. Crow, Donna Gabaccia, Lewis L. Gould, William E. Leuchtenburg, Arnita A. Jones, Ann Durkin Keating, the late Robert Kelley, James H. Madison, Martin Ridge, Lana Ruegamer, Naomi Rogers, Joyce Seltzer, and James Harvey Young. Two special friends and fine historians went beyond the call of duty—or friendship—and I can never thank them enough. David E. Shi and Bernard A. Weisberger read every chapter at least once, wrote unusually helpful (and long) critiques, and never lost their enthusiasm for the book's subject or its author. I am also grateful to literary agent Gerard F. McCauley for his interest in my work and for his expertise in placing my manuscript with Oxford University Press, which has a long and distinguished list in American social history.

My parents have been a source of love and encouragement—and, in one critical instance, financial support. In the middle of this project, when I had run out of research money and two institutions failed to fund my proposals, my mother and father generously gave me a grant that saw me through. But more than that, my father, Christopher J. Hoy, who made his career at the American Library Association, taught me to love books. I wish he could have remained well and lived a few more years to hold this book in his hands. My mother, Imelda O'Keefe Hoy, who insists that she cleaned while the rest of us read, showed me year after year the comforts of cleanliness. But this book is for Walter. To Walter Nugent, I extend a hearty and heartfelt thank you. For without him—my editor of the first resort, counselor, and sustainer—this book would not have been completed.

Dune Acres, Indiana   S.H.
November 1994

CONTENTS

INTRODUCTION

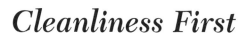

Cleanliness First

For a nation that judges other nations by their plumbing . . . .
—*LIFE* MAGAZINE, 1945[1]

Cleanliness has been on my mind in a serious way for nearly a decade. Not that I was dirty before then. It simply never occurred to me to give it any real attention. Only on those rare occasions when hot water was unavailable did it get a sustained, second thought.

Like many Americans who grew up in the 1950s, I lived in a middle-class suburban home where everything was clean, usually spotless. My parents, the children of Irish immigrants, knew the value of cleanliness; to them, it was as important as a good education. My brother and I went to school with our homework done and our necks clean—our underwear too, in case we fell on the playground and were rushed to the hospital. That's just the way it was with my family and most of my friends. Only rarely did something happen that made me think about the way we lived.

It happened one summer day in about 1957 at a swimming pool. I had recently begun shaving my legs, as had most of my girlfriends, and I noticed a woman in a beautiful bathing suit who didn't shave at all! I was shocked and repulsed. It made me wonder what was "wrong" with her; why didn't she shave her legs or underarms? Everybody said the woman was "foreign," and shaving legs and underarms was an "American" custom.[2]

A couple of years ago I was reminded of this incident on another summer day, when a well-traveled friend remarked at lunch that "Europe may have its castles and cathedrals, but America has its plumbing." That was the signal, of course, for everyone sitting around the table to begin stories about their first experience with European plumbing. The bathrooms were too small, and the showers were non-existent, except for those infuriating hoses and telephone-like gadgets that sprayed water everywhere. And, if the water pressure were adequate, then the supply of hot water was so limited that soap remained caked in their hair for weeks. One friend confessed that she visited a fancy hair salon in London simply to have her mane rinsed. Finally, in lavish detail, they took turns describing the wonderful showers that welcomed them home.

This book is not, however, about plumbing. Instead it is about us as a people, a people who developed and nurtured over a century and a half a love affair with cleanliness. This book is, in fact, the first general history of cleanliness in the United States. No one else has tried to answer what appears to be a simple question: How did Americans become so obsessed with cleanliness when, less than 200 years ago, Europeans found them dreadfully dirty and frequently disgusting?

The story is a complicated one, and everyone who reads it will bring personal memories and experiences to it. For that reason it is impossible to include every aspect of America's dirt-chasing saga in one volume. Yet the main lines of a large and important part of our history are here. I have traced with broad strokes American attitudes and practices regarding cleanliness from the early nineteenth century through the 1950s, and they reveal a startling transformation. Most pre-Civil War Americans were unclean— "filthy, bordering on the beastly"—if an English tourist is to be believed. Yet in 1958 the American people—now looking for "the cleanest clean possible"—spent about $200 million on products that made them smell better and took more than 500 million baths each week.[3]

How this happened is both fascinating and exciting. Among its most compelling episodes, chasing dirt meant ending life-threatening epidemics of cholera and dysentery, sewering a fast-growing country, eradicating hookworm, teaching immigrants and African-Americans along with the rural white majority about the dangers of dirt, and turning indoor plumbing into a national necessity. In short, this book documents the triumph of middle-class ideals and habits. It also highlights the critical role of women as agents of cleanliness—how they coped with the ever-increasing burdens and how they scored major victories, especially when it mattered most. From the perspective of a middle-class American woman (also a seasoned traveler) who has weighed the evidence, it is certainly better to be clean than dirty.

Chasing
Dirt

CHAPTER ONE

Dreadfully Dirty

... there was nutritiousness in the mud, and a man that drunk
Mississippi water could grow corn in his stomach if he wanted to.
—MARK TWAIN, 1883[1]

John Wesley, Benjamin Franklin, and Reality

In 1850, cleanliness in the United States, north and south, rural and urban, stood at Third World levels. Conditions we nowadays associate with peasant villages glimpsed on newscasts or educational television were common everywhere from the Atlantic to the Mississippi Valley (which was what effectively made up the settled United States at that time). More than four out of five Americans lived in pre-industrial, hygienically primitive situations on small farms or in country villages. Sanitation was not unknown, but the great majority felt no urgency about cleaning up. In the eyes of hardworking New England or midwestern farm families, dirt was seen as something positive, even healthy. Above all, it gave life and livelihood in the form of crops. The *idea* of cleanliness occasionally found ritual incantation in the words of John Wesley, about its being next to godliness, and in the precepts of Benjamin Franklin—but these were, as Hamlet said, "More honor'd in the breach than the observance."

Cleaning, washing, and bathing were laborious tasks and undertaken primarily for reasons of health or gentility. Despite widespread recognition of the Reverend Mr. Wesley's statement that cleanliness was a virtue "next to Godliness," this adage did not accurately reflect American thinking or practice (except for the Saturday night bath for churchgoers) in the mid-nineteenth century. Clergy of that time favored cleanliness to promote not piety but Christian respectability, and eventually, health.[2] People did not ordinarily consider themselves godly if they kept clean, nor ungodly if they remained dirty. Instead, commonly used words such as "neat" and "tidy" tended to describe orderly and polite individuals who were comfortably well off. Thus, in a very generalized Calvinist way, clean Americans may have appeared godly since they had the means to be so. For only those of some circumstance could regularly rely on the work of others—normally women who were wives, daughters, or domestic servants—to keep themselves and their surroundings clean. Domestics, in fact, did much to raise standards of cleanliness in the nineteenth century.[3] But that is getting ahead of the story.

Franklin's maxims were probably as well known as Wesley's famous phrase and, like his, were regarded with more piety than obedience. While old habits and ways of thinking did not entirely disappear, nineteenth-century Americans were adopting a new ethic of work, which was not the Puritan ethic "in modern dress." In the more secularized times from the American Revolution to the Civil War—more secular, that is, than seventeenth-century New England—Franklin's ideal of public usefulness had "all but nudged out God."[4] Industry, frugality, resolution, and cleanliness were becoming popular articles of middle-class faith.

Franklin listed in his *Autobiography* thirteen "Virtues" followed by "their Precepts." The tenth—between "Moderation" and "Tranquility"—was "Cleanliness"; he urged Americans to "tolerate no Uncleanness in Body, Cloaths or Habitation." He had lamented the condition of Philadelphia's streets, which were quagmires of mud after a rain and offensively dusty when dry, and at one point personally paid "a poor industrious Man" to keep "the Pavement clean, by sweeping it twice a week." Franklin believed personal cleanliness, even in small things, led to "Human Felicity." He said, for instance, that "if you teach a poor young Man to shave himself and keep his Razor in order, you may contribute more to the happiness of his Life than in giving him a 1000 Guineas."[5]

Franklin's devotion to cleanliness did not result from any lingering scrupulosity, however. He did not consider his virtues "as merely ideal ends without connection to real profit on this earth." As his successful career demonstrated, he saw "a direct link between the practice of these virtues and self-interest." Franklin "valued public spirit and philanthropy," not inner purity. His inspiration was secular rather than religious, respectable rather than redemptive. In fact his own family had been manufacturers of soap through most of the eighteenth century, "stamping the green cakes with a crown as a sign of quality."[6]

Yet despite Wesley's and Franklin's admonitions, colonial America was conspicuously unclean and continued so well into the next century. Before the Revolution only about 5 percent of the people lived in the handful of existing cities, with populations of about 15,000 to 30,000, and in the several dozen country villages of a hundred to a couple of thousand. Most Americans lived in rural independence, where sanitation was neither needed nor especially wanted. The few cities struggled to find enough water for private consumption and fire prevention. Philadelphia, the largest, boasted about 500 wells in 1771, of which only 120 were public. After yellow fever epidemics in the 1790s forced city fathers to install a public water system, fitful efforts at steam-powered pumps (some of which exploded) and cast-iron pipes (rather than earlier hollow logs) failed to keep up with population growth and civic needs. Only by 1840 could Philadelphia claim a dependable and adequate water supply.[7]

Boston and New York were no better off. Boston hardly possessed a public water system before 1790. Mains of hollow pine logs gradually reached the few hundred homes that could afford a charge of $10 a year, while the rest of the city relied on sporadic wells of uncertain purity. By the 1840s Boston and New York had opened large and distant reservoirs and began what quickly became an expensive urban necessity—laying miles of iron pipes and constructing massive aqueducts to convey water from afar. Even then the water did not always "smell right" but, far more serious, there was never enough. Within fifty years, both cities would find themselves in the midst of major water crises.[8]

Through the eighteenth century and well into the nineteenth, American standards, practices, and ideals about cleanliness were, in a word, pre-modern. If and when teeth were brushed, "it was with table salt and a chewed twig." And more often than not, medical remedies encouraged the sick to imbibe or smear on substances that would now be considered outlandishly loathsome. Take, for example, Ebenezer Parkman, who lived as the minister of Westborough, Massachusetts, from 1724 to 1782. He needed a painkiller to relieve a toothache and, on a neighbor's recommendation, concocted "cow dung fir[e]d in Hoggs Fatt—and lay all Night with my face on't despicable as it seems, it gave me relief."[9]

Americans began to think differently about dirt and to put their faith in prevention over cure as their country urbanized. As long as the United States remained predominantly rural, contagious diseases did not become menacing epidemics. Beginning in the 1820s, however, cities multiplied and expanded, and so did the risks of contagion. Americans who lived in port cities along the eastern seaboard or in the South, for instance, learned from their bouts with cholera that improved personal hygiene and public cleanliness helped combat the disease. As local officials began to enforce sanitary regulations during these epidemics, many discovered that a swept-up environment impeded the spread of cholera.

Those who took part in the religious revivals of the antebellum years began to prepare for the Second Coming of Christ by living more in accordance with the "laws of nature" and by distrusting the pills and drugs prescribed by would-be doctors. Charles Grandison Finney, one of the most popular religious revivalists of the pre-Civil War era, castigated physicians for dispensing one kind of medication to "one man and another to another man, without knowing whether it will kill or cure." Other Americans learned about ways to prevent illness by listening to lectures on physiology, visiting spas and water-cure establishments, or reading popular journals and advice books on health and hygienic living.[10]

Although most Americans still depended on farming in the mid-nineteenth century, market concerns began to intrude on isolated families and their self-sufficient, subsistent lives. Goods previously produced at home gradually appeared ready-made on the market. Even though whole families often went to work in factories during the beginning stages of industrialization, within a short period the inevitable separation of the workplace from the home occurred. Family roles, responsibilities, and expectations changed to accommodate these circumstances.[11]

The men who left their homes each day for work in shops and factories became more disconnected from domestic activities and acquired routines and habits that had not previously been a part of their everyday lives. In preindustrial America time and work moved at a pace more in tune with the seasons than the clock. During the late eighteenth century, farming fluctuated between days of long concentrated labor and shorter ones enhanced by visiting, fishing, and horse-racing. But by the early nineteenth century the tempo of farm life had noticeably increased. Many rural families in the East, for example, filled slack periods by producing shoes, hats, and woven cloth goods from materials put out by local wholesale merchants.[12]

Nevertheless, in antebellum America families owned far less clothing per person than they do today. Because shoes were so expensive, they were almost never worn in the countryside except in cold weather. When children and adults put on shoes, they often did not wear socks; and before 1840 they hardly ever wore underwear. It was "too expensive to buy, too troublesome to make, and . . . not considered necessary."[13] Instead men and boys usually wore long shirts, and women and girls dressed in "chemises." Their outer clothing was made of woven wool, leather, or felt. It could not be washed, but it was sometimes brushed. Shirts and chemises of linen or knitted wool were not washed either; when sweaty, they were hung out to dry. Eventually, cotton replaced linen and wool not only because it felt more comfortable but also because it washed more easily.[14]

All of this, however, is context and introduction. Changes in cleanliness practices between the days of Wesley and Franklin and the expansive 1820s were so slow as to be invisible. But from then until the Civil War, the speed of change accelerated; and the idea and practice of cleanliness were carried along by the inexorable shift toward urbanism and industrialism. Neither those two forces nor cleanliness, though, were more than partially in place by 1860. The majority of people continued living obliviously to the need or nicety of cleanliness. A visitor from abroad like William Faux, who accurately described American rural squalor as of 1819, could have said much the same in 1859. But by then, scarcely a generation later, city administrators and public health officials had begun holding "sanitary conventions" to seek solutions to common problems concerning sewerage, clean water, and the links between dirt and disease.

Certain key themes stand out in the history of cleanliness between 1820 and 1860: the persistence of preindustrial habits among most Americans; the popularity, at least among the urban upper middle class, of pleas for cleanliness; the idea of "home" as the center of virtue, and the role of "woman" as its guardian and protector, especially as men increasingly worked elsewhere; the belief that middle-class people distinguished themselves from the poor and countrified—that is, that "clean" and "classy" went together; and, finally, the need to take positive, concerted action to ensure public health. In short, Americans were beginning to grasp and accept the notion that to be clean meant to be respectable, publicly responsible, and healthy. By the 1850s they were also coming to see that cleanliness would be maintained in the family through the agency of the "true woman" and maintained in the community through public boards staffed by men who were leading citizens in a virtuous republic. Thus, when Americans (urban middle-class ones, at least) talked about being clean, their conversations generally focused on health, women's work and role, good social values, and the proper goals of public policy.

We will look at these changes and some of the individuals responsible for them. But first we need to comprehend how "dreadfully dirty" Americans of the nineteenth century really were.

The Filthy Farmstead

Early nineteenth-century Americans, whether on farms or in towns, lived in dirty, buggy, and smelly surroundings. Although they seemed unbothered by these conditions, travelers from other countries often found them disturbing. The English traveler William Faux, who visited Indiana and Illinois in 1819, described Midwesterners as "filthy, bordering on the beastly." He complained that water supplies were usually at a distance from sleeping quarters, and soap was "no where seen or found in any of the taverns, east or west"; he never grew accustomed to "dirty hands, heads, and faces every where." Even settlers, Faux grumbled, "seldom shaved" or washed their faces, and they almost never changed their linen. Another Englishman made a similar complaint about the availability of water: "In fact I have found it more difficult in travelling in the United States, to procure a liberal supply of water . . . , than to obtain any other necessity." Almost two decades later, English writer Harriet Martineau reported some improvement. She noted, for instance, that "the demand . . . for fresh air and soap and water" had increased. But she seemed disappointed that baths were "a rarity"—even in places less crude than the Wabash frontier that Faux described—and personal cleanliness was understood only in first-rate hotels.[15]

Faux paid a visit to yet another English emigrant pair, George and Eliza Flower, who built themselves a log cabin in Illinois in the early 1820s. Faux praised it as "the completest log cabin I have ever seen," with six or seven rooms; but the nearest water supply was half a mile distant. Eliza wrote home in 1833 that her large family (she had fourteen children of whom eight lived to adulthood) was "sometimes without any female servant for six months together—consequently I Cook, Clean, Wash, Recieve [sic] Company, Nurse my Children, Visit,—do all that comes to hand as a matter of course." Nonetheless, she found the Illinois backwoods "better than any place on Earth."[16]

The daily chores of farm women did not take them far beyond the confines of the house, yard, and barn. In the early decades of the nineteenth century, most farm families lived in small frame or log houses with one or two sparsely furnished rooms. Situated near a dirt road and next to a barn, stable, or piggery, these weathered dwellings often appeared "gray or dingy with neglect." Doors that did not shut tightly, windows without screens, mud floors without rugs or carpets, and large open fireplaces guaranteed that insects, barnyard animals, dust, dirt, and manure invaded the house. According to English agricultural reformer William Cobbett in 1818, there was "a sort of out-of-door slovenliness" around American farmhouses. Passersby saw "bits of wood, timber, boards, chips, lying about, here and there, and pigs and cattle trampling about in . . . confusion."[17]

Before that, in 1785 and 1786, a twenty-year-old English traveler, Robert Hunter, Jr., recorded his impressions of a long trip up the St. Lawrence River and thence southward through the newly liberated colonies to Charleston, South Carolina. Hunter liked Philadelphia, but otherwise found "scarcely a single town worth a European's notice." Richmond, Virginia, he said, was "one of the dirtiest holes of a place I ever was in." At Wilmington, North Carolina, he stayed at an inn where "the heat was so intense we were all obliged to dine without our coats and waistcoats, and our shirt collars open," and then "we retired to very disagreeable beds and dirty linen." But this was comparative luxury. A little later, outside Wilmington, Hunter was

> turned into an old barn that swarmed with rats and mosquitoes and, by way of a little variety, my bed (if you could call it one) was quite full of bugs and fleas. These, with the mosquitoes and the perpetual noise of millions of frogs, joined to the howling of the wild beasts in the woods, served at least to amuse me if I could not sleep. . . . I never remember to have spent so miserable a night. In the morning I was swelled all over with the bites of the bugs and mosquitoes.[18]

Not quite seventy years later, in 1853–54, the New Yorker Frederick Law Olmsted, just past his thirtieth birthday and soon to win the commission to design Central Park (and shortly after that to direct the United States Sanitary Commission), traveled for fourteen months through the South. What he saw confirmed the English visitors' reports. Olmsted found one miserable, disgusting stagecoach line and country inn after another. "Barbarous is too mild a term" for North Carolina's stagecoaches, he wrote; they and the "roads" had changed almost not at all since Hunter traveled them in 1786.

The bathing and toilet facilities had hardly changed either. In Norfolk, Virginia, Olmsted commented that "every clean towel that I got during my stay was a matter of special negotiation." At Gaston, North Carolina, he stayed at the only hotel, where he was "chummed up with a Southern gentleman, in a very small room. Finding the sheets on both our beds had been soiled by previous occupants, he made a row about it with the servants, and, after a long delay, had them changed." Bumping through South Carolina on a freezing stagecoach, Olmsted wondered why it had holes in the floor; he soon discovered "they were made with reference to the habit of expectoration, which . . . [was] very general and excessive."

Throughout South Carolina, the "better class" of country cabins had large porches, with "a wide shelf at the end, on which a bucket of water, a gourd, and hand-basin, are usually placed." But the water could be hard to get or hard to use. In western Louisiana, Olmsted asked a servant early in the morning for water: "we heard him breaking the ice for it outside. When we washed . . . the water was thick with frost, crusty, and half inclined not to be used as a fluid at all." And in east Texas,

> We were waited upon by two negro [sic] girls, dressed in short-waisted, twilled-cotton gowns, once white, now looking as if they had been worn by chimney-sweeps. The water for the family was brought in tubs upon the heads of these two girls, from a creek, a quarter of a mile distant, this occupation filling nearly all their time.

On several occasions Olmsted stayed in inns or cabins whose chairs were covered with deerskin. Invariably they were ridden with fleas. Of the many dirty lodgings he describes, one more should complete the picture. It was located in Woodville, in the southwest corner of Mississippi:

> I might have left Woodville with more respect . . . if I had not, when shown by a servant to my room, found two beds in it, each of which proved to be furnished with soiled sheets and greasy pillows, nor was it without reiterated demands and liberal cash in hand to the servant, that I succeeded in getting them changed on the one I selected. A gentleman of embroidered waistcoat took the other bed as it was, with no apparent reluctance, soon after I had effected my own arrangements. One wash-bowl, and a towel which had already been used, was expected to answer for both of us, and would have done so but that I carried a private towel in my saddle-bags. Another requirement of a civilized household was wanting, and its only substitute unavailable with decency.

A reformer at heart, and fundamentally an optimist, Olmsted later reflected (against much of his own evidence) that improvement was coming: "I congratulate myself that I have lived to see the day in which an agitation for reform in our GREAT HOTEL SYSTEM has been commenced." Commenced, perhaps, but not achieved for some time to come.[19]

Filthy houses and polluted surroundings recruited legions of flies, mosquitoes, ants, cockroaches, ticks, and bedbugs during warm weather. Unprotected by screens, which did not become available for home windows until after the Civil War, natives as well as visitors found no refuge and expressed their irritation with these disgusting and often painful nuisances.[20] Lavinia Stuart wrote her sister-in-law from Detroit in 1853 and described the flies "swarming about and tormenting" her "almost to death." She said her face pricked "as if some unseen spirit was sticking needles into it." On a trip through southern Illinois in the 1840s, William Oliver complained that no one ever enjoyed a complete and bloodless night's rest, even after removing the day's accumulation of ants and ticks, for a new and "combined attack" of mosquitoes and bugs kept everyone awake and embattled until the early morning hours. Only babies slept through the night, but even they had "clusters of flies parading over their mouths." Then, at breakfast, houseflies covered "everything on the table."[21]

According to a farm woman in Athens, Ohio, "those who were naturally clean and orderly" fought the flies at every meal. Determined not to let them "spoil everything" on their table, her mother always placed something tall at the center, spread a cloth over it, and slipped food under the cloth until everyone was ready to sit down. Later her sister acquired "little round-topped screens for every dish on her table." When guests were at table, par-

ents usually directed one of the children "to 'mind the flies.' " Fredrika Bremer recalled that during mealtimes in Charleston, South Carolina, black
boys or girls drove flies away with "a besom of peacocks' feathers."[22]

Travelers to America in the antebellum years remarked, without fail, on
the popularity of tobacco. On farms and in cities men usually chewed it,
while women sometimes used snuff or smoked pipes. However, it was the
almost universal practice of chewing and spitting that contributed so much
to the overall squalor. Men spat everywhere—in stagecoaches (as Olmsted
discovered), on the floors of boarding houses, the decks of steamboats, the
carpets of the Capitol, and on their own boots if they were poor marksmen.
Charles Dickens found this filthy and sickening custom "inseparably mixed
up with every meal and morning call, and with all the transactions of social
life." At a formal dinner party in Cincinnati, Frances Trollope remarked
that "the gentlemen spit, talk of elections and the price of produce, and spit
again." And to the amazement of Harriet Martineau, even the Shakers,
known for their fastidious wholesomeness, had spitting-boxes.[23]

Offensive odors naturally accompanied floors, rugs, and clothes soiled by
tobacco juice. In the countryside unpleasant and foul smells also emanated
from barnyards strewn with refuse and animal wastes, boots spattered with
manure and mud, and work and travel clothes drenched and stiffened with
perspiration. Neglected privies, unemptied chamber pots, and baby "napkins"
left drying by the fire or in the sun only added to a noisome environment that
modern Americans would have considered utterly unhealthy and distasteful.[24]

The arduous and dreaded chore of laundering, however, was what nineteenth-century women found loathsome. On wash day, housewives' spirits
fell "with the first rising of steam from the kitchen" and reached "a natural
temperature" only when their hot and heavy work had ended. Women usually washed on Mondays because their families dressed in clean clothes on
Sundays. And by doing the laundry weekly rather than monthly, they made
their chore easier. Not only did they reduce the size of the wash but they
believed they prevented dirt from injuring the clothes by hardening in the
fiber. One advice manual proclaimed the virtue of weekly washings compared with "the European custom of monthly or quarterly washes."[25] But
the cost to the farmwife was great. Eliza Flower's sister-in-law described a
typical day on an 1830s Illinois farm:

> up at daybreak, make the fire, call [the children]. . . . One day I wash, 2nd iron,
> 3rd make soap, 4th candles, 5th bake, 6th clean house. . . . Kitty [her small
> daughter] cleans the breakfast table and puts all the things that have been dirt-
> ied the day before into a large tub and it is Emily's [her other, smaller daugh-
> ter] business to wash them, whilst Kitty . . . wipes them and puts them in the
> right place.[26]

Farm journals and an 1862 Department of Agriculture report found that most farm women did not thrive under their regimen of back-breaking work and crude sanitation. Monday, or "Washing Day," was "the blackest day in woman's domestic calendar," according to *The Homestead*, a farm magazine. For much of that day, farm wives stood before a tub, lifting clothes and wringing them in harsh lime solutions. They may have been rewarded with clean laundry, but their efforts also produced "wrenched shoulders, arms, wrists, and scalded hands." The Department of Agriculture, for its part, reported that on three out of four farms "the wife worked harder and endured more than any person on the homestead."[27]

Towns and Cities, Dirty—and Dangerous

Life in villages and towns did not differ markedly from life in the country. Neighbors were usually closer and contacts more frequent, but the disorder and squalor common to farms also characterized in-town properties. Houses had the same unpainted, weather-beaten look, and they were surrounded by a similar array of barnyard animals, mudholes, rubbish, and weeds. The town's "business section" consisted of little more than a general store, post office, blacksmith shop, tavern, schoolhouse, a church or two, some shops for tradesmen, and offices for the local doctor and lawyer. All were tied together by a few rods of wooden sidewalks and hitching racks. In wet months, walkways, roads, and house surroundings were "apt to be a muddy combination of soil, dung, and dishwater."[28]

County seats were larger but not cleaner. In addition to what smaller towns displayed, the county seat had a courthouse, a jail, a newspaper, and stagecoach service, larger stores, and more houses and offices. It also suffered a greater number of animals on the loose, bigger piles of dung, and longer streets of dirt and mud. For the most part, antebellum travelers could find elegant hotels and shops or luxurious homes with manicured gardens only in the major seaboard cities of the Northeast. In the South, Frances Kemble Butler noted in 1838–39 that even planters' homes had an "air of neglect, and dreary, careless untidiness." When she scolded her slaves for their messy housekeeping, they retorted that "they had seen buckree (white) women's houses just as dirty, and they could not be expected to be cleaner than white women." Not surprisingly, then, most visitors to America seemed to agree that they found towns and villages "on the decay" as they went south of Philadelphia or west into the Ohio Valley.[29]

In the large cities, where foreign travelers generally felt more comfortable, there were also major pollution problems. Each horse, for example, daily deposited an estimated twenty-two pounds of manure on the streets.

Although hundreds of roaming pigs scavenged garbage thrown into fly-in-fested thoroughfares and kept them cleaner than they otherwise might have been, they too befouled the environment. In addition nearly every neighborhood had a peculiar stench, originating in its distinct arrangement of livery stables, slaughterhouses, and tanneries.[30]

While bothersome insects, ugly tobacco stains, and pungent odors could be found everywhere, an abundant supply of potable water could not be secured without some difficulty. In fact, one of the major differences between country, town, and city life revolved around the availability of water. In the country, farm families hauled water for home use from a spring, creek, well, rain barrel, or pump. In towns and cities without municipal water supplies, families drew their water from rain barrels or wells, and they sometimes made use of cisterns or a central spring or pump. Since plumbing was largely non-existent, water for washing, cleaning, and cooking almost always had to be carried from one place to another. If a family had the wherewithal and the know-how to install a small force pump that would bring water through a lead pipe into the house, they were considered especially fortunate.[31]

Those with running water inside their homes could wash themselves either in the kitchen or on the back porch. There they would find a wooden or tin basin, perhaps a stone sink, with a comb on a string and a looking glass hanging above. Those without such conveniences washed their faces, necks, hands, and sometimes feet outdoors, weather permitting.[32] By mid-century the washstand with pitcher, basin, and slop jar (for used water) became standard fixtures in bedrooms of middle-class homes. Thus many people in large cities and some small towns came to view outdoor washing as backward. In Susan Warner's best-selling novel of 1850, *The Wide, Wide World* (the all-time best-seller in England and America until *Uncle Tom's Cabin* broke Warner's record a few months later), ten-year-old Ellen Montgomery, obliged to leave her parents in the city and live with her aunt in the country, did not know what to do on the first morning of her stay when she could not find a wash basin. She was truly bewildered when, after asking several times about washing, her aunt gave her a towel and told her to go out the kitchen door and "down to the spout." Not knowing what a "spout" was, Ellen discovered a little stream of water pouring from the end of a pipe (which she later learned came from a spring at the back of the pig-field). Still she wondered what she should do without a basin. She tried to get her face under the spout but could not, since its water made the board she stood on so slippery that she nearly slid off into the mud. In the end she decided to be content "with the drops her hands could bring to her face."[33]

Those who "bathed" at washstands indoors also faced numerous difficulties, especially during winter in cold and temperate climates. Since houses lacked central heating and electric lighting, the first person to arise on a cold, dark morning usually found that the water obtained the night before "was chiefly broken ice." Lucy Larcom, who moved with her family to the textile mills of Lowell, Massachusetts, in 1835, watched her sister take a full bath every morning before work in a room without a fire and recognized that this "good habit" required "both nerve and will."[34]

Short winter days not only brought families in closer physical contact but also encroached further on their privacy. More often than not, those with the courage and determination to confront icy water on chilly mornings had to do so at the kitchen sink in the company of family members, overnight guests, or servants and help. Catherine Webb, the daughter of a successful New York City merchant who boarded for a short time with the Lyman Beechers in Litchfield, Connecticut, complained that she "could not take much of a bath" since the only place to wash was at the kitchen sink. At New England farmhouses, according to Francis Underwood, fortunate travelers would have use of "the 'sink' in the lean-to, next to the kitchen" and not have "to break ice" to wash their faces and hands. If they were truly lucky, they might discover that "a little warm water . . . from the kettle swung over the kitchen-fire" had been poured into the basin.[35]

The Tremont House in Boston, the nation's first "modern" hotel, opened in October 1829 and boasted eight water closets on the ground floor and eight bathing rooms in the basement. Seven years later, New York's Astor House installed a bath and water closet on each floor, and in 1844 the New York Hotel introduced the private bath.[36] Although water closets had become popular in luxurious English homes during the late eighteenth century, the majority of American homes did not have them or baths until they were connected to municipal water and sewer lines, which for many did not happen until late in the century. Most large cities in the United States built or expanded water supply systems during the 1840s and 1850s, but at the close of the Civil War only about 5 percent of American houses had running water.[37]

Since municipalities usually constructed water lines for those who could pay, only the wealthy could draw water from the mains. But compared with modern plumbing even the most advanced indoor piping proved technologically simple—usually a single faucet on the far kitchen wall or, less frequently, in the yard. Urban householders who could afford water closets (which, by the way, initially referred to the fixture rather than the closet-like space surrounding it) probably had them. These fixtures were initially pan closets, which received water through a valve on the supply pipe or later through an elevated cistern. Because ordinances prohibited connecting water closets to sewers, wastes from the closets flowed through wooden or brick drains to cesspools or privy vaults in or near the cellars of houses. As the number of water closets increased, so too did the quantity of fecally polluted water. When private contractors failed to empty overflowing cesspools or vaults, residents complained of backyards saturated or flooded "with stagnant and offensive fluids." Protests from the well-to-do, along with the fears of public health officials, who believed putrefying organic matter gave rise to disease-carrying miasmas, would eventually result in massive public works projects to replace cesspools and privy vaults with underground sewers.[38]

For the majority of Americans who did not have running water in their homes, habits of personal hygiene and housekeeping varied widely. In 1890 only 24 percent of all American homes had running water. And not until the 1930s would the entire urban population have running water, while most of the rural population would not until after 1945.[39] Thus, for a very long time, those who attempted to keep their families and homes reasonably clean found that the means to succeed lagged far behind their good intentions.

The Domestic Woman, Agent of Cleanliness

In the case of someone like Mary Todd Lincoln in Springfield, Illinois, cleaning was a daily chore that required a great deal of energy but offered little recompense. Like most American cities in the 1850s, Springfield had unplanked sidewalks and dirty streets, where "rooting pigs, roaming ducks and geese, homeless dogs, and escaped horses ate refuse and left their waste." The Lincoln's home had windows but no screens. In summer months, they and their neighbors, who lived in similar kinds of houses, could choose between fresh air swarming with insects or stagnant air without them. In the Lincoln's backyard was an outhouse behind a cistern pump. From it Mary Todd Lincoln and her sons drew water, carried it into the house, and boiled it to take care of their cleaning needs. These conditions, common to many Americans at mid-century, explain best why "most filth lay beyond the control of even responsible women," despite their fortitude and best efforts.[40]

Eliza Burhans Farnham of Rensselaerville, New York, is another case in point. Married in July 1836 to lawyer Thomas Jefferson Farnham, she began housekeeping in a village on the Illinois prairie in dreadfully dirty but mercifully short-term quarters. "Blistered hands and lacerated fingers were matters of no moment" to her, since she intended to turn their shabby, temporary residence into a home. When Thomas left for work on a Monday morning two days after their arrival, Eliza filled buckets with water and slaked lime and "put these cleansing agents to their duty." By evening their rented room was no longer "unequivocally filthy." Eliza had washed the

walls and window, scoured the chairs, and placed a carpet on the floor and
wild flowers in a broken pitcher. Tired from her labors, but elated with the
improvements, she anticipated her husband's surprise at finding "such a
snug, neat, little home."

Weeks later, when the Farnhams moved to their permanent house, Eliza
again found herself confronted by dirt. Unable to hire "a stout Irish or colored woman" to do the scrubbing, as she probably would have done had she
still been living in New York, and unwilling (she wrote) to sit down and cry
over the mess, she attacked it head on. With the aid of a broom and cloth,
she had by sunset brought order and "a comfortable degree of cleanliness" to
their home. Although dinner that night consisted only of cheese, crackers,
and water, the Farnhams rested well on a bed of straw. The following day
Eliza stepped up her "housekeeping operations" and once again cleaned the
place, but this time she did so with a "deluge of hot water and soap."[41]

Eliza Farnham's domestic experiences demonstrate the central role of
women in creating clean and comfortable quarters for their families. The
feminization of the middle-class home in the mid-nineteenth century made
it increasingly a separate and private place, one set apart from those public
places where husbands and fathers went each day to work. As the site of
male labor shifted from the homestead to stores, factories, and offices, the
house became "the place for another kind of work—specialized domestic
work—women's work." It transformed the house into a home, made it a
refuge as well as a dwelling, and produced an atmosphere that had not existed before. What had occurred in seventeenth-century Dutch households
happened similarly two centuries later in the United States. The husband,
who saw himself as the head of the family and led mealtime prayers, was
displaced as master in most household matters. And "it was the wife, not
her husband, who insisted on cleanliness and tidiness, not the least because
it was she who had to do the cleaning."[42]

Cleanliness alone did not create comfort, nor did it produce privacy, inti-
macy, or domesticity. But without a certain degree of cleanliness and order,
those feelings and values that the emerging middle class associated with a
good home and family and with genteel living and respectability could not
have developed. Had Eliza Farnham simply placed a vase of freshly cut
flowers in the midst of a squalid room, she would not have created a cozy
home for her husband's pleasure or her contentment. That much is obvious.
Yet modern Americans may not understand that in the antebellum years,
when water supplies were severely limited (indeed, to what one could carry)
and housekeeping tools were often little more than a "broom and a cloth in
hand," to be clean demanded the kind of hard work and persistence that resulted in "blistered hands and lacerated fingers" as well as aching backs and

early aging. However, the failure to be clean, as this nineteenth-century generation painfully learned, could be dangerous to one's health and even one's life.

If rural Americans—and women in particular—found it difficult to keep clean, the urban poor found it next to impossible. Washing and cleaning were extremely arduous tasks for working-class city dwellers. Families were crowded into tenements that bore no resemblance to the middle-class home. Except for those living in basements or backyard sheds, all water had to be carried long distances and up flights of stairs. And although house-keepers did not yet have to contend with the industrial dirt that would be-smirch them in the late nineteenth century, they did have to confront mud tracked in from unpaved streets, clogged chimneys, cracked plaster, and slop pails knocked over by children who had nowhere to play. But most poor women attempted to keep their lodgings neat and clean and took pride in whatever success they had. Even the Irish, whom Yankees sometimes confused with dirt itself, were proud of their "bits of carpits on their flures." Nonetheless, nativists argued for exclusion of the Irish from America in part because, they jeered, "the only water the Irishman used consistently was Holy Water."[43]

Of the nearly one million Irish who arrived in the United States between 1821 and 1850, the majority were landless and poor. Those who came in the worst years of the Potato Famine (1847–54) tended to be rural families. Once in America, they usually remained in East Coast and Great Lake cities, large and small. For the most part, the Irish wished to avoid farming, which had given them so few pleasant memories; but they also lacked the means to travel far beyond their ports of arrival. Cities too offered economic opportunities and friendly communities of other Irish immigrants. Fortunate men found good-paying jobs on public works projects, and women consid-ered themselves lucky when they were hired as domestic servants in middle-class homes, which they preferred to working in factories and mills.[44]

But the dirt-floor cottages in which these Irish women had grown up and the crowded tenements to which many of them had emigrated did not pre-pare them to become domestics in American households. Stereotypically referred to as "Biddy," Irish servants were sometimes described as "un-washed" and often said to perform housework "dirtily and shiftlessly."[45] Elizabeth Sullivan Stuart, who had grown up in Brooklyn and moved to the Michigan frontier in 1817, prided herself on the "standards of social deco-rum" she had established in her home during the subsequent thirty years. Although she was the daughter of an Irish patriot, her position as a "lady" seemed to blind her to the situation of her Irish servants. She complained bitterly about them and, in a letter to her daughter in 1852, described an encounter with one young woman ("an animal") whose hands were so greasy she could not turn a door knob. On this basis, she advised her daughter to rid herself of the "awful things" she had in her house and to hire Norwegians. They were, according to Stuart, "the best of all that are imported."[46]

There is little doubt that in some middle-class homes, like the Stuarts', standards of cleanliness rose in the 1840s and 1850s. But because of lagging technologies, the burden of new standards fell on housewives and servants alike. Although housewives shouldered all of the day-to-day responsibilities associated with a clean and comfortable home, they tended to do less of the actual work. Yet, firmly convinced that every part of the home "must be visited daily," they came to rely, often too heavily, on their servants.[47] When this happened, antebellum ladies began to tie their work as housekeepers to their role as women.

In the mid-nineteenth century, ladies imposed cleanliness on those around them. Mistresses concentrated on housework for comfort and appearance's sake; and before long "cleanliness, tidiness and the care and arrangement of possessions replaced domestic production as housewives' preoccupations." The upper-middle-class home of the 1840s and 1850s required downstairs a kitchen and a "wash house" behind it, and upstairs a bath as well as bedrooms and a nursery. But not much was said by ladies or gentlemen about toilets. For despite the growing bourgeois devotion to sanitation in person and in the kitchen, the outdoor privy was still the norm in polite society.[48]

Even before industrialization, men and women divided household labor in ways that seemed "to have no rhyme or reason." While both men and women (including children) carried water as needed, men nearly always chopped and hauled wood; women, for their part, washed and ironed clothes. Yet for a woman to spend all day at the wash-tub—making soap, boiling water, hoisting tubs, rubbing washboards, then rinsing, wringing, and hanging the clothes out to dry—demanded the same brute strength required in chopping wood.[49] In the preindustrialized world, women's work was by definition basically domestic.

In colonial New England, "good wives" defined their role by space (house and surrounding yards), a set of tasks (washing and cleaning as well as cooking, spinning, milking, and gardening), and a restricted area of authority (the internal economy of a family).[50] At various times and in a variety of ways, from the seventeenth to the mid-nineteenth century, women worked differently from their mothers or grandmothers. They gradually enlarged the role of housekeeper, mother, and nurse and relinquished or assigned to others menial tasks they no longer thought necessary or wished to do. Like their husbands who hired men and boys to ease their work when warranted and affordable, housewives often paid other women to help do the most onerous of their jobs. This practice, in fact, kept the sexual division of labor intact.[51]

During the antebellum years major changes in the production and distribution of goods along with a new work ethic affected the everyday operations of the home. While husbands and fathers became less actively involved in producing food and rearing children, wives and mothers spent less time milking cows, weaving cloth, and making candles. As economic and technological innovations reduced or eliminated male responsibilities at home—butchering pigs, cutting wood, and making boots—and freed them for work in town, women's "housework" (a term that dates from this period) increased. Although it is true that manufactured cloth made it unnecessary for women to weave, it did not do away with the need for them to sew. In fact, the availability of manufactured cloth seems to have stimulated a demand for more clothing. Since no shops sold ready-made clothes, women sewed more and, of course, laundered more.[52]

A short story in *Godey's* magazine described with unusual frankness the weighty burden of cleanliness and the possible consequences of bearing it alone. Mrs. Hamersly did her *own* mountain of wash until, in a moment of anger, she struck her daughter for making lumpy starch. Shameful and regretful, this overtaxed housewife accepted money from her husband to hire a washerwoman, young Biddy Macphersen. This solution was hardly open to every American wife. Yet even those housewives who could afford to employ domestics or "hired girls" remained responsible for household affairs. Thus to find a "good wife" in the seventeenth century or a "true woman" in the mid-nineteenth, one need only look at home.[53]

Preceptress of Reform: Catharine Beecher

Catharine Beecher, who wrote *A Treatise on Domestic Economy, for the Use of Young Ladies at Home and at School* in 1841, was the earliest and probably the most famous nineteenth-century promoter of the "domestic values" of efficiency, convenience, comfort, and cleanliness. Although a fervent abolitionist like her sister Harriet Beecher Stowe, Catharine was neither a radical nor a feminist. She believed, as did most of her generation, that women belonged at home. She was, however, unhappy with the inefficient and disorderly manner in which women carried out their responsibilities. Recognizing the confusion that industrialism had caused in home and community life, she offered in her *Treatise* a way to deal with these alterations. The home continued to serve as a refuge from an unfeeling world, but in Beecher's hands it also became a place of work for women, and for the nation an integral part of the larger community, where mainstream American values could be instilled and promoted. In fact, the overwhelming popularity of her *Treatise* seemed to rest on "its ability to combine a convincing domestic ideology with practical advice demonstrating how these ideals could be realized."[54]

Catharine Beecher was the oldest of the nine children of the well-known Congregationalist minister Lyman Beecher and his first wife, Roxana Foote. Several of Catharine's siblings earned fame, especially her sister Harriet and her brother Henry Ward Beecher, that "man of moods and impulses" whose congregations thrilled to his preaching.[55] When her mother died, the sixteen-year-old Catharine took charge of her father's household and later considered the years spent housekeeping as her true education. Her recollections of the experience, in fact, underlay her energetic campaigns to revise female education and her utilitarian instructions on how to care for families and organize housework.

Beecher was born in 1800 in East Hampton, Long Island, but spent a good deal of her adult life in the Midwest. She moved with her family first to Litchfield, Connecticut, and then to Cincinnati, where her father became head of a seminary. She subsequently founded several women's colleges in the Midwest. And it was here that she witnessed the impact of industrialism and technology on the American economy and home. It was hardly accidental, as she came to realize, that "the economy which mechanized wheat farming and meat packing would also turn to the mass production of domestic ranges and furnaces, of washing machines and mechanical carpet cleaners. . . ." However, in 1841, when Beecher's *Treatise* first appeared, technology had not materially altered the lives of the country's overwhelmingly rural population nor did Beecher accept the lack of mechanized tools as an excuse for haphazard housework. Her *Treatise* was reprinted almost every year until 1856 and it, along with a few other publications, eventually made her "a national authority on the psychological state and the physical well-being of the American home."[56]

Beecher believed that women should be educated for a profession as mothers, housewives, and teachers. In that sense, many of the arguments in her *Treatise*, along with the values she wished to instill, resembled those later articulated by Florence Nightingale during and after the Crimean War in an attempt to train women as nurses. Unfortunately for Beecher, however, her advice was given in peacetime and did not resonate with the same gravity and urgency. Nevertheless, in her crusade to define a new role for women, she increasingly emphasized their sphere of influence. In her *Treatise* she contended that no profession could be "successfully pursued" unless "superior and subordinate relations" between men and women were instituted. And, according to Beecher, women occupied the subordinate place *not* because they were inferior or dependent but rather because this arrangement contributed to "the general good of all."[57]

Beecher wished to inspire middle-class American women "with a sense of their high responsibilities" by convincing them of the importance of their work to families and the nation. She readily admitted how difficult it was to care for a home, but also reminded many of her readers of their English heritage (just as her father, a nativist, warned his congregations against Romish incursions). She saw the English as a people "distinguished for systematic housekeeping, and for a great love of order, cleanliness, and comfort."[58] Thus, whether in new western settlements or older eastern communities, Beecher especially encouraged these women to call on their inheritance and devote more attention to cleanliness, economy, and comfort by carrying out their housekeeping duties in a systematic and orderly fashion. For those willing to try, she offered practical suggestions on child-rearing, cleaning, training domestics, cooking, nursing the sick, sewing, and gardening. Nothing was too insignificant to keep families healthy and content.

At a time when plumbing and heating were largely unavailable to the middle class, Beecher's recommendations for a clean and comfortable home had obvious limitations. Frequently, when discussing specific household tasks, she encouraged "neatness" and "order" over "cleanliness." She tended to reserve the word "clean" for descriptions of things that could be made white (that is, clothes, walls, tablecloths) as well as for instructions on the care of the sick and one's skin. And she never asserted that cleanliness was next to godliness. Instead she offered another "grand maxim"—"A place for every thing, and every thing in its place."[59]

In Beecher's design for an ideal cottage, where every room had a wood-burning fireplace, only the kitchen had a sink. Although she emphasized the convenience of indoor running water and suggested that the kitchen sink have a drain, she likewise encouraged housewives to keep a slop-pail under the sink and two water pails near by. Knowing that clothes were more likely to be "clean and white" where there was "an abundance and frequent change of water," Beecher urged that wells and cisterns be located near the house to ensure the best results with the least effort. She merely mentioned that there were new ways of positioning wells and cisterns so that "by simply turning a cock, or working a small pump," water would flow directly to the place where it would be used. In this pretechnological age, when housework was exceedingly laborious, Beecher warned her readers that "every room added to a house increases the amount of sweeping, dusting, cleaning of floor. . . ."[60]

Nowhere in her *Treatise* did Beecher discuss bathrooms or water closets.

At one point, she remarked that privies were particularly hard on women and on the sick who must "go out of doors in all weathers." Yet, in the section entitled "On Cleanliness," she expressed great regret that the majority of Americans only washed the face, neck, hands, and feet; and she argued forcefully that they should remove dirt and perspiration from their whole body every day and dry themselves with a coarse towel. Eager to correct a popular notion that dirt was somehow healthy, Beecher pointed out that fresh air, exercise, and clean skin contributed to good health. Thus, like most mid-century promoters of bathing, Beecher encouraged more diligent use of the tin wash-pan, sponge, and towel. Almost no one recommended using soap or hot water—soap supposedly removed oils from the skin, and to heat water was so impractical that it ruled out daily bathing. Hence the typical bath meant a cold plunge or sponge.[61]

For at least two months of each year during the 1840s and 1850s Beecher took up residence in a number of the many water-cure centers recently established in the Northeast. Her sister Harriet often accompanied her. As a result of these visits, both became keenly aware of how an abundant water supply and daily bathing could improve one's living conditions and health. In an 1865 essay on the requirements of a healthful house, Harriet maintained that plentiful, accessible, and pure water was a "vital element." And four years later, when she and Catharine co-authored a new edition of the *Treatise on Domestic Economy*, they included a bathroom in their cottage design but admitted that a "full bath" was still a "great luxury."[62]

Toward the end of her life (she died in 1878), Beecher and other reformers of like mind had begun to change middle-class attitudes about cleanliness. They did this by explaining as best they could the links between dirt and disease, cleanliness and hygiene. But too many farm families still held dirt in too high regard. Not only did it give life, in their view, but it was also a sure sign of plain living, honest toil, and physical fitness. To be "dressed up" when there was work to do was simply "puttin' on airs." They cleaned up when they left home and appeared in public, but even then they washed only those parts of the body that could be seen.[63]

Beecher assaulted such notions. In her *Treatise*, she remarked on the "frequent washing and rubbing" horses received to keep them healthy. They were better groomed, she believed, than most of the farmers who owned them.[64] She was undoubtedly correct, but the elaborate care that farmers regularly gave to their horses provides another insight on commonly held beliefs about cleanliness. Since farmers considered horses special animals, they received special treatment. Farm families never lived off horses in the same way they lived off cows or chickens; they never ate horse meat, for instance. And, while horses worked by plowing the fields, they also carried families to church and into town. A well-groomed horse became a kind of status symbol that could occasionally be shown off to neighbors.[65] Thus for cleanliness to become an everyday concern, antebellum Americans needed to be convinced that dirt not only endangered their social standing but also their health. In short, they would have to believe that it could be dangerous not to wash.

Cleanliness, Health, and Virtue: Graham and Alcott

For health reformers like Sylvester Graham and William Alcott, the failure to bathe daily was only one of many bad habits that prevented Americans from enjoying good health. Graham, who is remembered for the cracker named after him, began his career for better personal hygiene as a temperance lecturer in Philadelphia. He remained largely unknown until 1832, when the United States' first major cholera epidemic catapulted him into prominence. Although there was little consensus among physicians or lay health reformers on how to prevent or cure cholera, a majority agreed that the intemperate and the filthy were most susceptible. Since cholera attacked the gastrointestinal tract, Graham argued against overstimulating the digestive system with liquor or greasy food. He encouraged those with mild cases to avoid damp air, keep clean, and abstain from coffee, tea, meat, and alcohol. When several of his ailing followers survived, Graham became known outside Philadelphia and more firmly convinced that individuals who ate properly, abstained from alcohol, bathed frequently, and lived in well-ventilated houses could avoid most illnesses.[66]

Today, when Americans spend a great deal of time and money on improving their bodies and their health, the significance of Graham's advice can easily be overlooked or underestimated. Yet a remarkable transformation took place in the United States between 1832 and 1866. During those thirty-four years, cholera, which had once been considered "a scourge of the sinful," was discovered to be "the consequence of remediable faults in sanitation."[67] This change of opinion, however, did not occur rapidly. It took years for middle-class Americans to realize that they could act in practical ways to prevent disease.

Along with Beecher and Graham, William Alcott became an influential advocate of healthful living. Born in 1798, a cousin and friend of Louisa May's father, Bronson Alcott, William published over a hundred articles, books, and essays between the 1830s and his death in 1859; all of them offered popular advice on such subjects as personal cleanliness, outdoor exercise, and a meatless diet. Passionate in the belief that sickness could be prevented by correct living habits, he became an enthusiastic missionary to the cause of preventive medicine and an elementary school curriculum that included training of the body as well as the mind. In the aftermath of the first great cholera epidemic (1832), he offered counsel similar to Graham's. Alcott did not completely reject medical aid, but he made it very clear that there was no specific cure for cholera. He encouraged plenty of fresh air, a simple diet, frequent washing and bathing, and a tranquil mind. He specifically warned against living in damp or stuffy quarters, mingling in large crowds, or becoming unusually tired.[68]

While Alcott's reputation grew and his publishing and speaking commitments increased, he found himself giving ever more attention to cleanliness. "Nothing in physiology or hygiene is plainer to the common mind," he argued, "than the great law of cleanliness." Neglect of this law appalled him. In 1850 he observed that a quarter of New England's population never bathed their whole bodies even once a year. Women and children were among those who did bathe occasionally, but just on Saturday night or Sunday morning. Men and boys, for their part, "washed" when they swam in a local pond or river. Only a very small number, he regretfully admitted, had adopted "on principle the practice of daily ablution."[69]

Alcott recommended the cold bath. He insisted it was the most invigorating, and conceded that it was the most accessible. For someone so convinced of the value of personal cleanliness, he must have been continually frustrated by his inability to persuade Americans to change their ways. He knew the effort and discipline demanded by regular bathing and, consequently, admitted that he wished that "the necessary apparatus" for taking baths was considered as indispensable as bedrooms and parlors.[70] But until it was, he had to content himself with trying to enlist parents, especially wives and mothers, in his cause.

Alcott explained to young mothers (as did Beecher) that dirt was not healthy for anyone, particularly children. Those who played in the dirt and were healthy could thank the open air and active exercise, not the dirt! At the end of his life, Alcott was still arguing against the healthfulness of dirt. He stated that "the strange saying that everyone, during his life, must eat his 'peck of dirt and his pound of tow,' had its origin in times of great ignorance. . . . To breathe dirt, or to eat it, would be equally injurious."[71] During summer and fall, when bowel complaints were common and thought to be somehow connected to dirt, Alcott warned mothers of the seriousness of neglecting to bathe their children completely and aid them in washing their hands thoroughly. Since he believed in a connection between cleanliness of body and strength of character, Alcott also told mothers that sons and daughters who were washed daily when babies and youngsters would continue these practices as adults and be better men and women.[72]

Like most health reformers of his day, Alcott accorded wives and mothers major responsibility for their families' health, appearance, and comfort. He shared Beecher's belief that what happened around the domestic fireside and in the nursery had significance far beyond a household's walls. While husbands and fathers were not completely absolved from responsibility in these matters, their role was ancillary. When it came to cleanliness, for example, husbands were told that they could do a great deal to help or hinder their wives' work; they could bring "more or less" dirt into the house, assist "more or less" in teaching their children to be clean, and haul "more or less" water and wood into their homes. All of these "almost nameless things of life," Alcott advised, could be done or not done in their wives' interest. But, more important, husbands were encouraged to provide their families with as many implements of bathing and ventilation as they could afford and to set an example for their children by taking baths frequently.[73]

In their crusade on behalf of cleanliness, the Beechers, Graham, and Alcott offered practical suggestions and prescribed helpful remedies to America's middle class. They showed little concern or compassion for the problems faced by the nation's expanding poor and immigrant population. In fact, they shared with most Americans the view that poverty was not an excuse for neglecting cleanliness. Alcott saw it simply as a question of self-control. "In order to find time for more washing, or money to pay others for the labor," he observed, "the poor must deny themselves a few things which they now suppose . . . are conducive to their happiness—but which are, in reality, either useless or injurious."[74] His sentiments typified the undaunted confidence of many antebellum reformers who believed that individuals could change and improve simply through an act of will.

Cleanliness as Public Policy: Griscom and Shattuck

By the 1850s the largest eastern cities contained ever-widening extremes of wealth and poverty. New York City, Philadelphia, and Boston had slums as filthy and as deadly as those in Paris and London. The squalid conditions of these slums and the fears they fostered resulted in new concerns about public health. Until then, city dwellers tended to become anxious about health matters only when they felt threatened by periodic epidemics. But the large numbers of poor working-class families that had appeared during the 1840s seemed to forecast an impending disaster. Various welfare organizations and leading sanitarians, most notably John H. Griscom of New York and Lemuel Shattuck of Boston, attempted to ameliorate these conditions and to turn personal and local concerns into a national public health movement.

Griscom, a physician who served briefly as a health inspector for New

York City during the early 1840s, underpinned his sanitary reform work with an avid interest in science and public welfare. He was also an influential member of the Association for Improving the Condition of the Poor, whose missionaries visited working men and women in their homes. Considering them the best-informed citizens on the living conditions of the poor, Griscom used their testimony as well as his own experiences in preparing his report of 1845, *The Sanitary Condition of the Laboring Population of New York*.[75] Perhaps for this reason he was able to understand what so many of his contemporaries did not.

In Griscom's view, poverty, not moral weakness or lack of self-control, generated the high incidence of disease and death among the urban masses. He knew that the rich, like the poor, were often "equally ignorant of the laws of life." Yet the rich had the means to obtain "greater comfort and more luxuries," which accounted "for their prolonged lives." Cleaner surroundings and better food, Griscom argued, could improve everyone's health and promote a more law-abiding community. He insisted that an educated child would be no better than his ignorant and unruly companions if he were "surrounded with dirt, foul air, and all manner of filthy associations." For Griscom the connection between morality and cleanliness was tenuous, indeed.[76]

It was not so for Shattuck. A Massachusetts legislator and statistician, he possessed attitudes more typical of his day. Worried about the debilitating effects of Boston's immigrants on the American native-born population, Shattuck could not free himself from the commonly held conviction that poverty was no excuse for neglecting cleanliness. However, since the immigrant poor seemed too undisciplined and complacent to improve their environment, he recommended a program of sanitary control in which the state and municipality would share the responsibilities of guardian, regulator, and educator of its citizens. Although Shattuck's general plan for improving the public's health was not implemented when he proposed it in 1850, many of its specific suggestions became standard practice by the early twentieth century.[77]

The reforms offered by Shattuck and Griscom embodied the crucial belief that disease could be prevented. In fact, prevention—"prevention of disease, prevention of suffering, prevention of sanitary evils of every kind"—became the cornerstone of their designs for promoting good health and long life. Shattuck, in his 1850 report to the state of Massachusetts, estimated that approximately half of the deaths in the commonwealth could have been avoided had more attention been given to personal hygiene and public sanitation. "Cleanliness in towns," he contended, was "of such immense importance to health" that the state and local municipalities had to make sure that it was not overlooked.[78] In this regard, Griscom called for the creation of "health police" who would have the power to enforce "a law of domiciliary cleanliness." Interestingly, he suggested that this law be written to make the owner of a tenement responsible for the cleansing rather than the tenant who was usually too poor to do it.[79]

Griscom's proposal for health police in New York City and Shattuck's for a state board of health and sanitary police in Massachusetts fell largely upon deaf ears. In general the public saw these recommendations as interfering with private rights. Many were alarmed by Shattuck's argument that, since "the most perfect cleanliness is necessary in all places" to prevent disease, "no person should be permitted to contaminate the atmosphere of his own house, or that of his neighbors, by any filth or other substance dangerous to the public health."[80] Strong sanitary measures could cause the destruction of profitable tenements and create a demand for the construction of large and expensive drains and sewers. Physicians, who should have been willing and able to argue on behalf of such measures, were not well respected or well organized in the 1850s. Furthermore, public attention was distracted from health matters by the debate over slavery and its impact on the nation.[81]

Sanitary Reform on the Eve of War

In May 1857, when Philadelphia hosted the first national quarantine convention, seventy-three zealous public officials and physicians attended. Not long after they convened, the group broadened the scope of its discussions to include issues of public hygiene as well as quarantine regulations and changed its name to "The Quarantine and Sanitary Convention." In April 1859, when the delegates met in New York City, they elected Griscom president and focused most of their attention on sanitary reform. Elisha Harris, later a founder with Henry W. Bellows of the United States Sanitary Commission, attended the 1859 and 1860 conventions.[82] All of these early public health reformers agreed that disease could be prevented and controlled by cleaning up the environment. Although the mechanisms by which diseases were transmitted (such as microorganisms) were not understood until late in the century, the connection between filth and disease was a powerful one. This idea had served local communities well during epidemics. It would soon prove to have lasting effects during wartime.

Popular behavior lagged behind bourgeois prescriptions in frontier-rural America. Wesley's and Franklin's maxims of the eighteenth century were not generally followed, nor were those of Beecher, Graham, Alcott, and Griscom or Shattuck in the mid-nineteenth century. Only with the onset of a national crisis—the Civil War—would urgency infuse the drive toward cleanliness.

CHAPTER TWO

A Wider War

The volunteers are now abundantly, yet far from wholesomely fed; they are lodged as well as the laws provide that soldiers shall be lodged; yet no sensible farmer lodges his beasts nearly as unwholesomely. . . . With typhus increasing, no means are available—at least none at all adequate—to keep them clean.

—FREDERICK LAW OLMSTED, 1861[1]

The Civil War provided public health reformers with a national laboratory in which to test their theories and apply their principles on hygiene. Unlike an epidemic, the war was neither local nor seasonal; but, like an epidemic, the Civil War created a full-blown crisis that captured everyone's attention. Far-sighted civilians mobilized a "sanitary" crusade in the North to guard the health of the fighting men by keeping their disease and death rates as low as possible. Women formed the shock troops who nursed Union soldiers amidst the filth and horror of hospital and battlefield during the bloody days of war and, with peace, headed south to minister to "contraband" former slaves. This shared purpose not only "brought home the idea of the value and economy of health and lives" but also contributed to "the wide extent to which the knowledge and principles of Hygiene" became "popularized . . . in civil as well as military life."

During the Civil War era, appreciation for cleanliness mushroomed. Stephen Smith, editor of the *American Medical Times* from 1860 to 1864 and later the first president of the American Public Health Association, recognized that by 1863 "the vocabulary of sanitary knowledge" and "the elementary facts of hygiene" had become "familiar in every household."[2] By the end of the war, most Americans had gained some new ideas about the meaning of cleanliness, and about "women's place."

Florence Nightingale's Good Example

In April 1861, with the bombardment of Fort Sumter and President Abraham Lincoln's call for 75,000 volunteers, Americans quickly recalled the recent experiences of the English in the Crimean War (1854-57). The massive outpouring of young male recruits, the uncertain preparedness of an army that had not been involved in a major conflict in some time, and the rush of untrained American women eager to follow Florence Nightingale's example created fears that the chaos and sanitary horrors of the Crimea would be repeated in the United States. In May 1861 the *American Medical Times* warned that the nation "must not wait to learn by bitter experience, what the Crimean war taught England and France." Instead, it urged Americans to "anticipate and provide against all dangers not essentially fortuitous." For the way "we save our citizen soldiers from preventible diseases and death," the *Times* contended, "is the most momentous question of this war."[3]

Of the innumerable individuals who offered instruction in the principles and practice of sanitary science during this period, none would become as well known and venerated throughout the United States as Nightingale, the Crimean War's "apostle of cleanliness." Although she never visited America, this "lady with a lamp" became famous for her much-publicized work in the Barrack Hospital of Scutari from 1854 to 1856. A year later her involvement in the investigation by the Royal Commission on the Sanitary Condition of the Army brought her more acclaim, as did her *Notes on Nursing* which, when published in London in December 1859, sold 15,000 copies within a month.[4]

When Nightingale joined the British forces at Scutari on November 4, 1854, she was responding indirectly to reports dispatched by William Howard Russell, special correspondent to the *Times* of London, and printed on October 9 and 12, 1854. He described the deplorable conditions in the British hospitals, where "there is not the least attention paid to decency or cleanliness" and "men die without the slightest effort being made to save them."[5] What Nightingale found in the Barrack Hospital confirmed Russell's observations. Supplies and furniture were inadequate or totally lacking, and sanitary arrangements were "inferior in point of crowding, ventilation, drainage, and cleanliness . . . to any civil hospital, or to the poorest homes in the worst parts of the civil population of any large town." But in late December, when Nightingale wrote to Secretary of War Sidney Herbert, she assured him that his instructions on washing and purveying would be carried out. Having already secured "the Turkish washing-house," she promised "to furnish every man in Hospital with a clean shirt twice a week."[6]

A powerful force for sanitary reform—especially because of Herbert's friendly support as well as her unusual personal popularity—Nightingale wasted little time in changing hospital policy within the British army. She assumed the duties of "Barrack Administrator" and devised various organizational plans so that the hospitals would run "upon a principle of centralization." Concerned about diet, supplies, and the patients' cleanliness (including their bedding, personal linen, and surgical appendages), she permitted few aspects of hospital routine to escape her notice. She usually described herself as "cook, house-keeper, scavenger . . . washerwoman, general dealer, store-keeper."[7] Nightingale had confidence in her principles and practices. In February 1855, for instance, she proudly declared that her hospitals had "no cholera" because she had placed "a sack of Chlor[ide] of Lime at the corner of every Corridor" and scrupulously saw to "cleansing out the places" that required it.[8]

Through use of "the wash-tub" at Scutari, Nightingale dramatically transformed hospital conditions. "It was upon the wash-tub, and all the wash-tub stood for," generations have been taught, "that she expended her greatest energies."[9] Her disciplined attention to cleanliness brought order out of chaos and reduced the number of deaths from disease. Portions of the Nightingale legend, at least, are true and account in many ways for her extraordinary influence in the second half of the nineteenth century. Her defense of cleanliness and hygiene rested on an obsolescent but popular view that "miasmas," or a noxious atmosphere, caused disease—a view that emphasized the importance of being clean. Although Nightingale was incorrect about miasmas, her beliefs nevertheless gave force and even efficacy to her practical suggestions regarding sanitation.[10]

Following the Crimean War, few were astonished when an investigation concluded that about three-fourths of all British casualties resulted from diseases such as dysentery, cholera, or typhoid, which had been contracted in the hospitals. Journalistic reports as well as evidence collected by the British Sanitary Commission graphically described sewers, "loaded with filth, untrapped, and without ventilating openings," whose emanations filled the air of hospital corridors and wards. Observers attempting to explain the high mortality rates cited clogged latrines, unemptied tubs, and naked men laying on floors in their own excrement. Nightingale recalled counting "as many as six dead dogs just under one ward window" in a muddy and filthy hospital yard. Admitting that approximately 4600 British soldiers died in Crimean hospitals during her tenure, she not surprisingly attributed their deaths mainly to "sanitary defects."[11]

Nightingale's Crimean experience fascinated American women, the majority of whom had attended sick family and friends. And many were mothers and housekeepers daily engaged in the act of cleaning. Catharine Beecher, who over the years taught middle-class women that there was "no one thing, more necessary . . . than *a habit of system and order*" in carrying out their "varied duties," had also advised them that good care for the sick involved "keeping a room neat, clean, and in perfect order, having every article in use sweet and clean. . . ."[12] But it was Nightingale's dramatic war work, "a marvel of womanly achievement," that inspired and created such intense interest "as to amount to a cult."[13]

American women took pride in Nightingale's recognized accomplishments in Crimea, and they relished the prestige it gave their work. Their satisfaction must have been considerable when they read her responses to written questions posed by the British Sanitary Commission as reported in the *New York Times* on March 11, 1858. Without equivocation, Nightingale told the royal commissioners that "the woman is superior in skill to the man in all points of sanitary domestic economy, and more particularly in cleanliness and tidiness." For this reason, she insisted, "great sanitary reformers . . . look to the woman to carry out practically their hygienic reforms." Since women have "a superior aptitude in *nursing*," she concluded that "the Anglo-Saxon would be very sorry to turn women out of his own house, or out of civil hospitals, hotels, institutions of all kinds, and substitute men-housekeepers and men-matrons."[14]

In 1860 Nightingale's *Notes on Nursing* appeared in the United States, where "its very extensive circulation" had important results. *Godey's* magazine, which reprinted portions of it, advised "every lady" to study and practice its precepts.[15] Large numbers obviously did. For in 1862 *Harper's Weekly* acknowledged Nightingale's wide-ranging influence; in North *and* South her name had become synonymous with nursing. A teenager in Mississippi, for example, demonstrated her patriotism by going to battle "in the capacity of Florence Nightingale," while numerous other women simply "threw open sickroom windows and dedicated themselves to cleanliness." Military and civilian medical people also admired Nightingale's work, and a few met with her in London.[16]

The First Women Volunteers

During 1861 thousands of resolute women in the North and South put aside their private household cares and offered their services, both as volunteers and as paid nurses. For the first time in the United States, women were to play a significant role in a major war. Working-class women, who had experience as laundresses and domestics, joined the ranks of middle-class women who had nursed family or friends but had never cared for strangers or worked for wages. They hoped that the skills they had acquired as mothers, housekeepers, and caretakers, along with the inspiration and instruction they had received from Nightingale, "could be put to useful and patriotic ends."[17]

Women were accustomed to volunteering their services for the public good. The 1850s had been a decade rich in humanitarian reform activities. In all parts of the country, institutions for the deaf, blind, insane, and orphaned had been built or expanded; the decade's economic uncertainties as well as its growing immigrant population and public health concerns had given Americans many opportunities to become involved in social welfare efforts. Very often middle- and upper-class women in cities had taken the lead in these benevolent causes and established extensive networks of voluntary associations.[18]

With the outbreak of the Civil War, women's organizations immediately directed their know-how, energy, and excitement to support the young men who had responded to the call of battle. These groups of women displayed the same heady enthusiasm and patriotism that characterized the army recruits. In Richmond, Virginia, Confederate Mary Boykin Chesnut wrote in her diary that every woman was ready "to rush into the Florence Nightingale business."[19] This was not news to the *American Medical Times*, which had already noticed that Nightingale's "example and practical instructions" were leading "thousands of American mothers and sisters . . . even before the first battle" to offer their services "for the relief of the brave men . . . so suddenly rushed to the field of conflict."[20] And wherever a man scurried to the front—in the South as well as in the North—there was certain to be "a Florence Nightingale at home, sitting in the rooms of the Ladies Aid Society, stitching on army shirts . . . and listening to [newspaper] items about the way the British Sanitary Commission was putting a woman's reforms into the British army."[21]

In the Confederacy, women were "knitting socks, making shirts, and stitching underwear . . . turning out everything from caps to sandbags, and sometimes supplying entire regiments." Up and down the South's class structure, from plantation matrons to ordinary housewives, women organized hundreds of relief societies to sew, raise money, make flags, and send off blankets.[22] They did much for their cause and would have done more, if the makeshift Confederate government had been better organized and funded. But it was unable to create a sanitary commission comparable to that of the North. Consequently these pages say much more about what happened in the Union than in the Confederacy, where the obstacles limiting the effectiveness of the South's women contributed to higher death rates from dysentery, malaria, pneumonia, and other diseases than from gunshots.[23]

Northern Ladies Aid societies also produced hundreds of articles, "some of them as fanciful as their ideas of war." There were quilts with embroidered lines of poetry, pillows stuffed with milkweed down, and havelocks (cloth cap covers, which hung down to protect the neck) modelled after those worn by the British in India. In anticipation of the summer heat, Ladies Aid societies began making these cap covers at a feverish pace and created a "Havelock mania," until it was discovered that soldiers received them "with incredulous merriment" and put them "to every manner of use except the one for which they were so honestly designed." The troops complained that "they kept the neck too hot," although the British invented them to prevent exactly that. It soon became apparent that too much "well-meant zeal" was being "fruitlessly expended" by wartime volunteers.[24]

Only a month after the Civil War began, Mary Bache Walker in Hoboken, New Jersey, speculated that enough havelocks, drawers, shirts, and hospital dressing gowns had been made "for both armies." But organization and distribution problems prevented many of these goods from reaching those troops most in need. A number of societies made articles for their favorite regiments, failing to send contributions "to a general depot for Hospital use without regard to particular regiments." Katharine P. Wormeley observed from Providence, Rhode Island, that "little circles and associations were multiplying, like rings in the water, over the face of the whole country; they were all in need of direction, information, guidance, and they felt it."[25]

In response to this obvious need, fifty-five women and a few men assembled on April 25, 1861, at the New York Infirmary for Women and Children in New York City. Elizabeth Blackwell, physician and friend of Nightingale, chaired the meeting and discussion centered on how to consolidate and direct the activities of aid societies around the country. Those present ended their deliberations by drafting an appeal, emphasizing "the importance of systematizing and concentrating the spontaneous and earnest efforts" of New York women, and by setting April 29 as the date for a follow-up meeting. The appeal, which appeared in the *New York Times* on April 28, warned that women "working without concert, organization, or head" were "liable to waste their enthusiasm in disproportionate efforts, to overlook some claims and overdo others. . . ."[26]

At the April 29 meeting, the Cooper Institute hall was "crowded with an earnest, enthusiastic, and patriotic assembly of women"—many of them from New York's most distinguished families. Numerous physicians well known to city residents also attended, as did the prominent Unitarian minister Henry W. Bellows. Together they organized the Woman's Central Association of Relief (WCAR) and elected surgeon Valentine Mott president and Bellows vice president. The group then discussed what it could do to supply goods and nurses to the army (which it did throughout the war, in cooperation with the Sanitary Commission). On the subject of nurses, the women pointed out that the Crimean War had proven "the total uselessness of any but picked and skilled women in this department of duty."[27]

Indeed, the Crimean experience overshadowed the deliberations of this organization, as it would those of the United States Sanitary Commission throughout the Civil War. Blackwell, who chaired WCAR's Registration Committee on Nurses, considered Nightingale one of her "most valued acquaintances" and shared her anti-contagionist views (the belief that disease spread through filth and "miasmas" rather than by contact with infectious organisms). Blackwell had recently visited Nightingale in London and become convinced that "sanitation is the supreme goal of medicine, its foundation and its crown."[28] She too believed in the unique capabilities women brought to nursing. Thus, even before creation of the Sanitary Commission, Blackwell's committee on nursing had joined with physicians at New York's Bellevue Hospital in providing one month's training to women before sending them to Dorothea Dix, recently appointed superintendent of women nurses in Washington, D.C. Unlike Blackwell, Dix did not know Nightingale personally, but she had traveled to Scutari during the Crimean War and inspected the famous Barrack Hospital. And, shortly after her departure, she had reported to the William Rathbones in Liverpool—close friends of both Nightingale and herself—that she found "the chief hospital . . . in excellent order."[29]

Such was not the case, however, in the federal capital in May 1861. When WCAR representatives—Bellows and Dr. Elisha Harris, together with physicians W. H. Van Buren and Jacob Harsen—arrived in Washington on May 16, 1861, they were aghast. Not only had "the country town" been "turned into a great, confused garrison," but even "quiet residential neighborhoods were in an uproar." Young soldiers, most of whom were away from home for the first time, crowded into the ill-prepared city and acted "as irresponsible as children." Having left mothers, sisters, and wives behind, they behaved as boys, whooping it up in the streets with their bugles and drums, getting drunk, firing weapons, relieving themselves in public, and neglecting to wash and "change their underwear for weeks at a time." Many of them had grown up on farms and had never been exposed to childhood diseases like measles; they promptly caught them. Almost a third of the troops got sick in 1861 before ever leaving their Washington staging areas, especially from gastrointestinal infections and the often lethal typhoid fever.[30]

These incidents of disorder and disease confirmed the WCAR delegates' determination to take charge and create a sanitary commission. The raw recruits in the neighborhood of Washington, numbering more than 30,000, were entirely unprepared for camp life; many had "enlisted as for a pastime, and went to camp as to a picnic." Although the best of the regiments built comfortable quarters, most volunteers were "entirely uninstructed in matters of hygiene, placed the tents too close together, did not provide drainage, and usually thought it unnecessary to dig latrines." The sanitary conditions of the city soon became disgusting.[31]

Most disturbing was that the army had made so few preparations to receive these young soldiers. Arriving in cattle cars from different parts of the country, they had waited in line for hours to ascertain where they would be sheltered and fed, "while their ignorant and inexperienced Commissaries and Quartermasters" learned their duties. Once in camp, regiments spent the night as they had en route to Washington, sleeping on rotten straw covered with shoddy blankets. The water supply at inland depots was not adequate for washing, and government rations were generally unwholesome and poorly cooked. Bellows and Harris feared that if these conditions persisted there would be disastrous results.[32]

Creating the Sanitary Commission

On the thirteen-hour train trip from New York to Washington, Bellows and his companions had talked at length about how civilians could serve their country during war. They all remembered "the frightful history of the British campaign in the Crimea," and Bellows admitted that he was impressed by "Miss Nightingale's labors" and "those of the English & French Commissions." Still uncertain about what they would do once they arrived in Washington, Harris suggested that they meet with the secretary of war and ask him to create a sanitary commission similar to the one that "had produced such happy results in the Crimea." By the time their train pulled into Union Station, they had unanimously agreed that they would urge the government "to establish a preventive hygienic and sanitary service for the benefit of the army."[33]

After a month-long struggle, on June 9, 1861, Secretary of War Simon Cameron gave his approval to a commission, but one that would restrict its "meddling" to the volunteer army. Several days later President Lincoln signed an executive order authorizing what he suspiciously called "a fifth wheel" to the coach of state. This new agency, the United States Sanitary Commission, immediately took action and shape, selecting Bellows as president, scientist Alexander Dallas Bache vice-president, and lawyer George Templeton Strong treasurer. Then on June 20 the commission appointed Frederick Law Olmsted secretary and chief executive officer.[34]

The motives of these New York and New England blue bloods—and there would soon be more—have been questioned and evaluated by historians for some time. Note that they very quickly took over the leadership roles from Blackwell and other women who formed WCAR. Through the war, many women would function in cooperation with, but clearly in subordination to, military or civilian men. It is unlikely today that this male assumption of wartime leadership would go as unremarked upon as it did then, but it was generally accepted that "man to man" discussions about government policy and battle tactics got better results. Dorothea Dix supervised the army's nurses, but she was the exception; the patrician Olmsted rather than the upwardly mobile and extraordinarily competent Blackwell ran the Sanitary Commission.[35]

Although skeletal, the commission's board was in place by the summer's end. In addition to founders Bellows, Harris, and Van Buren and officers Bache, Strong, and Olmsted, the board included New York physician Cornelius R. Agnew and chemist Oliver Wolcott Gibbs, Boston's well-known reformer Samuel Gridley Howe, and geologist John Strong Newberry from Cleveland. As a conciliatory gesture to the army's Medical Bureau, three army officers—George W. Cullum, Robert C. Wood, and Alexander Shiras—were also appointed to the board. Among the civilian members, the professions and the East Coast (especially New York) were better represented than business and the West. But as the number on the board gradually expanded to twenty-four, members from Ohio, Illinois, and Kentucky gave the commission broader representation as did the creation of regional branches and local auxiliaries.[36]

Whatever differences this representation may have signified, the commissioners shared a common strategy that centered on prevention. They maintained that the Sanitary Commission's primary objective was to contribute to the army's fighting effectiveness by reducing the incidence of illness as well as the number of deaths caused by preventable disease. It is nearly impossible to read any commission documents without encountering mention of the prevention of disease and the preservation of health through sanitary measures. From the beginning, the commission intended "to prevent the evils that France and England could only investigate and deplore."[37] Thus, in its inspection, publication, hospital construction, and statistical gathering programs, the Sanitary Commission continuously emphasized prevention over cure. Even when relief efforts began to consume large amounts of its resources, it insisted that preventive sanitary measures were "paramount to all questions of *relief.*" Motivated by the success of Nightingale, who through improved hygiene had significantly reduced the death rate in the British military hospitals, the commissioners were determined to demonstrate to the volunteer army and to the public that cleanliness was essential to their lives and to the survival of the republic.[38]

By wrapping cleanliness and order in the mantle of patriotism and victory, the commissioners defined a clear-cut mission: to teach the government, the medical bureau, the army, and the nation at home that "gunshots and cannon wounds, and death from battle, were not the enemies most to be feared in war." They had to learn that "the diseases of camp, arising from private ignorance, inexperienced officers, neglected or unknown sanitary police, the recklessness of raw soldiers, and the influences of exposure, unaccustomed food, and bad cookery" were the killers to guard against daily. For these reasons, Bellows and his colleagues had initially hoped they would be given "ample powers for visiting all camps and hospitals, advising, recommending, and if need be, enforcing, the best-known and most approved sanitary regulations in the army." But, in the end, the secretary of war made the commission simply advisory. Comparing it to its British model, Bellows complained that the United States Sanitary Commission had "been born paralytic" and was to be "endured" by government officials out of "deference towards a respectable body of supposed fanatics and philanthropists, backed by a large class of anxious and sympathetic women."[39]

Despite its disabilities, this group of health "fanatics" and philanthropists, supported by thousands of concerned women, devised an energetic program of action "to *prevent* evils to the health of the army." The commission began its work by inspecting camps around Washington and giving advice on "the choice of camp sites, the importance of drainage and police, and the character and cooking of food." Although the commissioners showed an early interest in preparing women for work on the battlefield, they and Dix agreed that "attention to hygiene in the Army [was] far more important than any present *added* efforts to assure nursing."[40]

Years of working on her own inhibited Dix from being able to "co-operate much" with the Sanitary Commission, but from the beginning she shared its concerns. She appeared "deeply depressed by the conditions of things" in Washington, D.C., in May 1861, and confessed that she worried a great deal about "provisions for the sick & for their proper care."[41] Besides her general uneasiness about hygiene among the recruits, Dix was particularly anxious about their diet. In fact she insisted that cooks were "much more necessary to the well being of the Army than nurses," arguing that ill-prepared food "creates more sickness than all the exposure and privations" to which the soldiers would be subjected. Fearing the possibility of a long war, Dix also urged the prevention of waste from the outset.[42]

When it came to matters of management, however, no one was more diligent than Olmsted. Bellows had hired him as the commission's general secretary largely for his "organizing powers [after] watching his operation & discipline at the Central Park" in New York City. Olmsted was a remarkable administrator. Fresh from his success as architect and superintendent of construction of Central Park—arguably the country's major municipal public work to that point—he had enhanced his reputation as a public administrator and broadened his interest in public health. He would go on to many more architectural and civic triumphs in his long career, but in 1861 he faced a huge challenge as inexperienced recruits poured into military camps (and before long, the hospitals). Olmsted accepted the the Sanitary Commission's day-to-day leadership because he saw in it "an opportunity to educate the common soldiers, who in turn would propagate such ideas among the American people."[43]

That task would not be an easy one. The majority of those who volunteered for service in the spring and summer of 1861 saw only the war's romantic aspects and felt only the excitement of leaving home. Departure celebrations took place everywhere, and when troop trains stopped at railway stations on the way to Washington, "soldiers were serenaded by brass bands, presented with silk flags, and inundated with speeches and prayers." If the officially powerless Sanitary Commission were to educate the large volunteer Union army in the realities of camp life and combat, it would have to cut through the hullabaloo of the recruits and their families, the chaos in the camps, and the inefficiency of the army's medical bureau. Olmsted's past experience as an organizer, his dedication to detail, his desire to hold a position of influence, and his commitment to providing care to as many soldiers as possible promised to make the Sanitary Commission "an effective instrument of benevolence."[44]

The need for instruction and supervision became apparent early on, as mentioned previously, since most volunteers were "as evasive of discipline as children and as unprepared for the work of war." On July 2, 1861, Olmsted wrote his wife from Washington that there was "a lot of fine material for soldiers here but no army." What he found instead were "seventy disjointed regiments of infantry under canvass." In too many instances, the individual in command had been elected by his soldier friends from home, and he knew that in a relatively short time his "subordinates" would again become his customers or clients. Not surprisingly, therefore, the discipline surrounding camp life resembled that "of a town-meeting or of an engine company." While the officers may have had "the best purposes," they did not know "how to control the diet, the personal habits, the ventilation and police of their quarters and camps." Instead they were "studying war *tactics*, intent on making *soldiers*"; and they inadvertently assumed that "intelligent men know how to take care of themselves."

Because many did not, camp dysentery took hold of "their regiments with a most threatening grasp."[45]

Despite a few quaint measures dating from General George Washington, when he required his Revolutionary War troops to bathe weekly, the United States Army had failed to institute any effective regulations on cleanliness before the Civil War. After temporary expedients in the War of 1812, the army had created a permanent Medical Department in 1818, which included surgeons and, begrudgingly, matrons to cook, nurse, and clean. But the Mexican-American War of 1846–48 exposed the department's inadequacies. Diarrhea and dysentery were rampant, maggots and gangrene festered in wounds, field hospitals became notorious as places to die rather than get better. According to an official army history of the Medical Department, "of the more than 100,000 soldiers who had left the United States to fight in Mexico, over 1,500 had been killed in action, but more than 10,000 had died of disease." It, once again, was "the great enemy"; the rate of death from disease of American soldiers in Mexico was "ten times that of civilians at home." Thirteen years later the army was set to embark on its bloodiest and grimmest conflict but, unfortunately, "a stubborn and unimaginative surgeon general" had learned nothing from the Mexican experience.[46]

Olmsted Starts Inspecting

In early July, when Olmsted and Harris examined the conditions of twenty camps around Washington, they were appalled and afraid. Every camp lacked "a system of drains," and "the sinks were unnecessarily and disgustingly offensive." They also saw that "cleanliness among the men was wholly unattended to," and their "clothing was of bad material and almost always filthy." A Dutch Reformed pastor in Brooklyn corroborated this in a letter to Commissioner Strong, reporting that men in New York's 47th Regiment were "dirty—covered with vermin and need a change of raiment for their health." The commission also learned that, even in places where water was available, few men bathed. As a result the volunteers appeared "really much dirtier than it can be believed they have been accustomed to be in their civil life. . . ."[47]

During the same month, Commissioner Howe investigated the sanitary condition of the troops around Boston for the governor of Massachusetts. He reported with astonishment that the government took better care of its war implements and its horses than the soldiers' health. What struck him most was the lack of cleanliness in the barracks and the privies. At Quincy, where Howe found the only camp privy near Boston "constructed with a view to decency," he noted that "even that was in a most neglected and filthy condition." Thus he recommended "more systematic and strict regulations" in all of the encampments, "especially [those] where women do not come." And he concluded that the army needed health officers and washerwomen—more than chaplains and nurses—and an urgent supply of "Soap! soap! soap!"[48]

These disgraceful living conditions help explain the Union army's defeat and rout at Bull Run in late July 1861. The extent of the panic and confusion provoked by the beating proved worrisome to all, but particularly to those who had expected a one-battle war. *Harper's Weekly* warned an anxious public: "From the fearful day at Bull Run dates war. Not polite war, not incredulous war, but war that breaks hearts and blights homes. . . ." On August 3, Olmsted wrote his father from Washington that the "best material for an army in the world has been ruined by bad management, inefficiency." The only solution, he believed, was to reorganize immediately, for the "sickly season" of the Potomac was at hand. To his wife, Olmsted confided that there was "but one Sanitary measure to be thought of now & that is discipline."[49]

Olmsted prepared the Sanitary Commission's official report on the troops' defeat at Bull Run. He drew his conclusions on their performance from "about two thousand items of evidence" collected by inspectors for the commission and physicians and examiners of life insurance companies. In a "General Summary," Olmsted pointed out that the volunteers had entered combat prepared "little better than a mob"; and those who fled to Washington, during or following the battle, looked like "wo-begone rabble." Many commissioners, besides himself, had seen them: "No two were dressed completely alike; some were without caps, others without coats, others without shoes. All alike were excessively dirty, unshaven, unkempt, and dank with dew."[50]

The volunteers were so terribly demoralized, Olmsted argued, because they lived in filthy camps, ate food of poor quality, and wore tattered clothing. He also emphasized that among the discontented and "soul-sick" volunteers, who were anxious about financial obligations at home and found war "all a muddle," there was "a growing want of confidence" between them and their officers. Convinced that the poorly administered army was at fault, Olmsted suggested that the Sanitary Commission should be more aggressive in carrying out its mission. He wanted the commissioners to "freely consider and determine the wants of the army" and "frankly represent them to the government and the people."[51]

Before the commission succeeded in orchestrating a campaign to reorganize and expand the army's antiquated Medical Department, it began inspecting camps. It hoped to "inspire officers and men with a sense of the nature and importance of sanitary laws, and with the practical application of hygienic principles." If successful, they would certainly prevent the spread of contagious diseases. But Olmsted, who believed slovenliness to be the nation's "most characteristic" vice, wanted more. He wanted to show these young men from mostly rural areas how to live healthy lives. "If five hundred thousand of our young men could be made to acquire something of the characteristic habits of soldiers in respect to the care of their habitations, their persons, and their clothing, by the training of this war," he wrote in December 1861, "the good which they would afterwards do as unconscious missionaries of a healthful reform throughout the country, would be by no means valueless to the nation."[52]

As preventive medicine, the Sanitary Commission's education and inspection program made significant gains. It developed manuals of procedure for field hospitals, proposed revampings to improve the Medical Department, and devised statistical forms to record levels of food supplies, camp drainage and sewerage, personal hygiene, and other sanitary matters. Its inspectors, the majority of whom had solid reputations as physicians or teachers, viewed their assignment as one of "suggesting, advising, and instructing the officers in camp" on ways to preserve the health of their troops. The inspectors tried not to cause unnecessary ill will when visiting camp sites, but they also knew that "the standard of the volunteers" regarding discipline should be "at least as high as that of the regulars."[53]

The commissioners and inspectors believed that the discipline found wanting in these young recruits had more to do with guidance or teaching than with punishment. Most of them had left their small towns or farms on a patriotic impulse and with little or no knowledge that "a man cannot be made a good soldier unless he is made to keep himself clean."[54] The stories they had heard at home from veterans of the Mexican War had not included such mundane subjects as hygiene, nor had the volunteers stopped to think how their daily lives would be altered once they were crowded into camps where few if any women were present. For those who did give these notions consideration, they probably concluded that their new routine would be adventuresome but would "remain in its essentials an extension of home life." Harriet Martineau, the contemporary English observer, contended that America's volunteer troops were not disciplined because the idea was new to them; they were of "a self-governing and unmilitary nation."[55]

But as the soldiers started getting sick, they realized that home's comforts had definitely been left behind. They may even have recognized how much "thought and labor" their mothers, wives, or sisters had expended in looking after their clothes, meals, personal comforts, and health. And they probably had an inkling that the freewheeling habits acquired on the road could be perilous. Those from rural areas who had never been exposed to the usual childhood illnesses quickly became victims of measles or mumps. Others, unaware of the relationship between dirt and disease, were introduced in camp to dysentery and diarrhea, typhoid, and malaria.[56]

The typical inductee, who had "felt as free as a bird" on leaving home, had also "lived like one" in camp. Nearly all the recruits urinated immediately outside their tents every morning. Most of them saw no reason to use the trench latrines, and those who did frequently "defile[d] the ground in various directions about the sinks" and rarely covered their feces with dirt. Even worse, those afflicted with severe cases of diarrhea dealt with their profuse and dangerous ejections "in the most perfunctory and careless way."[57]

Sanitary Commission inspectors tried to change these thoughtless practices. Armed with a form containing 180 questions, they moved through Union camps giving instruction and advice. They began their work by evaluating the character of the camp site (how it was selected, its precise location, the nature of the soil and subsoil) as well as the arrangement of the camp (the kind and extent of drainage, the source of water and its quality, the amount of space between tents and the number of men quartered in them, the condition of streets). From these general inquiries, they then proceeded to more particular ones concerning the care and habits of the troops.[58]

The inspectors examined bedding and clothing supplies, and they questioned officers about the soldiers' personal hygiene. They wanted to know, for example, if the men bathed frequently and if they were required to do so with an officer present. They also asked if each man washed "his head, neck, and feet once a day" and if evidence of negligence in washing was "looked for at inspection." In regard to the camps' cleanliness, the inspectors queried officers about the removal of garbage and rubbish, the distance between the tents and the men's privy, the actual size of the trench and whether it had a sitting rail or a screen, where the horses were kept in relation to where the soldiers slept and ate, and how often dung was removed. The inspectors, who were extremely interested in the kind of food that was served and how it was prepared, also urged that attention be given to "washing and scouring cooking utensils." And they inquired about the "preventive duty" of the surgeon: did he inspect the camp daily "with reference to its cleanliness"? Was he aware of "how the cooking was done"? Did he "report on these matters and urge remedies" to company or commanding officers?[59]

The Sanitary Commission received from the inspectors' written reports the information it needed to perform its advisory duties. At the same time, it knew that most officers would benefit from their association with this capable group of inspector-physicians (six permanent ones and fourteen who had been recruited to volunteer their services) and would welcome their suggestions and advice. New to their jobs, many officers recognized their ignorance of sanitary regulation and appeared eager to learn. Only in a few instances did some complain that they were not commissioned "to look after pots and kettles" or "to do the work of a housekeeper."[60]

In December 1861 Olmsted described the sanitary condition of the volunteer army in a report subsequently published by the commission. He relied primarily on the 200 regimental returns he had received from the inspectors. In regard to camp police and the attitude of many officers, he noted "a very marked and gratifying improvement." However, he expressed disappointment that a number of inspectors had found it difficult, even after an outbreak of typhoid, "to make the volunteer officers realize the actual military necessity upon which the army regulations, with reference to the personal cleanliness of the men," was based. Thus Olmsted again recommended "a strict enforcement of *Army Regulations*" and insisted that "each soldier . . . be provided with a clothes brush, shoe brush, tooth brush, comb, and towel . . . for which he should be required to account weekly." He also reiterated the commission's belief that whatever could be done to improve the volunteers' habits would be "amply repaid in their greater health and better spirit in their duty."[61]

By 1862 it had become clear that a much more vigorous inspection system was necessary if the troops' hygienic condition were to show much improvement. For this reason, as well as to secure the appointment of a surgeon general who would acknowledge the serious deficiencies in the army's medical services, the Sanitary Commission undertook and successfully obtained passage of an act to reorganize the Medical Department. On April 16, 1862, President Lincoln signed legislation that included a provision for commissioning sanitary inspectors and for appointing the surgeon general and his assistants on the basis of merit rather than seniority. This law allowed the commission to reduce the number of its inspections in 1862 and completely discontinue them in 1864.[62]

Since it had many other concerns, the Sanitary Commission was not left idle by the new law. It showed a real interest, for instance, in the needs of uncommissioned surgeons who worked under contract and also in the construction of military hospitals. Contract surgeons were frequently no more acquainted with the precepts of preventive medicine than were many of the regimental officers. In addition these surgeons were often required to treat wounds or diseases they had not seen in civilian practice. To assist them, the commission devised and disseminated a series of about twenty manuals or tracts, outlining the most up-to-date information on prevention and treatment of prevalent camp maladies and answering medical and surgical questions of a military nature.[63] Influenced once again by Nightingale's successes in Crimea, the commission promoted the building of commodious pavilion hospitals. In them, they thought, heavy concentrations of "poison" or "effluvia" from the large number of patients gathered under one roof would be dissolved in plenty of fresh air.[64]

For a commission that had had such a precarious beginning, the "Sanitary," as it became known among contemporaries, proved more popular and effective than anyone in Washington had predicted. Because of its expertise and influence, the Medical Department gradually improved, as did the officers; and even the men became "more ready to avail themselves of sanitary regulation."[65] Yet they continued to complain of inspections as well as carp about the time and effort that cleanliness required. Jenkin Lloyd Jones, a young recruit from Spring Green, Wisconsin, remarked in his diary that "washing day" had "duly occupied the afternoon." He probably spent that much time because he feared the "clothing inspection by Captain Dillon," who was "very particular" and "had little sympathy with his privates" who did not "look well." Nineteen-year-old James Newton from DePere, Wisconsin, grumbled in a letter to his parents that it took all of his "extra time to keep . . . clean." And Joseph Burt Holt wrote his wife from a camp in Washington that he wished she were there to do his clothes.[66]

As time passed, however, volunteers began to understand the relationship between dirt and disease. Having witnessed the deaths of sick friends, they now knew that disease killed more often than bullets. Chauncey Cooke, another Wisconsin native, wrote home that the "fear of bullets" did not bother him "half as much as the fear of disease." Convinced by the evidence, "veteran" recruits began to change their ways to protect their lives. William Prock Landon of Vincennes, Indiana, complained to a friend that his campsite, Harrison's Landing on the James River, was "an unhealthy place for sound men"; "dirty as pigs," they could barely find enough water "for cooking purposes and quenching thirst." To the same friend two months later, Prock groused both about the food and the fact that he had "but one shirt to his back—that a dirty one, and no time to wash it." As new habits formed, some soldiers seemed genuinely pleased with themselves. For instance, young Cooke told his mother that, although he had not previously assisted her in her work, he could now help "in so many ways." And John Brobst boasted that he could "wash, cook, sew, do anything as well as any of the girls."[67]

As a follow-up to its successful inspection program and the government's acceptance of its plans for model hospitals, the Sanitary Commission decided in September 1862 to take a look at the condition of general hospitals throughout the North. Since spring 1861 the army had nearly doubled in size, and the number of sick and wounded in the 184 general hospitals (many of them still makeshift) had quadrupled, but the medical inspection staff had remained the same. The commission reasoned, therefore, that "intelligent assistance from civil life would be acceptable." Under the leadership of Henry G. Clark, a Boston physician long interested in matters of sanitation, fifty-nine doctors "of established weight and character" agreed to visit these hospitals and examine their appearance, administration, and quality of care.[68]

In May 1863 Clark submitted a report of 2500 folio pages to the Sanitary Commission's Medical Committee. Without exception, the inspectors had been cordially received by the medical directors and surgeons. But hospital conditions, like their staffs, varied. One inspector found the hospitals he examined "in a most creditable condition." But in Cumberland, Maryland, another inspector visited a hospital that was "simply disgusting," with outhouses "filled with dirty clothes . . . soiled by discharges from sick men"; and the privy, consisting of a shed built over two trenches, was even more "filthy and offensive" since it had no seats, "simply a pole passing along each trench, for the men to sit on." Other inspectors complained about inadequate water supplies and the difficulties of washing and keeping wards clean.[69]

Despite the disheartening findings of many inspectors, the commissioners praised the medical staffs of half the hospitals they examined, rating 30 percent "Highly praised"; 20 percent, "Good"; 10 percent, "Adequate"; 40 percent, "Poor"; and none, "Terrible." One wonders whether 50 or 60 percent of the staffs were truly "adequate" to "highly praised," or whether the inspectors were being politic. For many in the army's Medical Department—and Secretary of War Edwin Stanton himself—had become irritated by the intrusion of civilian physicians posing as experts. At the end of 1864, Stanton banned commission inspectors from combat zones and closed patients' records to them; the "Sanitary" was "no longer completely indispensable."[70] But Stanton's action was at least a tacit admission that the commission had got results.

"A Woman's War"

Once the Sanitary Commission involved itself in army hospitals, it directed more of its attention to treating the sick and wounded. As a consequence a larger number of women became more intimately and practically involved in the Union war effort. When Stephen Smith reported on the Warehouse Hospital in Georgetown and Elisha Harris on the General Hospital at Fort Schuyler, both commissioners commented on the presence of female nurses. Smith observed that they appeared "to do their duties well," and Harris asserted that their "general influence" was "excellent."[71] As war broke out, patriotic women who had wanted to serve their country at the front found themselves employed in general hospitals. The army prohibited them from residing in camps or joining regiments on the march.

Most women, particularly at the beginning, had secured their places through Superintendent Dix. Afraid that the nursing experiment might fail if too many women of poor judgment secured hospital positions, Dix set about looking for women of character, good health, and some experience. She defined the kind of person she sought in this way: "No woman under thirty need apply to serve in the government hospitals. All nurses are required to be plain looking women. Their dresses must be brown or black, with no bows, no curls, no jewelry, and no hoop-skirts." Dix, who was well traveled, probably drew up this dress description after recalling the nursing successes of certain women's religious orders in Europe.[72]

One result of such scrutiny was that the title "nurse" carried cachet. Some 20,000 women served the Union army in all capacities, according to a good estimate, but only 2000 to 3000 were called nurses and were under Dix's supervision; these were "white women of the middle and upper classes." The other nine-tenths served as "matrons," "cooks," and "laundresses" and were African-American women (free or slave) and white working-class women. Thus class distinctions, though more rigid in the Confederacy, operated in the Union service as well.[73]

In the South, after slaves and servants left the premises, some upper-class women found themselves learning in a hurry to cook and clean. Sarah Morgan, for one, was "astonished that she 'could empty a dirty hearth, dust, move heavy weights, make myself generally useful and dirty, and all this thanks to the Yankees!' " Other women began nursing by volunteering to accept casualties into their homes, and later by raising funds and helping build field hospitals. The Confederacy had to depend much more than the Union on volunteers, and though "these women worked hard and long [they] did not earn enough money to be considered professionals." Unromantic drudgery, sickening smells and foul air, resistance from male doctors whom Mary Johnstone, in complaining to Vice President Alexander H. Stephens, regarded as "drunken political appointees," added up to bad working conditions. But the women achieved much; cleaner wards, more nutritious food, and better organization meant that their hospitals had a 5 percent mortality rate compared with 10 percent in male-run hospitals.[74]

One of the most famous nurses on the Union side was Massachusetts's Louisa May Alcott, who arrived from Concord at the Georgetown Union Hotel Hospital in December 1862. She had applied for a nursing position,

confident that she met Dix's requirements. Not only had Alcott nursed her
sister Elizabeth during a long illness, but she had also studied Nightingale's
Notes on Nursing and felt she "knew the canons of the profession." She was
thirty years old, in good health, and serious. And her made-over wardrobe
contained items of black and brown as stipulated by Dix.[75]

The Sanitary Commission inspectors who visited the Georgetown hospital only two months before Alcott's arrival reported that the old hotel building was "poorly adapted for a hospital." The basement kitchen was "dark,
damp, and dirty," and the sinks in the rear of the kitchen were "very offensive." Alcott later described this hospital as a "perfect pestilence-box . . . full
of vile odors from wounds, kitchens, wash-rooms, and stables." But here Alcott learned the duties generally assigned to female nurses: "the care of the
cleanliness of patients as to dress and person, the supervision, preparation,
and administration of extra diets and beverages, and such watching and
other care of the sick as the medical officers may direct."[76]

Hannah Ropes, matron of the Georgetown Union Hotel Hospital, taught
Alcott and her nursing companions to change patients' underclothes at least
once a week, wash their hands and faces with a strong brown soap, and
empty their bedpans whenever used. Convinced that a man could be transformed by washing him, dressing him in a clean shirt, and laying him on a
white bed, Ropes no doubt gave volunteer nurses some important lessons in
hospital hygiene. Thus, when forty wagons of wounded soldiers arrived
from Fredericksburg, Alcott was as prepared as most new nurses to do what
was expected.[77]

In *Hospital Sketches*, Alcott recalled the confusion of December 16,
1862, and the "wrecks of humanity" who filled the corridors of the Union
Hotel Hospital. After finding her way to her assigned post in Ward Number
One, she was given a "basin, sponge, towels, and a block of brown soap"
along with instructions "to wash as fast as you can." She hesitated at first but
then remembered her resolve to do what she was told. "[I] drowned [my]
scruples in the wash-bowl, clutched [my] soap manfully, and, assuming a
business-like air, made a dab at the first dirty specimen [I] saw." Having
successfully cleaned one old Irishman, she continued to scrub away "like
any tidy parent on a Saturday night." She later became known among patients as "'the nurse with the bottle,'" since she armed herself with lavender
water as a protection against "the vilest odors that ever assaulted the human
nose."[78]

Alcott and women like her joined with the Sanitary Commission in providing "humane and efficient care for wounded, sick, and dying soldiers."[79]
Nightingale's well-publicized lessons in the basic principles of sanitation,
now reinforced by their own wartime experiences, made these female

nurses forceful agents of cleanliness. But if they had had any notion that cleanliness reflected a certain godliness, their work as nurses removed it. For example, Alcott described an incident in which she tried to care for a " 'red-headed devil' " from the Confederacy who had been shot in the foot. He refused her assistance; but he so vigorously performed his ablutions "in a sea of soap-suds" that he reminded her of "a dripping merman, suffering from the loss of a fin." Amazed and amused, Alcott reflected: "If cleanliness is a near neighbor to godliness, then was the big rebel the godliest man in my ward that day."[80]

Since these volunteer nurses had no formal training and no experience other than tending the sick at home, their ideal was not the well-ordered hospital but the well-managed home. Those who had left the hearth to nurse the boys in blue brought with them knowledge of mothering, house-keeping, and caretaking as well as an informed sense that their particular skills could alter the despicable conditions so characteristic of military hos-pitals. In many instances they did. Sophronia E. Bucklin, a young nurse as-signed to the Thirteenth Street Hospital in Washington, had charge of the linen room. One day, upon investigating the wash-room with the hospital steward, she discovered hundreds of pieces of wet and dirty garments on the floor. Saddened by what she found, she asked the steward's permission "to undertake a revolution in the department." Bucklin and seven black women proceeded to clean up the mess and several days later provided the patients with "a supply of clean clothing, and clean beds."[81]

Despite their exhausting labor on behalf of the patients, Bucklin noticed that officers and doctors "threw out hints that women were a nuisance in war." She and a good many others were unhappy and annoyed by these signs of ingratitude, but they continued their back-breaking work, satisfied that "many a poor wounded fellow blessed in his heart the women who pro-vided sheets, fresh from the purifying scent of water, for his beds." While some of these women no doubt were incompetent or insubordinate, most volunteer nurses wanted to be put to good use and to please those in com-mand as well as those in their care. They "quietly and patiently worked, doing, by order of the surgeon, things which not one of those gentleman would have dared to ask of a woman whose male relative stood able and ready to defend her and report him."[82]

According to Georgeanna Woolsey, an energetic volunteer nurse from New York who worked for the Sanitary Commission on its hospital ships during the Peninsular campaign in 1862, these pioneer women performed their assigned duties for two reasons—"to gain standing ground for others" and to see "sick and dying men comforted in their weary and dark hours." Woolsey had been among the select group of women admitted to the

WCAR training program in New York City. Through Blackwell's influence Woolsey and her sister, Eliza, secured positions in army hospitals in the Washington area during the winter of 1861–62. Although both women later served with Olmsted on the commission's hospital transports, it was "Georgy" who made the lasting impression. Almost thirty years later, Olmsted said he believed that Georgeanna Woolsey "would, upon orders, take command of the channel fleet; arm, equip, man, provision, sail and engross the enemy, better than any other landsman I know."[83]

Woolsey proved to be one of many women who flourished during her wartime service. In October 1861 her mother commented that she had recently seen "Georgy" in Washington and that she looked "better and certainly fatter than when she left home." Yet, despite her enthusiasm, she sharply criticized those she felt did not measure up. Like many others in Washington, she found Dix difficult and overbearing. Acknowledging her "splendid" career, Woolsey remarked that Dix would have greater success "with more graciousness of manner." However, she reserved her strongest criticism for the army and its medical staff. The uncaring army appeared as a "a cold spectre," whose unfortunate presence was felt "everywhere"; and the Medical Department was "an absolute Bogie." It stood proudly and "continually in one's path," keeping "shirts from ragged men, and broth from hungry ones . . . and quietly assert[ing] that it had need of nothing."[84]

The Woolsey sisters considered themselves lucky in April 1862 when Frederick Knapp, Olmsted's assistant, offered them positions as "nurses at large" on the government steamboats the Sanitary Commission would use to transport the wounded from combat areas on the Potomac and James rivers to general hospitals in the North. These ships, "stripped of everything movable but dirt," had been lying idle until the secretary of war authorized what proved to be "the most arduous and harassing duty performed by the Commission during the war." During the eleven weeks that Olmsted personally supervised and assisted his staff on these steamers, they had one "distinct" plan—"that every man had a good place to sleep in, and something hot to eat daily, and that the sickest had every essential that could have been given them in their own homes." Thus before the *Daniel Webster* and the *Wilson Small* set sail on April 30, a dozen "contrabands" (former slaves) had worked "night and day scrubbing and cleaning" them in preparation for the commission's first thirty-five patients who, upon arrival, were "tea'd and coffeed . . . undressed and put to bed clean and comfortable."[85]

This small group would, however, be the last. Within days the transports received over 300 "very sick" and "horribly filthy" patients. No longer could the commission staff and nurses treat all these patients as they had the first thirty-five—as if they were "alone in a private family." For during the course of the summer, these ships removed 8000 sick and wounded soldiers from the Peninsula. While doing so, Olmsted grew increasingly frustrated with the medical officers' negligence, callousness, and inefficiency. Yet the women aboard showed themselves to be "in every way, far beyond" what he had expected.[86]

The genteel women who worked such long hours on commission transports appreciated Olmsted's "wise, authoritative, untiring" supervision. Although Katharine Prescott Wormeley described him as an "autocrat and aristocrat," she admitted to liking Olmsted "exceedingly," for "he would protect and guard in the wisest manner those under his care." Georgeanna Woolsey, another admirer, reported how Olmsted "would come quietly" into wards, when there was "no one round to look at him." On one occasion she found him "on the floor by a dying German, with his arm round this fellow—as nearly round his neck as possible—talking tenderly to him." A stickler for organization, discipline, and efficiency, Olmsted was also kind and humane. Neither hardhearted nor sentimental, he was a demanding administrator with a large vision of what the Sanitary Commission might accomplish. And through his commanding leadership and relentless concern, the commission not only led the way to cleanliness but saved lives.[87]

During the Civil War it was not uncommon to hear it said that "whitewash and women" were "the best disinfectants."[88] This bit of mid-nineteenth-century wisdom probably originated with the more glamorized accounts of Nightingale's sanitary efforts and then gained credence through popular reports on American nurses such as Clara Barton or Mary Ann "Mother" Bickerdyke. Although these women did "a little of everything," as Wormeley related, most of their work was "very much that of a housekeeper." On the commission's transports, for example, they laundered the patients' bed linens and clothing, managed a pantry and storeroom, prepared and cooked food, and had "general superintendence over the condition of the wards." Yet because they were on or near battlefields, their responsibilities had an urgent and dramatic aspect. When an influx of wounded soldiers arrived unannounced, women nurses left their usual work, rushed to the men, and quickly made them "clean and comfortable" before turning them over to other hands. Through repeated crises and in the face of so much suffering, they learned the value of discipline. "No one must come here," counseled Wormeley, "who cannot put away all feeling." "Do all you can, and be a machine," she continued, "that's the way to act; the only way."[89]

On April 5, 1864, the New York *Herald* stated, "All our women are Florence Nightingales." Impressed as the newspaper may have been with the unusual activities of northern nurses at the front, most women in fact remained at home. But few sat idle. Instead they supported the Union cause through the efforts of their local aid societies—a couple even bore the name of "Florence Nightingale." In churches, schools, and parlors, 7000 groups of women participated in the Sanitary Commission's auxiliary relief program. These local units made, purchased, or collected goods that the army needed and then sent them to regional or branch offices, where they were sorted and repackaged. Once repacked, the supplies moved through central distributing stations in Washington or Louisville on their way to hospitals or field relief agents. Since the commission refused to accept contributions for specific individuals or units and since it encouraged work that was "abundant, persistent, and methodical," women at home too learned lessons in discipline and efficiency.[90]

The British journalist George A. Sala, who traveled in the United States during the Civil War, believed that no other conflict "in ancient or modern history . . . was so much of a 'Woman's war' as this." Bellows, who aside from Olmsted had the best view of the Sanitary Commission's many activities, agreed; he observed that "never in any war in any country" had there been "so universal and so specific an acquaintance on the part of both men and women, with the principles at issue, and the interests at stake." The credit for this accomplishment belongs jointly to the commission, which entrusted its relief activities to the Woman's Central Association and its branches, and to able women like Louisa L. Schuyler in New York City and Abby W. May in Boston, who made the Sanitary Commission "as much their protege as their patron." Together they succeeded in collecting and distributing supplemental supplies valued at approximately $12 million.[91]

Schuyler and May explained the commission's objectives vis-à-vis the volunteer army in issues of the *Sanitary Bulletin* and in published association reports. Emphasizing its concern for the soldiers' health by inculcating habits of cleanliness and discipline, the New England Women's Auxiliary Association learned, for example, that inspectors had been engaged to urge "rigid attention to the minutest details of each man's care of his person, his clothing, and his dwelling place." And executive committee chairman May explained that the individual "who is clean, orderly and mannerly" will be a better man and fighter "than he who is unclean, slipshod, minus some buttons, strings and straps, with a filthy tent, and brutish habits in general." Thus, while appealing for items such as soap, sponges, towels, bandages, sheets, and undershirts, May also encouraged her readers to apply "the good old New England custom of 'spring and fall cleaning'" to the nation. For it was now, she insisted, that "the great national house . . . must undergo a thorough cleaning." If these kinds of solicitations were not sufficiently convincing, the twelve segments of Nightingale's *Notes on Nurs-*

ing that appeared in the *Sanitary Bulletin* from December 1863 through August 1864 probably were.[92]

By 1862 thousands of northern women had become directly involved in the commission's work. Information and goods "moved back and forth between Washington, the military outpost, and the most distant households of the United States." The active participation of so many women ensured the interest of whole families. Except for exchanges of personal letters, the connections most civilians had with the army during the Civil War were largely made and continued through "Sanitary" agencies. According to a contemporary, "the mere fact that the word 'Sanitary' was brought into every hamlet, and played its part in all conversation, was a very important fact," especially in educating or persuading those who had been ignorant or unconvinced of the importance of cleanliness. For "prominence given to a word gave, of necessity, prominence to an idea."[93]

The South and the Freedpeople

Women in the South had their "Florence Nightingales" in Fannie Beers and Kate Cumming, but they did not have the good fortune to participate in a national organization committed to the health and welfare of the volunteer army. Nor had there been reformers proclaiming the "gospel of cleanliness" in the prewar South—or so, at least, said Olmsted and Harriet Beecher Stowe, after visits there. One astute Confederate veteran explained in simple language why the South had no Sanitary Commission: "We were too poor; we had no line of rich and populous cities closely connected by rail. . . ." In southern communities, he said, "every house was a hospital." Thus, while circumstances did not permit such an operation, neither did sentiment. The states' rights philosophy of the region encouraged donations to particular individuals and regiments. Southern women who supported the Confederacy through their local aid societies generally collected goods and distributed them to their own.[94]

Nevertheless, an unusual cleanliness campaign got under way in New Orleans after its capture in April 1862. Threatened by an outbreak of yellow fever, the Union General in charge, Ben Butler—a Yankee who later admitted he knew nothing about "Yellow Jack"—ordered a war on dirt in the hope of saving his troops. Studying local accounts of an 1853 outbreak and recalling that Moses had "enforced the most thorough, careful and minute cleanliness in regard to all dead or decaying animal matter," Butler began a massive public works program. He first established a tight quarantine on the Mississippi River below New Orleans and paid 1100 unemployed poor whites, "contrabands," and prisoners "to clean the city from all deleterious emanations of animal matter"; he then ordered households to clean up their yards and employed inspectors to visit every ten days. Butler's clean-up thwarted "Yellow Jack" and lowered the incidence of certain endemic diseases. Intensely disliked for his despotic methods, he nonetheless won the gratitude of many for his successful sanitary experiment.[95]

But it was those generous women working with former slaves who played a key role in encouraging cleanliness for purposes of health, progress, and acceptance. (Booker T. Washington never forgot their advice, as we will see in the next chapter.) Beginning in 1862 thousands of female teachers, most of them Northerners, moved to the South and served as agents of freedmen's aid societies. For the most part, these volunteers taught school and dispensed relief, but they also gave innumerable lessons on cleanliness. Yankee women who left home for short or extended periods of service had various motives for doing so, yet they shared a view of the freed population "as culturally backward but not inherently deficient." And they believed they could narrow the cultural gap and improve the lot of former slaves by teaching them how to read and write *and* how to be thrifty, industrious, disciplined, and clean.[96] In less formal ways, the "contrabands" in their camps and schools received instructions similar to those given to young army recruits. Among African-Americans, however, cleanliness was emphasized as being important to their health as well as for their advancement and acceptability.

Nearly everyone who worked among the former slaves remarked on their unsanitary residences. Cornelia Hancock, a volunteer nurse from New Jersey, spent the winter of 1863-64 at a contraband hospital and camp outside Washington. "The situation of the Camp," she wrote to her brother, "is revolting to a degree." Since it had only one well, which was often broken, water for nearly a thousand people had to be carted from Washington. Her solution was simple—"a national Sanitary Commission for the Relief of Colored Persons . . . would save lives and a great deal of suffering."[97]

Laura Towne, who left Philadelphia for Beaufort and Port Royal Island in April 1862, found the blacks in South Carolina in much the same condition. Shortly after her arrival in Beaufort, she visited a home of former slaves where she met "a dirty family and two horribly ugly old women." She knew that they had "got a lesson from some one," for they said, "'We got to keep clean or we'll all be sick.'" But, as she wrote in her diary, "they were not putting their lesson to use." To her chagrin, the streets of Beaufort were full of "dirty and ragged" children. Recognizing the "hard task" ahead, Towne renewed her commitment to "anti-slavery work" and vowed "to do it earnestly."[98]

Slave quarters had always been deprived of things a middle-class person of the time would regard as necessary, and when slaves became sharecroppers after the war, the number of conveniences did not increase appreciably. Houses were cramped, without plumbing or running water, and everyday living "took place in one room where 'stale sickly odors' inevitably accumulated." This does not mean, though, that former slaves had no standards of their own. In what was probably a carry-over from West Africa, for example, African-Americans in Georgia and elsewhere regularly swept their front yards—partly to keep away snakes and insects, partly to be able to cook or do the washing outside the cabin. For several generations, in fact, "the swept yard was the most important 'room' of the household, the heart of the home." Slavery and sharecropping did not mean *no* cleanliness, but rather, achieving it against great odds. The problem was compounded further in the immediate aftermath of emancipation, when many former slaves traveled about the lower South seeking better lives. A Mississippian wrote in October 1865 that "Vicksburg has been unusually sickly this season—on account of the crowded state of the town—especially the number of negroes congregated in small houses, & living without any cleanliness."[99]

Committed to improving the situations of these poor and desperate people, northern women (with very different standards of cleanliness) worked long days sorting, repairing, washing, and distributing clothes sent to them by their aid societies. They also helped African-American women and children "patch their rags" and "make bed-ticks for themselves," in a sincere attempt "to teach them cleanliness." Since these Northerners found the former slaves "a very imitative people," they believed they could instruct "by example as well as by precept." Susan Walker, a Midwesterner, wrote home in March 1862: "Visited cabins and preached industry and cleanliness. Mrs. J. had done much to induce the last, already at her insistence whitewashing and scrubbing have commenced and imitation is large in the negro. I am hopeful." And a young woman in Mitchellville, South Carolina, told the New England Freedmen's Aid Society that "at first the children came to Sunday school in the same dresses they wore on a week day." However, "once they saw their teachers dressed a little better on Sunday," they came the following week "with some change in their apparel, if it was nothing more than a clean apron."[100]

Determined to help the former slaves make their way in American society, these Yankee teachers consciously promoted their cherished values— "sobriety, cleanliness, industry, thrift, and fidelity to contracts." In school, more than in any other place, African-American children learned "habits of neatness and cleanliness" along with "reading, writing, spelling, and Arithmetic." Elizabeth Hyde Botume, who taught in Beaufort, South Carolina, contended that "needles and thread and soap and decent clothing were the best educators, and would civilize sooner than book knowledge." To inculcate practices of personal hygiene, teachers offered prizes to those with the "neatest, best written" copybooks. As a result, youngsters at Ladies Island, South Carolina, usually came to school "with clean hands, that they might not soil their books." Those who did not found "a pail, a wash-basin, soap, and towel" in the corner, where they were made "to perform the necessary ablutions."[101]

Teachers used whatever reading materials and textbooks they could find. Lydia Maria Child's *The Freedmen's Book* (1865) proved one of the more popular. A white abolitionist who had given up her career as a novelist and author of children's stories to advocate freedom, Child included in her text biographies of prominent African-Americans such as Benjamin Banneker, Phillis Wheatley, and Frederick Douglass as well as poems, anecdotes, and essays. In "The Laws of Health" Child encouraged African-Americans to wash often, especially if they lived near a pond or river, explaining that troublesome sores "might be prevented by frequent bathing." But in an essay entitled "Advice from an Old Friend," she gave former slaves an additional reason for taking care of themselves and making a good impression—"it is one of the best ways to prove that you are not inferior." Child did not hesitate to tell her black friends that they would be respected as freedmen if they wore "working-clothes that are clean and nicely patched" and lived in "a white-washed cabin, with flowering-shrubs and vines clustering round it."[102]

More of this kind of advice reached freedmen through textbooks published by the American Tract Society. Isaac Brinckerhoff's *Advice to Freedmen* and J. B. Waterbury's *Friendly Counsels for Freedmen* were unconventional in that they were directed to adults and did not attempt to teach literature or history; they simply offered practical advice on how to live as free men and women. Unlike Child, ministers Brinckerhoff and Waterbury did not link cleanliness to health. Instead they emphasized solely the civilizing force of middle-class values. They advised former slaves that "the surest way to improve one's condition" was "to improve one's self." In their opinion, "even a poor person" could be clean since soap and water were not expensive. Thus, with cleanliness available to all who sought it, a clean body, washed clothes, and a tidy home clearly indicated one's growing respectability and acceptability.[103]

Like the army recruits tutored by the Sanitary Commission and its emissaries, many African-Americans schooled by Yankee women made improvements in their appearance and living quarters. They did so because they wanted to adopt ways more consonant with their new freedom and because they received some means and instruction to assist them. Their teachers, who had come to the South to lift African-Americans "out of the defilement of . . . slavery," responded enthusiastically to these changes.[104] In letters and diaries they related how much cleaner their "scholars" were, even when "wearing the same garments," and how "uniform neatness, taste, and cleanliness" characterized their Sunday outfits. One New England woman, who had been "endeavoring to instill habits of cleanliness" into her servant, proudly described her success in a letter home in September 1863. Rose, who had been unconcerned about hygiene, now changed "her 'linen' twice a week," took "a warm bath every Saturday," and kept "her head and feet in a condition to which they were strangers previously."[105]

Bringing Cleanliness Home from the War

When Billy Yank came marching home in spring 1865, he too appeared "more spruce" than before his encounters with inspectors and volunteer nurses. By the war's end, many veterans had learned "how to take care of themselves." They knew it paid "as a sanitary measure" to select "high, sandy ground" instead of "low, swampy country" for a campsite, and they would never sleep on the ground if "as many as two poles" were available.[106] They had also come to relish baths that soothed their aching feet after long marches and to rely on tubs of boiling water that removed lice from the seams of their clothes. And they grew dependent on large quantities of soap, which to Europeans seemed extravagant. While it is impossible to say for certain that these veterans acquired better habits of hygiene as a result of their wartime experience, it is reasonable to believe that they did. For many former Union soldiers would have probably agreed with the veteran who remarked that he had learned lessons "never afterward to be forgotten" and picked up habits which were "not readily shaken off."[107]

New York City sanitarian Stephen Smith, who served as an inspector for the Sanitary Commission, was not alone in testifying to "the wide extent to which the knowledge and principles of Hygiene" had "become popularized . . . in civil as well as military life" during the war. A decade after its end, John Shaw Billings, then assistant surgeon general of the United States Army, contended that "the recent military experiences" had "done more for the cause of Public Hygiene in this country than any other agencies." He said that there were physicians everywhere who, due to their "army experience," possessed a living faith "in the efficacy and necessity of pure air and water, and of cleanliness." But equally important were people outside of "military lines" who, according to Massachusetts health official Henry I. Bowditch, also learned "by dire experience, or by the urgent appeals of experts in sanitary matters, the all-important rules of cleanliness."[108]

What then was the impact of the Sanitary Commission and the men and women who worked through it? They saved many lives and helped shape postwar behavior, despite Secretary Stanton's disapproval and the army's less than full cooperation. Olmsted, who always prized statistics, in 1861 employed the Boston actuary E. B. Elliott to analyze the Bull Run casualty figures and other data. In 1863, at the Fifth International Statistical Congress in Berlin, Elliott reported that in the first two years of the Civil War the Union army "had suffered distinctly lower rates of disease than had European armies in wars earlier in the century," as a result of the commission's preventive efforts. These, he acknowledged, were modeled after British initiatives during and after the Crimean War.[109]

In 1862 the Union army's rates of sickness and death had soared in comparison with the prewar years, with diarrhea, measles, typhus, typhoid fever, malaria, various fevers, and scurvy the leading afflictions. This occurred before the Sanitary Commission's reforms took effect. As the war wore on, the diarrhea plague diminished. The Sanitary Commission and its nurses did not eliminate disease in the Union army, any more than Nightingale had done in the British; more men continued to die of disease than from battle. But their work greatly reduced disease mortality. The ratio of disease deaths to battle deaths for the Union in the Civil War was about three to two. In the Mexican-American War of 1846–48, the ratio had been more than six disease deaths to one battle death.[110]

While it is true that the volunteer organizations that came to life during the war failed to discover "any important hygienic or medical principle that altered the basic assumptions of sanitary science," they effectively directed the attention and enthusiasm of large segments of the American people to support their cause. Calling on the Crimean experience and the much-publicized work of Nightingale, its apostle of cleanliness, sanitarians instructed military personnel and civilians alike about the relationship of dirt to disease. Subjects rarely whispered earlier in mixed company became everyday topics of discussion at breakfast tables and in parlors. Those who had seen the actual war knew all too well "the filthy spewings of it. . . . War may be an armed angel with a mission, but she has the personal habits of the slums." This "bit" of knowledge, combined with the sanitarians' wartime successes, provided the foundation for the struggle to bring sanitation to American cities during the 1870s and 1880s.[111]

CHAPTER THREE

City Cleansing

To keep the world clean—this is one great task for women.
—HELEN CAMPBELL, 1897[1]

The Sanitary Lessons of the War

In 1865, most sanitarians agreed that "immense strides" had been made in matters of public and personal hygiene during the Civil War. But their crusade did not end with Appomattox. As they turned their attention to problems at home, they recognized enormous new threats to the nation's well-being. The "Filth Diseases," so dreaded by soldiers, were now perceived as serious "foes of life and health" for the citizenry as well. The phenomenal growth of cities and towns after the war forced survivors in both the North and the South to confront these old enemies that had already brought so much sickness and death. The country's health and welfare were seen as being "dependent upon the cleanliness" of its people. Thus, sanitarians urged Americans to do battle once again. This time they were asked to make "warfare against uncleanness."[2]

Neighborhoods in the nation's largest cities became the first new battlefields. Although beliefs regarding the causes of disease had not changed appreciably since 1861, wartime mortality statistics demonstrated that the programs of the United States Sanitary Commission had indeed saved lives. These facts strengthened the convictions of sanitarians that cleanliness often prevented the outbreak of disease and ordinarily stopped it from spreading quickly or widely in densely populated areas. Not surprisingly, those who had been in the war saw striking similarities between urban neighborhoods and army camp sites. Physician Stephen Smith, a former Sanitary Commission inspector and later a founder of the American Public

Health Association (1872), observed that New York City's poor were "an immense army in camp, upon small territory, crowded into old filthy dwellings without the slightest police regulation for cleanliness."[3]

The Civil War experience unquestionably shaped the sanitary reform movement in the critical decades of the late nineteenth century. By 1865 the war's lessons were widely known; physicians along with the public had generally come to understand that disease could be prevented. This concept had been central to the public health recommendations offered by John H. Griscom and Lemuel Shattuck in the 1840s and 1850s. But professional apathy and public indifference had discouraged any action leading to a national movement.[4]

In the postwar years, however, the rush to the cities brought new vitality. Billowing smokestacks and shrieking factory whistles beckoned a better life, and they attracted a record number of strangers from the countryside and abroad. But rampant growth produced shocking and life-threatening conditions that challenged urban Americans and ultimately transformed their physical environment and everyday habits. In fact, from the end of the Civil War to the close of the 1890s, the contours of American society probably changed more than in any other period of comparable length in its history.

Although America's bustling cities and towns may have appeared inviting to those seeking wider opportunities, late nineteenth-century urban areas were always crowded, noisy, dirty, and smelly. These conditions probably surprised newcomers upon their arrival. As they settled in, however, they tended to become accustomed to living in congested neighborhoods that disgusted and discouraged middle-class sanitarians. Life on a small farm in the United States or on a peasant holding in Central Europe hardly set the standard for cleanliness or civility; but, then again, neither did life in the modern American city. Along with growth, opportunity, and new fortunes unfortunately came congestion, noise, filth, and stench. And the sheer crowding into compact spaces of people used to living in rustic surroundings multiplied the threat of contagions of all kinds. Urban density, like cramped army camps, promoted disease—often in epidemic proportions—far more efficiently than rural isolation.

Epidemics had devastating effects on the local communities in which they occurred. During the nineteenth century periodic outbreaks of cholera, typhoid, and yellow fever terrorized whole sections of the nation every few years. They forced businesses to close and families rich enough or well enough to leave their homes and take refuge in the countryside. Epidemics also left hundreds, sometimes thousands, dead in their wake. Because these scourges now seemed preventable, they could no longer be taken for granted. Thus, in many parts of America, epidemics—or, more accurately, the threat of them—proved to be "life savers." They created a crisis situation, not unlike war, in which entire communities, frightened and demoralized, willingly accepted restrictive measures aimed at preventing or controlling the onslaught of disease. And in almost every instance, those in positions of authority and influence recommended city cleansing.[5]

During most of the late nineteenth century Americans commonly believed that filth and bad smells caused infectious disease. What had finally taken hold in the popular mind during the Civil War and its aftermath was the relationship of dirt to sickness. Filth, usually in the form of noxious odors or "miasmas" arising from decomposing organic wastes, became largely blamed for epidemics of cholera, yellow fever, and typhoid as well as typhus, scarlet fever, and diphtheria. Recognition of dirt as the source of disease made stagnant water, saturated ground, and smoke-filled air equally suspect. Thus, in their battles against "offensive odors and filthy things," sanitarians of the day preached cleanliness as "the first element of health."[6]

New York City was home to the founders of the Sanitary Commission and many of its most active members. During the closing months of the Civil War, it also became the focus of the first major confrontation for improved sanitary conditions and the birthplace of what was later described as "the fundamental movement for environmental sanitation in the United States."[7] On February 13, 1865, Stephen Smith appeared before a joint committee of the New York state legislature and reported the findings of a metropolitan sanitary survey conducted in 1864 by the Council of Hygiene and Public Health of the Citizens' Association. Smith had been the principal organizer of the survey; Elisha Harris, his colleague and former secretary of the Sanitary Commission, had prepared the final report. The investigation, conducted by a staff of thirty-one physicians, adopted procedures similar to those used by the Sanitary Commission when it inspected military camps and hospitals. Inspector-physicians gave an account of their districts "mainly in terms of cleanliness and filth."[8]

Smith's testimony and Harris's final report presented graphic descriptions of New York's miserably dirty neighborhoods and accused municipal authorities of gross negligence. Both men believed that the health and well-being of a locale could be "measured by its cleanliness." They were not surprised, therefore, that such outright neglect—which could have been "prevented by sanitary regulations"—resulted in "a fearfully HIGH DEATH RATE" and the social degradation of those living in them. Smith and Harris felt, in fact, that the city's draft riots in July 1863 would not have occurred had these conditions not existed. For these reformers and others, cleanliness provided a practical solution to many of the bewildering social problems facing urban America. Hence they confidently urged immediate and city-wide sanitary improvements.[9]

The filthiness that existed in New York City at the war's end was neither new nor unique to that metropolis. Hectic cleanup campaigns followed yellow fever outbreaks in the 1790s and cholera visitations in the 1830s and 1840s. In 1845, twenty years prior to publication of the Citizens' Association's report, Griscom had described similar scenes of squalor and neglect in *The Sanitary Condition of the Laboring Population of New York*. Since then, other individuals had continued as best they could the arduous campaign for sanitary reform. Even during the Civil War public-spirited citizens had introduced health bills into the state legislature each winter. Although none passed, daily newspapers, popular journals, and Smith's influential *American Medical Times* had steadfastly supported them. But during the war years, New York and other municipalities undertook almost no public improvements in sanitation, and most urban conditions grew worse because of the war's dislocations. In the end it was pressure from the press, sanitarians, and a certain enlightened public—urged along by another terrifying cholera threat—that resulted in passage of the Metropolitan Health Bill of February 1866.[10]

Epidemics and the Urgency of Water and Sewers

Cholera, the "classic epidemic disease" of the century, appeared initially in the United States in 1832, returned in 1849, and came again in 1866. Even though it almost always attacked the poor, who lived in the most crowded and dilapidated parts of New York City, everyone was frightened by its approach. Unsure of the causes of cholera, people knew well its horrifying effects. Victims at first simply felt sick. Then very quickly they began suffering from severe vomiting, diarrhea, and dehydration that turned their faces blue and their hands and feet an icy cold. They could and often did die within hours or days.[11]

The suddenness and unpredictability of cholera made it terrifying. Tuberculosis, which was a common and massive killer in the nineteenth century, caused a slow death. But cholera killed with unusual speed. Individuals who seemed healthy one morning could be dead the next—and no one really knew why. Equally debilitating to victims and their families were the disease's manifestations, especially the relentless vomiting and defecating. The fear that one could be struck by the disease while on the street or at work was also alarming.[12] For good reason, those who could do so usually fled to places that were dry, open, and clean.

Yellow fever visited the United States nearly every year during the nineteenth century, and no cities suffered more than New Orleans and Memphis. In 1873, almost thirty years before it was discovered that the *Aedes* mosquito transmitted yellow fever, the disease took the lives of 2000 of the 5000 Memphis residents who contracted it. Five years later, when another yellow fever epidemic ravaged the Mississippi Valley, 8100 people died in New Orleans and 5100 in Memphis. Effective sanitary measures helped prevent a large loss of life in New Orleans when the plague returned in 1879, but another 600 people died in Memphis. It was this sad series of events that gave "an impetus to city sanitation heretofore unknown" in Memphis. George E. Waring, Jr., the sanitary engineer who would design and supervise the construction of its sewers in the early 1880s, credited these epidemics with infusing "a new and vigorous impulse" into the sanitary movement in the United States.[13]

Every day newspapers and magazines carried vivid accounts of the 1878 and 1879 epidemics. New Yorkers, among others, wondered if they were safe and often criticized officials in Memphis and New Orleans for permitting large areas of their cities "to go badly drained and uncleaned." Yet, as they looked around at some of the tenement houses nearby, they knew that their immunity to yellow fever was due principally to their northerly latitude, where earlier frosts killed the *Aedes* larvae sooner. For if the presence of filth posed difficult health problems for northern cities, lack of sanitary conditions was even more formidable for a southern city like Memphis. Not only was it flooded annually by the Mississippi River, but its summers were also terribly hot and humid. And in the ten years between 1860 and 1870 its African-American population had increased from 3000 to 15,000. Since Memphis provided no accommodations for these former slaves, they lived in the streets and built "rude and wretched hovels" for themselves on the outskirts of the city. They, along with Memphis's Irish immigrants, suffered the most from the yellow fever epidemics.[14]

In each case—yellow fever in Memphis or cholera in New York—disastrous epidemics quickly led to massive cleanup campaigns. In the spring of 1866, when cholera threatened New York, the Metropolitan Health Board initiated such a huge effort that by summer's end New Yorkers had in large degree conquered an epidemic. Stephen Smith contended that because the board had adopted energetic, preventive measures it deserved the public's confidence and should become a model for other communities.[15] Although Smith's analysis may not have been entirely correct, it certainly appeared so to contemporaries.

Within weeks of its creation, the Metropolitan Health Board had swung into action. It organized the city's police into a kind of sanitary squadron and quarantined all personnel on the steamer *Virginia*, which had cholera

patients aboard. Bands of physicians made house-to-house visits to tenements and moved victims out of the worst apartments to neighborhood dispensaries. Round-the-clock disinfectant squads reported to premises where
cholera cases were found. And volunteers distributed circulars giving advice
on personal hygiene and bulletins outlining the epidemic's progress. The
board, enlightened by experiences with camp hygiene during the Civil War,
strove to demonstrate that public and personal cleanliness prevented the
spread of infectious diseases. And with the enemy at its door, the Metropolitan Health Board did not toy with halfway measures. It proclaimed a state
of emergency and assumed authority to make and enforce whatever regulations were necessary to halt the deadly cholera.[16]

These quick and determined actions prevented a major onslaught. About
600 persons died of cholera in New York City in 1866. From today's perspective, 600 is no small number. But Americans of the mid-nineteenth
century had become resigned to thousands dying during seasonal outbreaks
of cholera, typhoid, or yellow fever. New York's triumph should be attributed to the Metropolitan Health Board's aggressive sanitary program. It
takes nothing away from that victory to realize, as we now do, that rising living standards and advances in sanitary science in western Europe as well as
in North America also played a part in subduing cholera's attack during the
spring and summer of 1866.[17]

The Metropolitan Board of Health's success prompted other cities to establish municipal health boards, which were often followed in time by the
creation of state agencies. Virtually every major city and state would have a
health department by 1900. While not all of them were equally effective,
they demonstrated a growing sense among urban populations of the importance of expert authority and concerted action. In matters of public health
Americans were learning that they had to be their "brothers' keepers." In
fact, personal health and comfort forced private individuals to take an interest in their neighbors' sanitary condition. And when epidemics "burst upon
a community," they could rely on the advice of government health officials
to limit the "sphere of disaster" and offer some protection.[18] The power of a
plague was such that, while it almost always wreaked havoc among the poor,
it almost never completely spared the rich.

During epidemics, therefore, rich and poor alike witnessed the value of
cleanliness. It alone seemed to work, while quarantines almost never did. If
dirt and disease were synonymous—as they certainly seemed to be and as
sanitarians insisted they were—then the need for more water could hardly
be questioned, for water was "the most necessary of all the means used to
secure cleanliness" of person and place.[19] Thus, in a prodigious attempt to
obtain water to protect people's lives, cities would make unprecedented in-

vestments in vast systems of public works during the last decades of the nineteenth century.

The largest cities, including Philadelphia, Boston, New York, Cincinnati, and Chicago, had begun addressing their water supply problems before the Civil War. But by the war's end supplies that city officials and public works engineers had once figured would be ample for decades no longer were adequate. None of them had foreseen how enormous their cities would become. In 1860 only sixteen cities had populations over 50,000; by 1910, well over eighty did. To keep pace with this burgeoning growth, many cities continued to invest large sums in water projects even during the 1873–78 depression. In Boston, where officials were authorized to expend $5,250,000 on the Sudbury River between 1871 and 1879, residents thought that "a good supply of clean water would make Boston a healthier place to live." They also hoped it would provide them with better fire protection.[20]

During most of the nineteenth century, communities sought water for civic purposes. They needed plentiful supplies to fight fires and to cleanse streets of dirt and debris. For those trying to protect the public's health, city streets and walkways were always worrisome because their care was so sporadic. Individual citizens remained responsible for cleaning their premises as well as the thoroughfares in front of their homes or businesses, and these areas were nearly impossible to keep clean simply by hand sweeping, the most commonly used method in 1880. Basil March, who figured prominently in William Dean Howells's novel, *A Hazard of New Fortunes* (1890), described how uneasy a New York City street made him feel at the end of winter with its "frozen refuse melting in heaps ... with the strata of wastepaper and straw litter, and eggshells and orange peel, potato skins, and cigar stumps." In summer, when it rained, pedestrians like the fictional March often waded through beds of slime. Thus as cities grew in size and the fears of epidemics became more widespread, water usage for street flushing substantially increased.[21]

Water for household use, however, did not surge in the immediate postwar years. Only the wealthy had running water in their homes. Not until the 1880s and 1890s did the idea become prevalent that running water was a household necessity. A survey conducted in 1880, for example, showed that five out of six Americans had no means of washing or bathing themselves except for pails and sponges. This fact confirmed what Michigan's Board of Health discovered in 1877 after an unusual investigation of bathing practices. Most people in the state, who admitted to sponge-bathing only infrequently, were "very little accustomed to the general ablution of the body,—in other words, [they were] not clean."[22]

Water for streets rather than for baths motivated city officials in the

1860s and 1870s. They hoped that by flushing streets, especially in hot weather, they would wash away what was foul and stagnant, thereby preventing those vapors dangerous to the public's health. However, the increase in water usage for civic, industrial, and some household purposes created new problems of drainage and disposal. The answer was an even larger investment in public works for a society generally convinced—and frequently reminded by recurring epidemics—that the causes of most disease lay in an unclean environment. Borrowing heavily from the experiences of Europeans, American engineers constructed extensive and expensive networks of drains and sewers, particularly in the years following the devastating yellow fever epidemics in the Mississippi Valley.[23]

George Waring and the Sewering of America

These terribly destructive outbreaks during the 1870s aroused in the whole country an interest in sanitation and hygiene unmatched since the Civil War. Enthusiasm for sanitary reform was always difficult to sustain at the national level. But, outside war, nothing stirred Americans to action more quickly than an epidemic. Thus, in the wake of the yellow fever epidemic of 1878, Congress created a National Board of Health with largely investigatory and advisory responsibilities; it was to assist state and local health officials in devising quarantine regulations and sanitary measures to check the spread of epidemics. Memphis was its first real assignment and test. Residents had concluded that in the face of yellow fever they needed less heroism and more drainage.[24] In response, the National Board of Health sent the colorful and flamboyant sewerage expert Colonel George E. Waring, Jr., to Memphis in 1879.

Labeled by a contemporary as "the greatest apostle of cleanliness," Waring became the most conspicuous anti-contagionist, environmentalist, and propagandist of the late nineteenth century. His reputation and influence in the United States would eventually equal and, in some quarters, surpass that of Florence Nightingale during the 1860s. In the mid-1870s, in articles on the sanitation and sewerage of houses and towns published in the *Atlantic Monthly* and *Scribner's Monthly*, he crusaded against dirt, filth, and sewer gas. In fact, he was said to have made New Englanders so afraid of sewer gas that they "feared it perhaps more than they did the Evil One."[25]

While Waring preached the dangers of sewer gas, he also built sewers. By 1874 he had constructed them for Ogdensburg and Saratoga Springs, New York. Two years later he completed the first "separate" sewer system (using two sets of pipes that separated sewage from storm water) in the United States for the small resort town of Lenox, Massachusetts. In each instance he defended the huge sums of money spent on these projects by pointing to their sanitary benefit, namely better community health. By 1879 Waring had decided that the devastation of Memphis and New Orleans was due to the simple fact that "they were not kept clean" and that they lacked sewerage. In contrast to northern cities, he contended, southern cities had simply failed to appreciate "the importance of municipal and domestic cleanliness."[26]

Waring began his unusual career as a sanitarian in 1857 when he became agricultural and drainage engineer for New York City's Central Park. Hired to install a system of drains in the park, he remained on the staff of Frederick Law Olmsted and Calvert Vaux's pioneer public works project until its virtual completion in 1861. During this period, Waring and Olmsted began a lifelong friendship. When the Civil War broke out, Waring enlisted almost immediately; he left New York in May 1861 for Washington as a major in New York's 39th Regiment, sometimes known as the Garibaldi Guards. At the end of June, when Olmsted arrived in Washington to consider a position with the Sanitary Commission, Waring met his former boss, showed him around the camps, and gave him his tent to sleep in. As they toured the makeshift arrangements in and around the Capitol, they probably noticed the lack of drains and the unkempt appearance of the volunteers. But since Waring ended up spending most of the war years as a colonel in the Missouri Cavalry, he and Olmsted seemed to have had little contact until later when they both returned to New York.[27]

Immediately following the war Waring took up the farming he had left when he joined Olmsted's staff at Central Park. As manager of the Ogden Farm near Newport, Rhode Island, and as a writer on technical aspects of his work, he developed a reputation as an expert on scientific agriculture. He also began writing popular horse stories and taking fashionable trips to Europe. *Scribner's Monthly* and *Atlantic Monthly* magazines, which published Waring's pieces on plumbing in the mid-1870s, initially carried accounts of his European tours to Americans who could not travel. Thus, when Waring went to Memphis as a commissioner of the National Board of Health in November 1879, he was known not only to agricultural and engineering specialists but also to the general reading public.[28]

The energetic and enterprising Waring arrived in Memphis with two colleagues and a plan to cleanse the city "of all objectionable accumulations" of filth. While the other two commissioners from the National Board of Health organized a sanitary survey of the city, Waring designed a sewer system and promptly convinced his colleagues, the rest of the National Board, and Memphis officials of its merits. He then hired himself out to the city to supervise construction of the "Waring separate system." Although some of its design features caused controversy among engineers, the project helped transform Memphis from one of the dirtiest cities to one of the cleanest by 1890. And Waring's talent for publicizing his success made him and his sewer system famous. Between 1880 and 1892 at least twenty-two American communities built sewers modeled after those in Memphis.[29]

Cities constructed thousands of miles of underground sewers in an attempt to handle the ever-increasing wastes that fouled the urban environment and threatened the public's health. Tanneries and slaughterhouses, for example, created huge amounts of liquid byproducts, and most neighborhood cesspools and privies were overflowing with household and human wastes. The introduction of public water supply systems had added immeasurably to the quantity of wastewater to be disposed of, and citizens pressured local governments to be allowed to use storm drains to rid their premises of household wastes. With more abundant water supplies had come the development of indoor plumbing and bathtubs. The flush toilet, first invented in 1809 but hardly used until the 1880s, further boosted wastewater volume. In the end municipalities resolved their drainage problems and overcame opposition to using storm sewers for household wastes by constructing large combined sewers or Waring's smaller separate ones.[30]

His reputation as a practical and decisive sanitarian spread as a result of the Memphis venture. With more offers for work than he could possibly accept, Waring began traveling as a consulting engineer to many cities in the United States and Europe. He also served as a special agent responsible for the social statistics of the Tenth Census (1880), and in 1883 he appeared before Congress in support of continued funding for the National Board of Health. More fearful of the idea of federal intervention than of the outbreak of some future epidemic, Congress allowed the board to die quietly. Waring, for his part, continued his mission against defective drainage and filthy surroundings.[31]

Waring believed, as did most sanitarians, that "spasmodic cleanliness in municipal affairs" could be likened to an individual who bathed and changed clothes merely once a year. Therefore, during his travels and in his writings, Waring urged constant and scrupulous attention to sanitary matters. If cleanliness successfully warded off disease, then it was foolish and useless to clean up only when yellow fever or cholera threatened. Waring counseled his audiences to remember that yellow fever was a "minor" disease and that "far greater mortality and infinitely greater disability" resulted from "the constant operation" of a host of illnesses, which sanitation could also help prevent.[32]

Since death records were not required by law in most states until after 1900, more is known about the sheer rates of death prior to 1900 than about its causes. But this much is fairly certain. Cancer was low on the list of

major killers before 1900, because it mainly strikes the middle-aged and el-
derly; many people died of other diseases first. Despite the absence of
motor vehicles, accidents claimed many victims (as a percentage of population), because of appalling (and largely uncompensated) risks taken daily by
railroad, mine, and factory workers. Strokes and heart disease led as causes
of mortality, but they cut down a smaller percentage than today since an
array of lethal diseases, now minor or nonexistent, were then so common.

Pneumonia and "flu," the second leading category of deadly diseases,
claimed seven times more victims than they currently do. And the third-
and fourth-ranked causes have since become insignificant: tuberculosis,
which took more lives than cancer does now, and gastrointestinal infections,
which were close behind even without counting diarrhea and dehydration
in newborn infants. A variety of "children's diseases," which have been no
worse than annoyances since the 1920s, took significant numbers of lives
every year—whooping cough, measles, scarlet fever, and the dreaded diphtheria. Typhoid and related illnesses rounded out the list of major killers,
disposing of a higher proportion of the population than now die in motor
vehicle accidents.

These death rates held for 1900 and for those parts of the country that
kept statistics. In the 1880s, death rates were even higher from the pul-
monary diseases (including tuberculosis and pneumonia)—the direct results
of cramped quarters, poor ventilation, and polluted air—as well as diseases
resulting from impure water (gastrointestinal upsets and typhoid). While
cholera no longer wiped out whole districts as it had through the mid-nineteenth century, serious outbreaks of typhoid, diphtheria, influenza, and
other contagions remained all too common.[33]

In view of these facts, it is understandable why Waring and his fellow sanitarians, whose knowledge of the causes of disease was admittedly "frag-
mentary and imperfect," clung to the one known means of reducing the incidence of sickness.[34] Cities in the 1880s were bewildering and perilous
places. While neighborhoods retained some of the flavor of small-town life,
urban areas generally lacked the familiarity and stability that made country
people feel comfortable and enterprising. Instead, as city dwellers, they
often felt besieged by forces they did not comprehend. Thus epidemics,
fires, or child mortality, "matters that previously would have been considered separate incidents, or even ignored, were seized and fit into a frame-
work of jeopardy, each reinforcing the others as further proof of an immi-
nent danger." This sense of emergency prompted individuals with
experience and influence to fall back on measures they knew had been effective. Since cleanliness had a proven record, sanitarians embraced it as a
means of controlling their world.[35]

They instructed a nation bent on progress that filth bred chaos and bar-
barism, while cleanliness ensured order and advancement. Confident and
determined, sanitarians convinced large numbers of middle-class Americans that cleaning the environment of its most offensive nuisances would al-
leviate the major sources of urban danger. The optimism of their message
insured its success, even at a time when French and German discoveries in
bacteriology were demonstrating that germs rather than filth were the true
cause of disease. But Americans accepted the germ theory only gradually—
and for good reason. The original theory "was difficult to understand and
even more difficult to prove."[36] And when it was finally verified, it simply
provided the Civil War generation of sanitarians with yet another rationale
for cleansing the city.

In the battles against filth, urban Americans concentrated their attacks on
the "two great nuisances"—sewer gas and uncollected garbage. While the
staggering mounds of refuse in streets and alleys would eventually pose
more difficult problems, most city dwellers feared sewer gas as "the dead-
liest and most insidious foe" of all.[37] No doubt these worries were the natural accompaniments of the sewer-building craze that took place nationwide during the 1880s and 1890s. They also resulted from the cautionary
and perplexing advice of sanitarians who warned incessantly of the life-
threatening dangers of leaking drains. Much of what alarmed the public is
contained in an 1885 ode to "Modern Sanitation":

> Our sanitation! Tis the art
>   Of filling up our homes with drains.
> Ah! sewer-gas acts well its part
>   By conjuring up man's aches and pains.
>
> The beauteous scarlet fever skips
>   With typhoid hand in hand.
> While sweet Diphtheria gayly trips
>   O'er stationary washstand.
>
> The cholera doth laugh to see
>   Its comma bacilli.
> Old dysentery's microbe
>   Is out upon the fly.
>
> Malaria with its poisonous dart
>   Lurks 'neath the water-trap.
> Measles upon its round doth start,
>   Small-pox wakes from its nap.

The crafty plumber makes his bill,
    The sewer-gas ascends.
The doctor gives a sugar pill
    'Tis thus we lose our friends.

The undertaker says 'tis well,
    The funeral corteges pass.
The letters on the tombstone spell
    Hic Jacet, Sewer-Gas.[38]

This poem demonstrates how the germ theory enabled leading sanitarians, the majority of whom remained anti-contagionist in their thinking, to trumpet the threat of sewer gas. Although they used words such as "bacilli" and "microbes," sewer gas remained mysteriously responsible for illnesses of every kind. The plumbing and drainage systems that had been installed to safeguard the public's health now seemed themselves to generate contagious diseases. One puzzled physician admitted publicly that if he were building a house he would not "have it connected in any way with a sewer"; instead he would construct "a sort of annex" in which he would gather "all the pipes and fixtures, water-closets, baths, and wash-basins." Charles F. Chandler, a chemist in New York City's health department, recalled that the public "seemed to think that the only protection necessary for their families from contagious and infectious diseases was a large plumber's bill."[39]

Statements from Waring, the chief proponent of the poisonous nature of sewer gas, also fed the nation's fears. According to him, poisonous sewer gas could not be "clearly defined," but since it was known "chiefly by its effect," the danger was thought "to lurk not so much in those foul stenches . . . as in the odorless, mawkish exhalations which first announce themselves by headache and debility." Waring himself admitted that household plumbing "has led to a great increase of risk." Yet he urged cities to continue to make these "essential improvements." His faith in the willingness of individuals and communities to engage in sanitary action probably best explains his optimism in the face of possible hazards. Thus he campaigned tirelessly to involve groups of citizens—especially plumbers, women, and school children—in the work of city cleansing.[40]

Like so many of his contemporaries, Waring believed that the state of each neighborhood's health rested largely in the hands of its plumbers. They, after all, repaired or replaced the faulty pipes and drains that emitted the perilous sewer gas. Waring insisted more than once that "good plumbing work . . . is the sanitarian's best aid." But because plumbing was a new trade and most plumbers were as confused about the dangers of sewer gas as the public they served, they often decided simply "to ventilate anything and everything!" And their customers, who sometimes characterized them as little more than "tinsmiths," regularly accused them of making "extraordinary blunders" for excessive profits.[41]

For these reasons, sanitarians across the country supported the beginnings of a "plumbers' movement" in the early 1880s. It eventually resulted in the creation of a National Association of Master Plumbers as well as local sanitary associations for plumbers. These groups advanced the cause of "scientific plumbing" through education and licensing programs; they also improved the public image of plumbers by encouraging them to cooperate with state and local health departments. Within twenty years bacteriologists in these health agencies would disprove the sewer-gas thesis—microorganisms, not the mysterious gas, were the problem. But as late as World War I most Americans still considered sewer gas a source of disease, and fears about it heightened the ardor for cleanliness.[42]

Women as Municipal Housekeepers

In 1885, when the sewer gas theory raged and the germ theory pleaded for a hearing, Harriette M. Plunkett called on women to join with plumbers in a line of defense against dirt. Plunkett had become interested in sanitary reform in the 1870s through her husband's involvement with the Massachusetts state board of health. Although household sanitation was the main focus of her book, *Women, Plumbers, and Doctors* (1885), Plunkett's practical suggestions for keeping homes healthy showed women how outside pollutants threatened their families' lives. Sewer gas and germs alike could enter private living quarters through "overlooked channels of infection" that included leaky sewer pipes, contaminated wells, broken drains, impure ice, and unclean milk. Mindful of Florence Nightingale, who forged "the first link in a great chain of events," a new generation of American housewives needed to "rise above the beaten paths of cookery and needlework" and extend their activity beyond the front door.[43]

Few would have disagreed with Plunkett that women were primarily responsible for maintaining a clean, healthy, and comfortable home. At the turn of the century most people believed that women had "certain intuitive convictions" when it came to matters of "order and cleanliness." Home sanitation and village improvement were "congenial to the feminine temperament," it was said, "even as the intimate connection between a woman and a broom-handle is an obvious and natural fact." These widely held beliefs ensured that the increasing burdens of cleanliness would fall, as they always had before, mainly on women.[44]

Although middle-class housewives had expanded their sphere of responsibilities during the Civil War, they had not relinquished any of their traditional obligations. In the postwar years they continued to stretch the boundaries of the home, but more and more they assigned the daily chores of cooking and cleaning to live-in domestics. So even though a good deal of housekeeping changed hands, it remained woman's work. Yet, freed by servants of their most taxing burdens, more affluent women were able to take on the duties of municipal housekeeping.

City cleansing was "especially woman's work," as George Waring recognized as early as 1877. It required "the sort of systematized attention to detail" that developed "more naturally out of the habit of good housekeeping than out of any occupation to which man is accustomed." Women probably agreed with Waring, particularly the few who were already members of village improvement societies along with the many who had become active in the fast-growing Woman's Christian Temperance Union. For them municipal housekeeping was just another aspect of "home protection."[45]

Frances Willard, the dynamic and innovative WCTU leader, had attached the concept of home protection to women's demand for the ballot as early as 1876. Then, in the 1880s, when she was in full control of the WCTU, she masterfully turned home protection into a slogan and used it to encourage women to get involved in activities *outside* the home to protect the home. Temperance recruitment motivated Willard, to be sure; but the notion of home protection went a long way toward convincing middle-class women that they were still good mothers and devoted wives despite their participation in public affairs.[46]

The movement for sanitary reform attracted women who were satisfied with their roles as wives, mothers, and homemakers. And by broadening the traditional definition of home to include more than "four square walls," Willard gave them an exciting, new mission—"to make the whole world homelike." Municipal housekeeping would unite women of many backgrounds, but the most articulate resembled the leaders of the WCTU, who were white, upper-middle-class, educated, and native-born Protestants of Anglo-Saxon ancestry. Motivated by a desire to protect their homes and nurture their families, they came to believe that they, as the nation's homemakers, could improve the deplorable housekeeping practices of their cities and towns. And so they did. These custodians of cleanliness not only awakened their communities to the lackadaisical ways in which municipalities were being managed and kept, but they were also responsible for significant public health initiatives.[47]

Village improvement proved to be the precursor of municipal housekeeping. Women first organized to perk up the appearance of their surroundings in the 1850s in rural New England. They acted primarily in response to the demands of summer visitors who wanted such popular amenities as porches or bay windows and appeared "shocked by old-time country makeshifts." The founder of the first improvement society, Mary Hopkins of Stockbridge, Massachusetts, formed the Laurel Hill Association in 1853 after overhearing some tourists "commenting on the intelligence of a population willing to live" in a place "devoid of any attempt at sanitation or adornment." Within a few years, the Laurel Hill Association changed Stockbridge from "a rough, shabby village" to "a handsome orderly town."[48]

In the antebellum years civic pride drove village improvement societies more than any other factor. The example of new suburbs, which touted well-drained and spacious yards with large trees surrounded by uniform sidewalks, provided additional incentives. By supporting the activities of their improvement societies, New England townspeople hoped to prevent decline rather than to control growth as would be the case in cities in the decades following the Civil War. Health was occasionally mentioned as a reason for local betterment, yet it was usually associated with drainage and sometimes with Olmsted's work in New York City.[49]

But in the aftermath of the Civil War, when sewer gas and miasmas became life-threatening specters, New York City women took to the streets for reasons of health to remove the ever-increasing amounts of garbage, manure, and rubbish. The Ladies' Health Protective Association, founded in 1884, was the earliest women's organization formed to clean up an urban environment. New York City had become, according to newspaper accounts, the dirtiest and unhealthiest municipality in the nation largely as a result of a surging population that seemed to have no bounds. People had begun to wonder, in fact, if a city as large as New York could be kept clean at all.[50]

Fifteen women from the exclusive Beekman Hill section of the city believed it could. Angered by an enormous, foul-smelling pile of manure allowed to accumulate in their neighborhood and by the dust that dirtied their houses, clothes, and faces, this group of women decided to organize themselves into the Ladies' Health Protective Association and go to court. Despite the owner's contention that the nuisance was fertilizer and harmless, they successfully forced its removal. In an 1887 appeal for cleaner streets, these same women told Mayor Abram S. Hewitt that men had been "derelict in the matter of street cleaning," probably because it did not directly affect them. Yet, they pointed out, too much of women's time and energy was "spent in removing from floors and walls, furniture, utensils and clothing, the dirt and soil" that invaded "the household at every hour" and threatened their families' survival. It was for this reason—and because they had reached "the climax of aggravation"—that they had become involved in street cleaning.[51]

The Ladies' Health Protective Association also made specific recommendations to the mayor for improving the condition of New York City's streets. It asked that the annual appropriation for street cleaning be adequate for the work; that street-sweeping machines be used late at night; that neither ashes nor garbage be allowed to accumulate in front of residences; that homeowners be required to purchase galvanized iron receptacles; that crematories be built to dispose of house ashes, garbage, and street sweepings; and that the city be divided into sections managed by foremen, responsible to a street commissioner, and cleaned by laborers, who should be paid by the piece and not by the day. One of the association's boldest proposals urged the mayor to appoint women as inspectors, since "keeping things clean, like the training of children and the care of the sick, has ever been one of the instinctive and recognized functions of women."[52]

In its street-cleaning campaigns, as well as in others related to slaughterhouses and schools, the Ladies' Health Protective Association described the need for city cleansing in a way that ordinary people could understand and champion. The women members of this organization were undoubtedly influenced by the emerging public health movement even though their proposals, like those of most civic groups, lacked medical or scientific explanations. Instead they spoke largely in domestic and esthetic terms. If arguments based on home protection were not persuasive, they resorted to ones they considered more basic—ones that reflected a culture of cleanliness that they assumed civilized people shared. In their street-cleaning appeal to Mayor Hewitt they had said that "even if dirt were not the unsanitary and dangerous thing we know that it is, its unsightliness and repulsiveness are so great, that no other reason than the superior beauty of cleanliness" should compel New Yorkers to do what was necessary to achieve a level of comfort and self-respect. For municipal housekeepers, a city could not be attractive or beautiful unless it were clean.[53]

Aside from creating greater public awareness, the Ladies' Health Protective Association achieved few remarkable results until Waring was appointed street cleaning commissioner in 1894 by reform Mayor William L. Strong. But new women's organizations such as the Sanitary Protective League, the Street Cleaning Aid Society, and the Women's Health Protective Association of Brooklyn became active in 1890 and also helped New Yorkers understand the seriousness of the city's sanitary problems. Then in 1892 in Chicago, soon after it was selected to host the 1893 World's Fair, another group of women established the Municipal Order League "to promote the healthfulness, cleanliness, and beauty of Chicago." Its first objective or "main business" was street cleaning.[54]

Ada Sweet and a Cleaner Chicago

Chicago's Municipal Order League modeled itself after the Ladies' Health Protective Association in New York City. Anxious that Chicago might not appear attractive to out-of-town visitors during the World's Fair, the Chicago *Tribune* called on local women to "imitate the action of their sisters in New York" and accomplish what the men of the city had failed to achieve—clean streets and alleys. Chicago's thoroughfares were "held captive" by private contractors and their scavenging companies, regularly hired by elected officials and frequently accused by the general public of doing little or nothing except to draw money from the city's purse. Administrators preferred the contract system, which they claimed was cheaper, to a municipally operated street-cleaning service. But because contract terms were difficult to enforce, companies and the officials who employed them provoked fierce criticism. Reformers, who feared for the public's health, favored more efficient municipal services, while boosters worried about possible embarrassment during the World's Fair.[55]

At a mass meeting on March 27, 1892, in Central Music Hall, Ada Celeste Sweet, the able first president of the Municipal Order League, declared war on Chicago's filthy streets and alleys. Under Sweet's direction, league members did as well as the New York women in informing neighborhoods and their elected representatives of the need for sanitary improvements. Street-cleaning aid societies sprang up around the city, and volunteers signed up to serve as inspectors in their voting districts, where they kept watch over nearby streets and alleys during the spring and summer months. Their good work paid off on July 15 when the Chicago City Council passed an ordinance creating a new Department of Street Cleaning and the office of street-cleaning superintendent. Stunned by this victory, the press gave appropriate credit to league members but reserved its highest praise for Sweet, the organization's "prime mover." To "her intelligent zeal and remarkable force of character" Chicagoans owed this triumph.[56]

While the new ordinance did not completely abolish the contract system in Chicago, it was a major step in that direction. It also attempted to deal with a problem intimately connected to that of dirty streets and alleys—garbage disposal. After an inspection visit to a local incinerator where garbage was burned, Sweet commented that she would like "sweepings from the streets cremated." In the 1890s incineration appeared to Sweet and others as the perfect disposal method; the burning of garbage at extremely high temperatures seemed to offer an efficient, "scientific," and sanitary way for cities to rid themselves of polluted waters, reeking dumps, and sordid landfills. The new ordinance, therefore, authorized the building of several municipal incinerators. Those who had been uneasy about Chicago's appearance during the World's Fair now had reason to believe that visitors would find their "municipal house swept and dusted."[57]

Had Sweet and her Municipal Order League succeeded where scores of civic-minded citizens had previously failed? It certainly appears so. Sweet told Elizabeth Cady Stanton, America's foremost woman's rights advocate, that public opinion in Chicago had "never been so strong . . . in favor of public cleanliness." No doubt Sweet was an exceptional person, and the zeal and force of her character were fortified by her personal contacts and political experience. As a young woman in her twenties, she had accompanied her father, Colonel Benjamin Sweet, to Washington, D.C., when he was appointed deputy commissioner of Internal Revenue in 1872. When he died two years later, Sweet accepted an appointment as head of the United States Pension Agency in Chicago from the Republican Grant administration. Because of her efficient management, she was reappointed by Grant's two Republican successors. In 1885, when the Democratic commissioner of pensions in the Cleveland administration sought to replace her, she waged an intense and successful battle to retain her position. The petitions signed on her behalf give evidence not only of her political know-how but also of an influential corps of friends and acquaintances.[58]

Since Sweet apparently left no diaries and few letters, an assessment of how she went about furthering the cause of city cleansing is problematic. By 1889 she had established her own claims office in downtown Chicago and conducted day-to-day affairs under the motto "Despatch is the Soul of Business." Dedicated to efficiency and in touch with "the local state of public feeling," Sweet obviously capitalized as best she could on preparations for the 1893 World's Fair. This event, more than any other, contributed to the short-term accomplishments of the Municipal Order League in the spring and summer of 1892. Most Chicagoans wanted their city to look good to out-of-town guests. They also hoped to prevent an outbreak of cholera or typhoid among the millions of visitors who would travel to Chicago—many during the hottest months of 1893—and generate a voluminous amount of additional dirt and garbage.[59]

Yet, despite these concerns, Sweet and the Municipal Order League could not sustain their success. Soon after passage of the July 15 ordinance that some had hailed as a victory, property owners balked and eventually prevented construction of incinerators in their neighborhoods. In August Sweet complained publicly that the city fathers had begun to renege on their promises, and the contractors and inspectors were doing little or nothing in areas outside the central business district. Mincing no words, she blamed the contract system for creating "plague spots" in parts of Chicago, where typhoid fever was epidemic. Disappointed by these relapses, the league turned its attention to a related issue—the establishment of free public baths. Sweet ultimately concluded that real sanitary improvements would occur only when citizens elected individuals who would abolish the contract system and prohibit the political appointment of inspectors. At the close of 1892, speaking to the Chicago Woman's Club, Sweet took satisfaction in the City Council's $75,000 appropriation for garbage crematories and the start of a municipal bath system; still she feared that Chicago was not spending money in the neighborhoods that needed it most. The club's president agreed, saying simply "the city needs a housekeeper" and "women will have to take hold & do the work."[60]

Although only partially successful, Sweet and the Municipal Order League—and the abundant newspaper coverage they received—increased public awareness of the need for cleanliness during the Chicago World's Fair. While outlying streets and alleys remained cluttered and dirty, the downtown appeared clean and orderly. And visitors spent most of their time at the Fair itself which, by 1890 standards, was a sanitary wonder. In this "White City," as the exposition came to be called, over 3000 water closets were installed (in contrast to only 250 at the 1889 Paris Exposition and 900 at the Philadelphia Centennial Exposition in 1876), the drinking water was filtered, and the paved streets were cleaned and swept nightly.[61] Whether Sweet and her friends believed their municipal housekeeping efforts were responsible for these conditions or the pleasure guests took in them, it is impossible to know. Nor can we know their reaction a year later when George Waring, popular sanitary engineer and outspoken advocate of city cleansing, became New York City's street-cleaning commissioner. New York may have benefited more immediately than Chicago did from its own White City.

Waring Cleans Up New York City

Waring's appointment was "ideal," and he owed it to Eleanora Kinnicutt. Although she left even fewer traces than Ada Sweet, Kinnicutt is remembered for her effective involvement in New York City's street-cleaning affairs during the 1890s. As leader of the Street Cleaning Aid Society, she refused membership to women who themselves did not have clean cellars; she wanted activists "who practiced what they preached," she said, not "mere shouters." Demanding and persevering, Kinnicutt played a critical role in securing approval for a plan that reorganized the city's street cleaning department in May 1892. And after the 1894 election of Mayor William L.

Strong, the reform candidate, she used her influence to secure the office of street cleaning commissioner for Waring.[62]

His accomplishments in this position were so dramatic and so appreciated that they have been described in detail by contemporaries and historians alike. As all these accounts attest, Waring transformed the streets of New York from among the dirtiest in the nation to the cleanest during his three-year term. He also removed politics from the day-to-day operations of the street-cleaning department. In a warm letter to his old friend, Frederick Law Olmsted, five days after becoming commissioner, Waring pledged that he would "never give in to any influence, whether of politics or of friendship," and "appoint the second best man for any place." This was "big talk" but not "brag," he said, promising to succeed in cleaning up New York's "streets and system both."[63]

Waring's ammunition in his great war against dirty streets and dirty politics was public interest and "printers' ink." He knew, as he told Olmsted, that public sentiment was in his favor. The sanitary reform movement of the post-Civil War decades, which Waring had helped create and shape, now gave him a stage on which to perform. On horseback, amid martial band music, he annually paraded about 3000 street-cleaning employees in white duck uniforms before an audience of cheering New Yorkers and envious nonresidents. He also boasted of the department's new competence to awed journalists. His men, well trained and disciplined, were nothing less than "soldiers of cleanliness and health . . . fighting daily battles with dirt." To prove his point, Waring took the press and city officials on tours of improved neighborhoods; he also met regularly with volunteer civic groups, especially women's organizations. While he needed their continued support and cooperation, he no doubt recognized that their municipal housekeeping had produced a good share of the public sentiment to which he masterfully appealed.[64]

Waring also enlisted children in his public relations campaign. Convinced that "cleanliness is catching," particularly among the young, he had organized forty-four juvenile street-cleaning leagues by late 1897. Members acted as "eyes, ears, and noses" for the street-cleaning department by reporting unsightly nuisances, and Waring presented badges, certificates, white caps, and prizes to about 2500 children to keep them involved in his war against pesky litter. They in turn took pledges, sang songs, cleaned up school yards, instructed parents and relatives in the ways of sanitation, and marched with Waring's "White Wings" in the annual parades. While these youngsters captured the public's heart, no one—including Waring—seemed to know how effective they were. What the city had gained, he claimed, was "the neutrality of thousands of children" who by their league participation were kept from making neighborhoods dirty.[65]

When Waring became street-cleaning commissioner, he vowed a tough fight against the dirt on New York City's streets. A showman, to be sure, Waring was also an environmentalist. But, like so many of the people who appreciated him, his environmentalism rested on the filth theory of disease. Not trained in science or medicine, Waring accepted what the health experts of his day believed—"that filth and decay in every form were a serious menace to health, both from the disease germs which they contain, and the poisonous gas which they give off." Taking no chances when it came to germs or sewer gas, the "apostle of cleanliness" sought to remove anything that was dirty or smelly. Since he had begun to consider the role of bacteria in causing specific illnesses, he probably would have embraced the more sophisticated contagionist theory had he lived beyond October 1898.[66]

Waring's "can-do" message reached civic-minded Americans, especially those who were trying to adjust to an urban society that lacked the familiarity and stability of the countryside. The depression of 1893 had left them unnerved and even more lacking in the confidence they needed to solve the overwhelming problems posed by city life. Waring gave them hope. He accepted New York City on its own terms without questioning the rate of its growth or the nature of its economic activity. Although he was naive about the ultimate benefits city cleansing could contribute to the nation's health and well-being, he demonstrated that community action could make profound and lasting improvements in the quality of human life. His fans saw in his success "the final solution to all of [their] other problems of government." If they could "clean the streets of the Republic," said one New Yorker, then they could "accomplish other cleanings that have in the past seemed hopeless of accomplishment."[67] Ironically and regrettably, Waring's life was cut short in late 1898 by yellow fever, contracted in Havana where President William McKinley had sent him to establish a sanitation system in the aftermath of the Spanish-American War.

New York reformers continued Waring's cleanliness crusade and broadened it to include prostitution. By 1900 numerous urban communities had established vice committees or social hygiene societies; however, in New York City, where brothels seemed to be everywhere, the campaign against them was unusually militant. For married men and bachelors who frequented houses of prostitution, they signified liberation. But to others, who knew the dark side of this "social evil" and descried it as dangerous and unclean, brothels stood for nothing more than disease and sin.[68]

Progressive reformers joined the purity movement to rid the city of its "dirt," moral as well as material. Local governments wanted their streets free of vice and crime, or at least out of sight. Sanitarians, concerned about the public's health, hoped to regulate prostitution as a preventive measure against venereal disease. Vigilance groups, who came together to fight the "white slave traffic" by their own means, sought to abolish prostitution, as did many women's organizations; they campaigned hardily for a single standard of morality (meaning a change in male behavior). Their work at home may have taught them that matters of cleanliness demanded more than regulation.[69]

By World War I New York reformers believed they lived in "the cleanest city in the world." Unbeknownst to them, though, they were not as responsible for this condition as they liked to believe. More important than all of their efforts were the new skyscrapers and high rise apartments that replaced the old houses of prostitution. And during World War I the federal government led a fierce attack on venereal disease. Posters and pamphlets reminded American troops that it was the "Kaiser's best friend" and that "German bullets [were] Cleaner than Whores." After the war, immigration laws radically reduced the number of transient men and women; prohibition forced prostitutes off New York's streets and into speakeasies; and states passed laws making prostitution illegal. Yet the initiatives of anti-vice campaigners had succeeded in making social cleanliness a vital part of city cleansing.[70]

Caroline Bartlett Crane Tests the Waring Model in Kalamazoo

Waring's success had a phenomenal impact on American cities. It seemed to ignite a new civic consciousness. Women's groups especially came to recognize that their "historic function" had always been "along the line of cleanliness" and ultimately accepted more responsibility for securing a cleaner environment. In the North and South, as well as the East and West, women championed *public* cleanliness. Many worked to increase community awareness and personal commitment to city cleansing; others—like Mary McDowell, Chicago's "Garbage Lady"—took on the more difficult task of persuading elected officials to improve inefficient municipal housekeeping practices. In African-American communities, too, women's clubs became involved in local improvement efforts. Atlanta's Neighborhood Union, organized in 1907 by Lugenia Hope, counted among its achievements several ordinances that eliminated outhouses and provided regular garbage collection for black residents.[71]

Of all these women, it was Caroline Bartlett Crane, the most unusual self-made "sanitary expert" of the twentieth century, who acquired a national reputation for municipal housekeeping. She began in 1904 by successfully adapting Waring's street-cleaning methods to six blocks of Main Street in Kalamazoo, Michigan. Between 1905 and 1917, at the invitation of elected officials and volunteer organizations, she inspected the sanitary conditions of sixty-two cities and fourteen states, becoming "America's public housekeeper" par excellence.[72]

Crane came to Kalamazoo in 1889 as minister to its First Unitarian Church. Motivated more by the Social Gospel and settlement house movements than by sanitary science or public health concerns, she wanted her church to be "an experiment station in social progress." Before long she ran a range of social services that included a kindergarten, a Frederick Douglass Club for the community's African-American population, manual training classes for young men, and study groups for adults. In 1896, when she married a local physician, she resigned as minister and focused her extraordinary energy on community matters.[73]

She first turned her attention to Kalamazoo's slaughterhouses. Several years *before* Upton Sinclair published *The Jungle*, the book usually credited with raising slaughterhouse regulation as a major issue, Crane and several women investigated seven slaughterhouses that supplied meat to local shops and markets. Shocked by what they found, the group appeared before the city council and disclosed its findings. The buildings and grounds were unbelievably dirty; and interior surfaces were coated with "blood, grime, grease, hair, mold, and other quite unmentionable filth." The slaughterhouses made no distinction between healthy and diseased animals—both were cut and delivered to Kalamazoo's butchers. The council responded that it could regulate only those slaughterhouses within the city limits, so Crane appealed to the state board of health. When it refused to interfere, she made a study of meat inspection laws in other states, drafted a model bill granting Michigan municipalities the right to inspect meat sold within their corporation limits, and then consulted the assistant state attorney general on its constitutionality. As soon as the bill was introduced in the legislature, Crane traveled to Lansing to lobby for its passage and was rewarded for her determination when it became law in May 1903.[74]

The meat inspection battle convinced Crane that municipal housekeeping was "the most vitally important function of city government." On several occasions she told the community that "our common house" must be kept clean—the air, individual houses and premises, schools, places of public assembly and trade, factories, and stores where food is prepared. Determined to act as well as talk, Crane founded the Women's Civic League of Kalamazoo in 1904. One of its first projects was street cleaning. Before approaching the mayor and city council for permission to take charge of six blocks of Main Street for a three-month period, Crane studied the street-cleaning practices of other cities. She discovered that many streets and sanitation departments had adopted methods advocated by Waring, and she decided to imitate his experiment in Kalamazoo.[75]

Crane began by outfitting the street sweepers in white duck uniforms. She then assigned each man to a particular section of the street, which was systematically swept and periodically flushed. Immediately following their sweeping, the workers bagged the dirt and refuse and removed them in horse-drawn carts. In the beginning, the sweepers were reluctant to change their ways; they did not like to use bags and frequently ignored an important injunction—"sweep with the bricks and not across them." Crane, however, refused to give in. Throughout the experiment she personally inspected the sweepers' work each day. She dismissed those who refused to follow her directions, and she increased the wages of those who adapted and were industrious. Kalamazoo's "White Wings" eventually took pride in their work and became advocates of Waring's methods.

In addition to the actual street cleaning, Crane and her league friends obtained an ordinance against spitting on sidewalks. They also visited Main Street merchants and asked them not to sweep or throw anything from their stores into the streets; and they took photographs of filthy alleys and showed them first to the adjacent property owners and then, if the alleys were not cleaned, to an interested public. They placed galvanized-iron and aluminum-painted cans on corners; and they furnished the Junior Civic Improvement League with handouts for distribution to residents, requesting them not to litter. At the end of the three-month period, Main Street was cleaner than it had ever been.

Crane had accomplished for Kalamazoo what Waring had achieved in New York City. His system, she had proven, was sanitary, efficient, and economical. By quickly bagging the dirt, it did not blow into nearby homes and businesses, nor did sweepers waste their time gathering and handling the same dirt. No longer were two-horse wagons used, with two men stopping to pick up bagged dirt and rubbish; one-horse carts, driven by one man, not only proved adequate but also saved time and labor. Even though the sweepers were paid higher wages under Crane's administration, the city saved money each day. Despite this saving, Kalamazoo only partially adopted Waring's methods in 1904. But three years later, following a street-cleaning study by an all-male civic committee, the city council implemented the practices previously advocated by Crane and the women's league.[76]

Crane became a national figure as a result of her street-cleaning work. Women's clubs across the country invited her to speak at their meetings, and municipalities wanted her to inspect their slaughterhouses and counsel them on street-cleaning methods. As the demand for her services increased, she devised procedures for examining cities of different sizes and in 1909 formally began a career as a sanitary consultant. Before agreeing to conduct a survey of a city or state, Crane made sure her visit was supported by government officials along with local women's groups. On one occasion she rebuked Mrs. C. G. Higbee, president of the Minnesota Federation of Women's Clubs, for failing to involve "men quite as much as women." Crane, like Ada Sweet and George Waring, knew that the campaign for municipal sanitation was "not a woman's campaign alone."[77] In Nashville, the initiative for Crane's visit was taken by the Tennessee Federation of Women's Clubs; yet before she accepted, the state, city, and county boards of health, the mayor and city, the board of trade, the Centennial Club, and the Anti-Tuberculosis League had to join in the invitation.

Another important part of Crane's preparation was the questionnaire. Before investigating a city, she required that eighty-two "Questions about Your City" be answered. She wanted to know population size, form of government, property valuation, tax rate, system of municipal accounting, bond issues for public improvements during the previous three years, charter amendments passed and defeated during the past five years, methods of supplying and treating water, miles of streets and sewers, and municipal provisions for cleaning and repairing pavements as well as for the collection and disposal of refuse. She asked for a map showing the location of the city's parks, playgrounds, schools, and recreation centers. She inquired about smoke nuisances and efforts to abate them, if they existed. And she requested copies of municipal ordinances concerning meat, milk, and market inspections. Once a prospective city had responded satisfactorily to these questions, Crane had its daily newspapers delivered to her for a two- to four-month period before her arrival.[78]

When she reached a particular city—such as Rochester, New York, or Montgomery, Alabama, which she visited in 1911 and 1912 respectively— Crane was escorted to the facilities and institutions she wished to see by individuals well acquainted with their operations. On the final evening of her stay, she gave a public address in which she reported on the community's sanitary conditions and offered specific suggestions for improvement. Crane always asked that the "largest and best place" be used for her talk "to the people"; she did not want a church or a courthouse that would seat only a select few. "The people will come," she said, "when they learn what [the talk] is about, and when the selection of a large and popular auditorium makes it plain that they are really *expected* to come."[79] She charged $100 a day plus expenses for her services, and she sometimes asked a higher fee if officials wanted a lengthy, written report.

Crane was particularly suited to her work as a municipal housekeeper and sanitarian. Like Waring, she knew the value of press coverage. It was not unusual for her to prepare a series of news releases on a forthcoming visit and then distribute them to the sponsoring organizations for their own publications and to the local newspapers. And, as a minister, she had learned to speak before large audiences. Thus, when she assembled an entire community to hear the closing address of one of her investigations, it was difficult to distinguish the sanitary expert from the civic revivalist. But her message was clear. Cleanliness was a crucial ingredient in the "making of an ideal city."[80]

Although few ideal cities resulted from Crane's efforts, permanent civic improvements followed from her sanitary surveys. A year after her visit to Calumet, Illinois, a public official claimed that the citizens counseled by Crane had changed Calumet from a mining camp to a beautifully clean city. In Uniontown, Pennsylvania, her condemnation of the public water supply caused the state board of health to make an independent investigation, which confirmed her findings; shortly thereafter the town eliminated the hazardous conditions. The year following her survey of twelve cities in Kentucky, the state legislature passed more health legislation that it had in its entire history. And, in at least twenty cities, municipal improvement leagues were created to correct deficiencies noted by Crane during her visit or in a final report.[81]

Following in the footsteps of Waring, who had taken great pride in freeing his department from the influence of local politicians, Crane contended that sanitary improvements could best be made when partisan politics were removed from municipal housekeeping. In her public addresses, she repeatedly emphasized that mayors, aldermen, commissioners, and street sweepers, one and all, should be elected or appointed on the basis of their ability to direct or carry out city business and not for reasons of party loyalty. Unfortunately, Crane did not demand a place for herself in city hall. Although an advocate of woman suffrage, she and most female sanitarians sought ways to influence politics "without touching the sources of their inequality." Their organizations continuously adopted goals that were conservative in nature: "to educate members, mentally and morally; to create public opinion; to secure better conditions of life." Products of their age, they characteristically employed the three-pronged Progressive method of investigation, education, and persuasion to achieve their ends. Yet, even though their part in sanitary reform was "chiefly suggestive or cooperative," they were major players in creating cleaner and healthier cities.[82]

Public and Private Cleanliness in the Progressive Era

During the first two decades of the twentieth century, the sanitarians' efforts gradually became institutionalized, and the anti-miasma rationale finally (though gradually) gave way to the germ theory. In this Progressive era, a time when reform and improvement touched virtually every aspect of American life, the American railway network—including street railways—came into being above ground, while the infrastructure of clean water and sewerage lines continued to spread below ground. New types of urban government, notably the city manager and commission reforms, were adopted in all regions of the country, and with them came experts, bureaucrats and civil servants, to whom anything less than efficient and clean cities were professionally outrageous. Order, efficiency, scientific principles, and professionalism became the watchwords of progressive America. What were innovations in the days of Waring and Crane came to be expected and commonplace by the 1920s; nothing less would do. Public and private cleanliness were the American norm, ubiquitously honored if not everywhere faithfully practiced.[83]

As cleanliness became the national expectation and its scientific basis ever more firm, the disturbing possibility lurked that not everyone would share or practice it. Like other features of progressivism, public sanitation and personal cleanliness retained a lingering middle-class, indeed upper middle-class tincture. Would these laudable standards become normal also for "outsiders" or "newcomers," that is, the large African-American minority as well as the millions of European and Asian immigrants who began arriving in great numbers in the 1880s? The whole campaign to make cities clean, and therefore safe, would fail if they did not. How then did these marginalized people become convinced of the "American Way" of cleanliness?

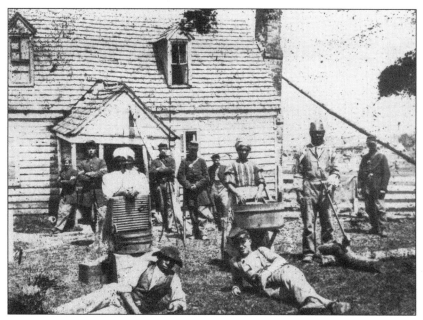

As "contraband of war" in a Union army camp in Yorktown, Virginia, in 1862, black women did the washing. Courtesy of The Library of Congress.

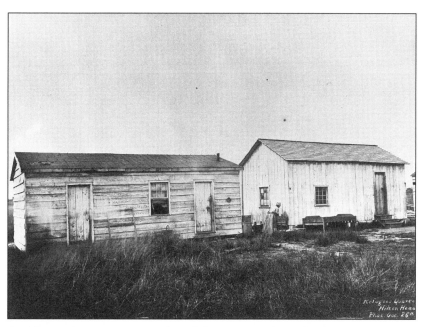

An African-American woman chased dirt unassisted at refugee quarters in Hilton Head, South Carolina, 1864. Courtesy of The National Archives.

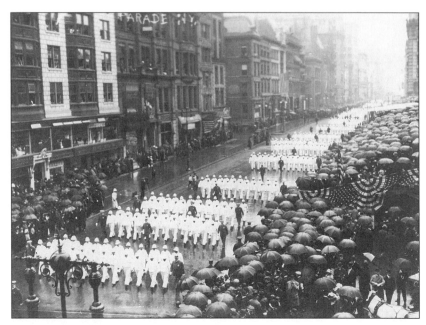

New York City's "White Wings" on parade, c. 1900, symbolized the importance of city cleansing. Courtesy of The Library of Congress.

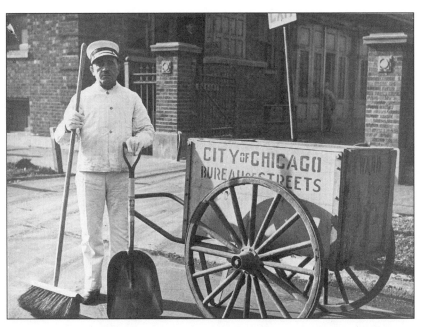

Chicago also outfitted its street-cleaning employees in white duck uniforms. Courtesy of the Public Works Historical Society.

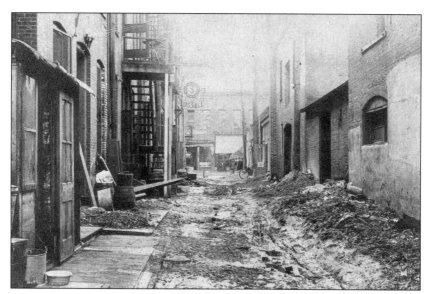

Caroline Bartlett Crane directed Kalamazoo's attention to its dirty streets and alleys, and their cleanup. Courtesy of the Archives and Regional History Collections, Western Michigan University.

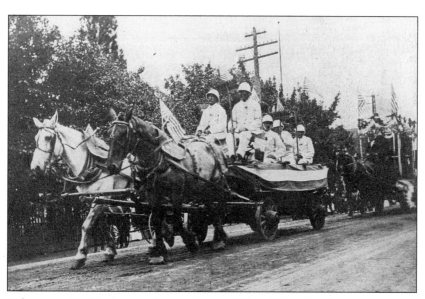

Kalamazoo, Michigan, proudly paraded its "White Wings," c. 1904. Courtesy of the Archives and Regional History Collections, Western Michigan University.

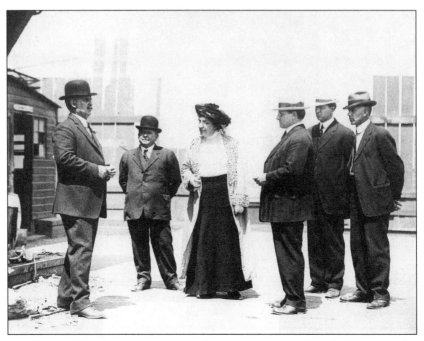

Caroline Bartlett Crane inspects a garbage incinerator in Seattle. Courtesy of the Archives and Regional History Collections, Western Michigan University.

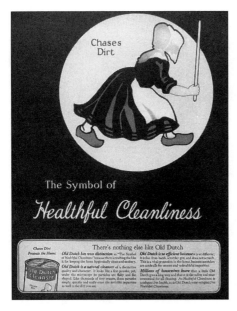

For decades good health motivated Americans to keep clean, as shown in this 1920 Dutch Cleanser ad. Courtesy of Ladies' Home Journal.

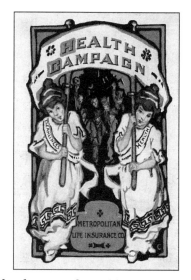 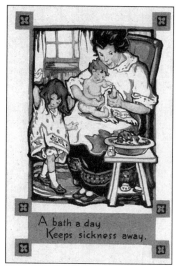

"Cleanliness" and "Health" formed the foundation for Metropolitan Life's "Health Campaign" pamphlet. In the last panel of the pamphlet, families are told that a "bath a day keeps sickness away." Courtesy of Metropolitan Life Insurance Company Archives.

A winning poster in a 1925 contest sponsored by Hygeia *magazine gave the first reason for cleanliness. Courtesy of* Hygeia.

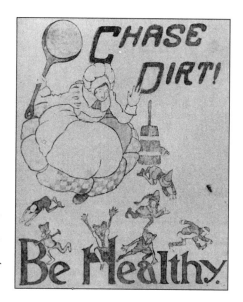

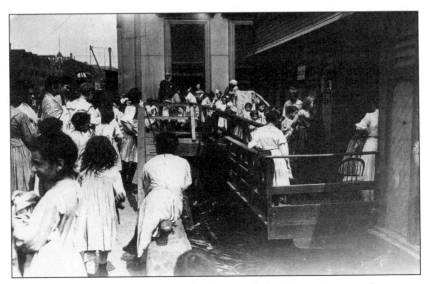

In cities, where working-class families frequently lived in quarters without bathrooms, young women and girls relied on public bathing facilities on "Ladies Day" (c. 1910). Courtesy of The Library of Congress.

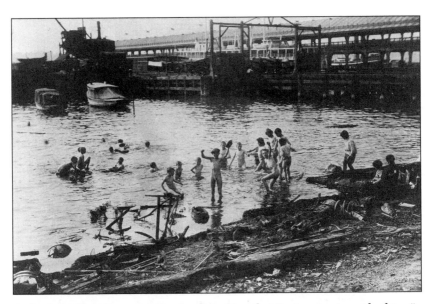

Despite the Cleanliness Institute's admonition that "swimming is not bathing," rivers and streams proved to be popular places for cooling off and cleaning up. This photo is from New York City, c. 1910. Courtesy of The National Archives.

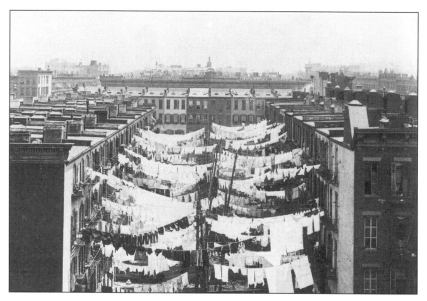

Doing the laundry was a particularly onerous job for women who lived in tenements without "modern" conveniences and with no help other than their children (Detroit, c. 1900). Courtesy of The Library of Congress.

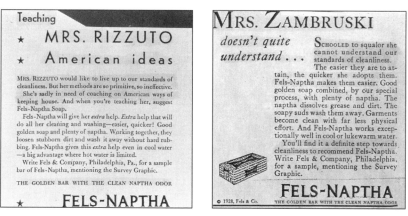

Teaching

★ MRS. RIZZUTO

★ American ideas

MRS. RIZZUTO would like to live up to our standards of cleanliness. But her methods are so primitive, so ineffective.

She's sadly in need of coaching on American ways of keeping house. And when you're teaching her, suggest Fels-Naptha Soap.

Fels-Naptha will give her *extra* help. *Extra* help that will do all her cleaning and washing—easier, quicker! Good golden soap and plenty of naptha. Working together, they loosen stubborn dirt and wash it away without hard rubbing. Fels-Naptha gives this *extra* help even in cool water—a big advantage where hot water is limited.

Write Fels & Company, Philadelphia, Pa., for a sample bar of Fels-Naptha, mentioning the Survey Graphic.

THE GOLDEN BAR WITH THE CLEAN NAPTHA ODOR

★ FELS-NAPTHA

MRS. ZAMBRUSKI

doesn't quite understand ...

SCHOOLED to squalor she cannot understand our standards of cleanliness. The easier they are to attain, the quicker she adopts them. Fels-Naptha makes them easier. Good golden soap combined, by our special process, with plenty of naptha. The naptha dissolves grease and dirt. The soapy suds wash them away. Garments become clean with far less physical effort. And Fels-Naptha works exceptionally well in cool or lukewarm water.

You'll find it a definite step towards cleanliness to recommend Fels-Naptha. Write Fels & Company, Philadelphia, for a sample, mentioning the Survey Graphic.

© 1928, Fels & Co.

FELS-NAPTHA

THE GOLDEN BAR WITH THE CLEAN NAPTHA ODOR

Not satisfied with the cleaning efforts of immigrant women, the makers of Fels-Naptha urged social workers through a series of ads in Survey *magazine during the 1920s and 1930s to teach women like Mrs. Rizzuto and Mrs. Zambruski the American way of cleanliness. Courtesy of* Survey.

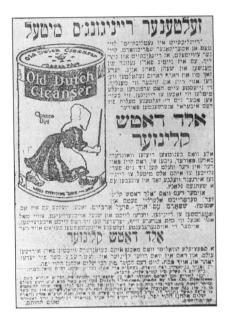

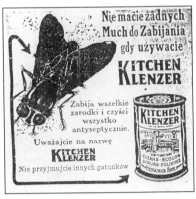

Fitzpatrick Brothers promoted "Kitchen Klenzer" and warned Polish families in Milwaukee and Chicago about the dangers of flies. Courtesy of Kuryer Polski.

Jewish immigrants quickly became acquainted with the dirt-chasing Dutch lady who spoke to them from the pages of Yiddishes Tageblatt. *Courtesy of* Yiddishes Tageblatt.

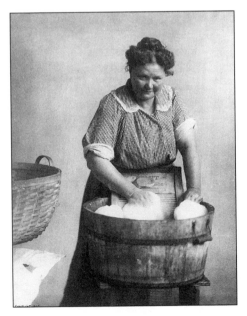

Despite the arduousness of the task, many immigrant and black women became laundresses because they could do the work at home. Courtesy of The Library of Congress.

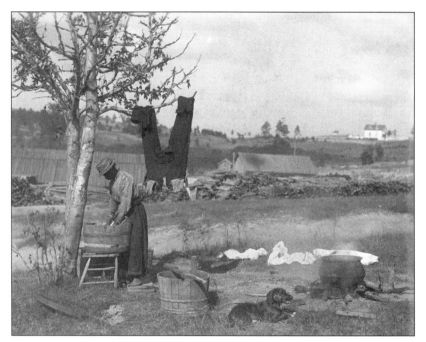

A working woman alone near Tuskegee, Alabama, in 1902 demonstrates how difficult washing could be. Courtesy of The Library of Congress.

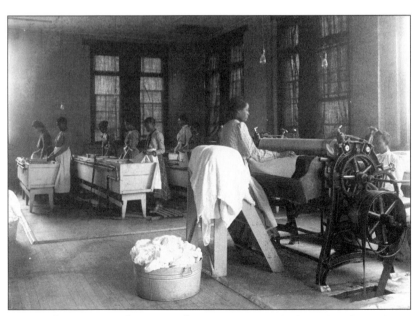

In 1902 the women students at Tuskegee Institute worked together doing the laundry, which had to meet Booker T. Washington's high standards of cleanliness. Courtesy of The Library of Congress.

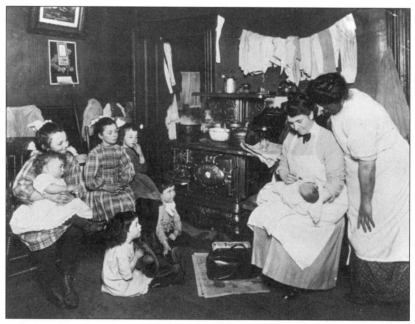

Settlement workers, visiting nurses, and domestic educators were among the many reformers who instructed mothers and children on the "right living" that led to good citizenship. Courtesy of the Metropolitan Life Insurance Company Archives.

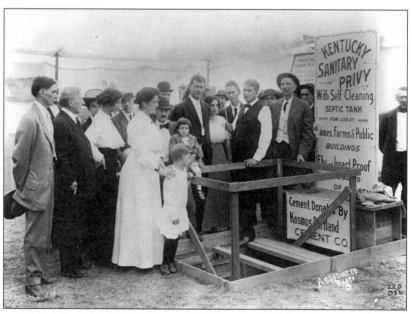

In 1913, during the Kentucky campaign to eradicate hookworm, about 12,000 people viewed an exhibit on the sanitary privy. Courtesy of the Rockefeller Archive Center.

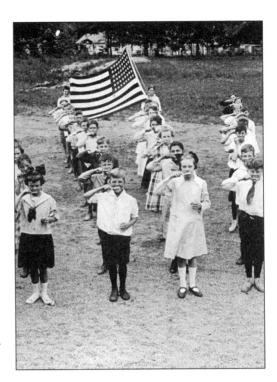

The students at the Tennessee Coal, Iron, & Railroad Company school in Fairfield, Alabama (c. 1915), learned how to become better Americans by joining together in the fight against tooth decay. Courtesy of The Library of Congress.

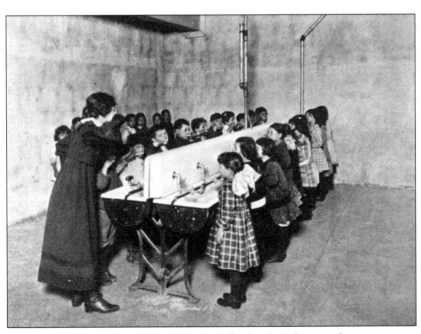

School teachers conducted "toothbrush drills" for their first-graders in Kansas City (c. 1915). Courtesy of the State Historical Society of Missouri.

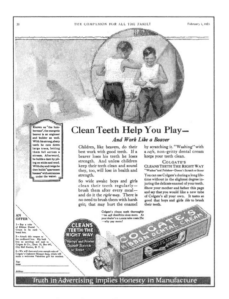

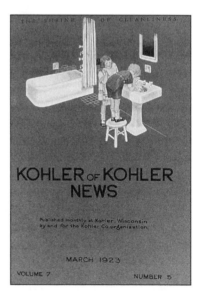

Top Left: Colgate claimed its toothpaste cleaned teeth "the right way" and made its users more successful workers and players. Courtesy Ladies' Home Companion.

Top Right: During the 1920s, middle-class Americans in cities generally lived in homes with white bathrooms that were nothing less than "shrines of cleanliness," according to the Kohler Manufacturing Company. Courtesy of the Kohler Company Archives.

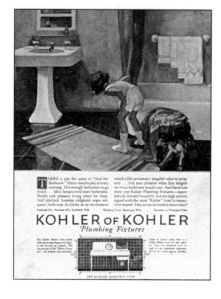

By the 1930s, middle-class city folk saw the need for more than one bathroom. "Health and pleasant living plead for them," in the words of Kohler. Courtesy of the Kohler Company Archives.

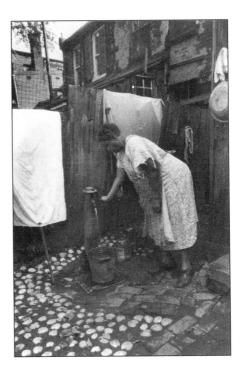

In low-income neighborhoods (Washington, D.C., 1935), residents continued to rely on outdoor water supplies. Courtesy of The Library of Congress.

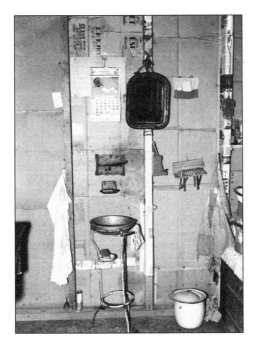

Farmhouses fared little better than slum residences during the 1930s. This one is in southern South Dakota, 1937. Courtesy of The Library of Congress.

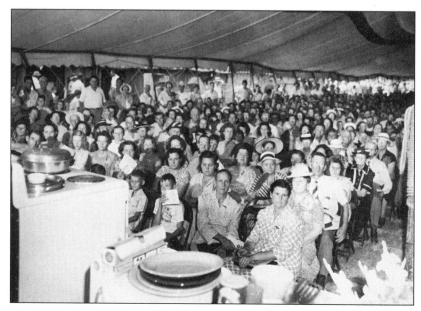

Farm women attended annual meetings of the Rural Electrification Administration in the late 1930s, wanting indoor plumbing and electrical appliances to ease their workload. Courtesy of The National Archives.

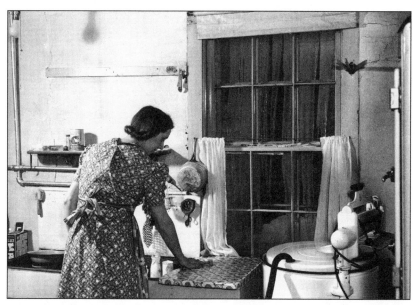

By 1940, this Vermont farm woman, with Lux and Old Dutch at her sink, had added running water, electric light, and a washing machine to her kitchen. Courtesy of The Library of Congress.

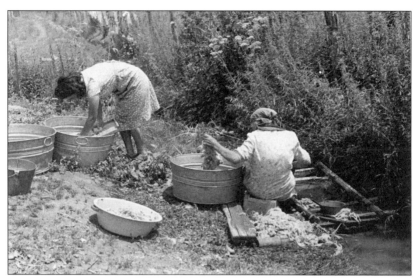

As late as 1940 these women in Chamisal, New Mexico, did their wash along an irrigation ditch. Courtesy of The Library of Congress.

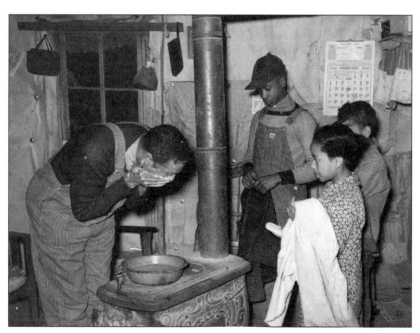

In 1940, in Creek County, Oklahoma, a tenant farmer and his children stood in line to wash up the "old-fashioned" way. Courtesy of The Library of Congress.

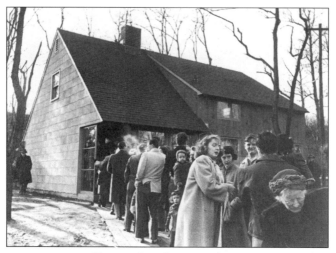

In 1949, potential buyers, largely veterans and their families, stood in line to inspect a model house that sold for $7,990 in Long Island's Levittown. Courtesy of The Library of Congress.

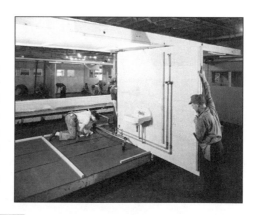

Popping the bathroom in. After World War II, pre-fabricated houses with bathrooms and modern appliances became the order of the day. Courtesy of The Library of Congress.

She who waits for her knight must remember . . . she will have to clean up after his horse.

In recent years, women have been reminding themselves as well as the men in their lives that chasing dirt is an equal opportunity pursuit. Courtesy of Northern Sun Merchandising.

CHAPTER FOUR

The American Way

She told us that by those Americans, everybody in the family had a toothbrush and a separate towel for himself, "not like by us, where we use one torn piece of shirt for the whole family, wiping the dirt from one face on to another."

—ANZIA YEZIERSKA, 1925[1]

Becoming American

A collection of efforts to improve personal cleanliness paralleled the public health and municipal housekeeping campaigns of the late nineteenth and early twentieth century. Municipal housekeeping and health matters involved civic-minded women and sanitarians as leaders; the drive for personal cleanliness expressed the moral leadership of private individuals like Booker T. Washington and settlement-house workers (chiefly female), who tried to inculcate middle-class standards of hygiene among the African-American and immigrant minorities. In the process, cleanliness became something more than a way to prevent epidemics and make cities liveable— it became a route to citizenship, to becoming American. It was, in fact, confrontation with racial and cultural outsiders that transformed cleanliness from a public health concern into a moral and patriotic one.

Personal cleanliness became a matter of keen public interest as soon as Americans realized how dirt and disease threatened their way of life, even in times of peace. Now convinced that cleanliness was fundamental to the nation's well-being, these recent converts preached their gospel to all who appeared not to have heard it, especially those who had passed "through a whole season without a bath, and possibly [had] never been completely immersed." Most Americans considered the "unwashed" to be the millions of immigrants from southern and eastern Europe who recently arrived in the country's newly plumbed cities. Seeking employment and opportunity, they were quickly told that "Good Health is Wealth," which could be obtained by keeping clean.[2] Thus, while public cleanliness remained urgent, especially in cities, personal hygiene acquired greater immediacy. And newcomers—first those from the peasant lands of Europe and later those from the rural South—received special attention.

Cleanliness for health's sake impelled reformers to teach immigrants certain basic facts about American life. Their beginning lessons on how to find work, become citizens, and learn English frequently included advice on how to keep clean in an urban environment. Although hardly dirtier than poor whites fresh from the countryside, most immigrants soon caught on that prosperous Americans cared about cleanliness. Not wishing to appear inferior or recalcitrant, these newcomers tended to agree that "the American way was the best way."[3] With few resources and great difficulty, they adopted American habits of hygiene as best they could—not only to stay healthy but also to be accepted and "get ahead."

By the turn of the century middle-class Americans idealized cleanliness as their "greatest virtue." They no longer simply believed that sick people died of dirt; they now professed "the inestimable importance of keeping clean." Cleanliness was a "sanitary safeguard" against contagious diseases (whether caused by filth or germs—many were still not sure) that had been learned by hard experience; and as Americans became increasingly enamored with the notions of progress and enterprise in the decades following the Civil War, they also grew to value cleanliness as "one of the characteristics of high civilization." In this context it is not surprising that many old-stock Americans were alarmed by the arrival of the "huddled masses" from Italy, Russia, Greece, Poland, Austria-Hungary, and the Balkans. In 1907 over 80 percent of the 1,285,000 new immigrants who came to the United States were from these countries, as compared with only 13 percent in 1882. Thus, despite the need for unskilled laborers, most city dwellers were bewildered by these people who not only looked different but seemed so ignorant of American manners and customs.[4]

In response to these widespread fears, social workers, educators, and employers attempted to help immigrants adjust to their new surroundings by teaching them American ways. Americanization programs insisted that training in hygiene begin as early as instruction in English. In fact, since these Americanizers tended to believe that the foreign-born did not appreciate sanitation, they used English lessons to teach adults as well as children how to bathe (with soap and warm water), when to bathe (preferably every day but at least every week), and where to bathe (first in public baths, then in bathrooms). Within months of their arrival, immigrants learned that "there was an American way to brush teeth, and an American way to clean fingernails, and an American way to air out bedding." By linking the tooth- brush to patriotism, Americanizers clearly demonstrated that becoming American involved a total makeover of personal habits and loyalties.[5]

Booker T. Washington—Toothbrushes and More

Cleanliness had first been wrapped in a mantle of patriotism by the United States Sanitary Commission and the Freedmen's Bureau during the Civil War. Young northern recruits from the countryside learned that personal hygiene and Union victory were closely linked, and former slaves were taught habits of neatness and cleanliness along with reading, writing, and civics. In the years following emancipation, cleanliness became even more intricately tied to patriotism through the freed slaves' desire for social ac- ceptance. Booker T. Washington, the most influential African-American leader of the late nineteenth century, preached the "gospel of the tooth- brush" whenever the occasion permitted him to do so. He insisted that one of the most helpful lessons he received at the Hampton Institute was "in the use and value of the bath."[6]

General Samuel Chapman Armstrong, who had commanded a regiment of African-American troops during the Civil War, founded the Hampton Normal and Agricultural Institute in Hampton, Virginia. Located on a large contraband campsite across Hampton Roads from Norfolk, it opened in 1868 under the auspices of the Freedmen's Bureau and with generous sup- port from the American Missionary Association. The school began with only twenty students, but it grew in less than a decade to over a thousand. These students, along with friends and supporters, would be reminded regularly of the importance of cleanliness through Hampton's monthly publication, the *Southern Workman*. "Remember," it instructed its readers in May 1875, "that the thing above all others which Society insists upon is 'cleanliness,' and that this cleanliness must begin with your skin and the clothes which you wear."[7]

Armstrong, the son of New England missionaries to Hawaii and a gradu- ate of Williams College, believed that deficiency of character could be traced to ignorance and bad habits. As a student at Williams he took a sponge bath every day, even on cold January mornings. Later, as an officer of the 9th Regiment of United States Colored Troops, he was known for his daring as well as his neatness. He admitted to being a "poor housekeeper" but insisted that he was a "good camp-maker"; in February 1864 he said that everything in his tent at Camp Stanton was "neat, tidy, comfortable, and homelike." Six months later, when the 9th Regiment was stationed near Petersburg, he boasted that his camps were "not only the cleanest, but the handsomest in the brigade."[8]

As Armstrong developed plans for Hampton Institute, he was continually reminded of the Hilo Manual Labor School in Hawaii that he had inspected on tours with his father in 1851. Like Polynesians, African-Americans were not innately inferior, Armstrong believed, only backward, and since they too were "in the early stages of civilization," they needed training along with their education. Thus, besides requiring African-American students to learn manual skills, he forced them to acquire "habits of regularity" and self-discipline. In many respects, Hampton resembled an army camp except that most of its teachers were women. Armstrong found their influence "more refining" than men's.[9]

In Washington's case, however, it was Armstrong who proved the most inspiring. In him, Washington found a father, teacher, and guide for his entire life. From him, Washington learned a trade and how to teach; he also became well versed in the reputedly Yankee virtues of thrift, industriousness, cleanliness, and abstinence.[10] Although he had grown up as a slave on a Virginia plantation, he had already been exposed to New England ways by the time he reached Hampton in 1872. For about a year and a half following the war, Washington had worked as a houseboy in the home of General Lewis Ruffner and his wife Viola in the West Virginia mining town of Malden.

Mrs. Ruffner, a former Vermont school teacher, recalled that young Booker was always "more than willing" to follow her instructions. He appreciated the precise commands she gave him, especially in matters of neatness and cleanliness. In *Up from Slavery*, Washington later confessed that because of her example he never saw scraps of paper around a house or in the street but that he wanted "to pick them up at once"; nor could he see a filthy yard, an unwhitewashed house, or a grease-spot on a person's clothes without wanting to call attention to it. He also knew that had it not been for Mrs. Ruffner he might never have been admitted to Hampton.[11]

In 1872 when Washington arrived at the institute following a long walk, he was dirty and resembled a tramp. As a kind of test of the young man's character, the head teacher asked him to sweep a nearby recitation room. He confidently grabbed the broom, remembering what Mrs. Ruffner had taught him. Since he identified the head teacher as a " 'Yankee' woman who knew just where to look for dirt," Washington swept the room three times and dusted it four times. After he finished, the head teacher carefully inspected the room; finding no dirt on the floor or dust on the furniture, she told him he could stay and offered him a job as janitor.[12] During his three years at Hampton, he cleaned the academic building.

Despite the time spent under Mrs. Ruffner's tutelage, Washington's daily life at Hampton was "a constant revelation." Having meals served at regular hours, eating on tablecloths, using napkins, sleeping on sheets, and taking baths were all new to him. He liked these practices and quickly adopted them; for a lifetime, he followed and advocated them. Even when he traveled he tried to bathe each day. If he were a guest in a single-room cabin that lacked bathing facilities, he often slipped away "to some stream in the woods." When Washington left Hampton and returned to his former home in Malden, where he taught from 1876 to 1878, he required his students "to keep their clothes neat and clean, and their hair combed every morning, and the boys to keep their boots cleaned." He accomplished this by initiating a morning inspection patterned after Hampton's, where he had learned that "cleanliness, quiet colors, and well-brushed boots" characterized a gentleman's dress.[13]

Washington opened Tuskegee Institute in Alabama in July 1881, and Hampton provided the model. Like General Armstrong, Washington wanted to educate young people *and* build character. Since most of the students came from homes with few conveniences, he taught them how to bathe and care for their teeth, clothing, and rooms. He demanded that "everywhere there should be absolute cleanliness"; and what he required was enforced by inspectors who looked for "the soiled collar, the loose button, and the unpolished boot." Armstrong's "gospel of the toothbrush," Washington was fond of saying, was part of the Tuskegee creed. But in a more serious vein he acknowledged that, while African-Americans might be excused their poverty and lack of comforts, they would not be forgiven their dirt.[14]

Washington attempted through his educational methods to "resolve the antagonisms, suspicions, and aspirations" of freed people, white Southerners, and white Northerners. This task grew exceedingly difficult by the 1890s, however, since most African-Americans saw no improvement in their living conditions and suffered new restrictions upon their economic opportunities and political rights. In response to such harsh realities Washington encouraged patience, cooperation, industry, discipline, and cleanliness in the belief that these virtues would eventually win the sympathies of conservative Southerners and rich northern capitalists. To begin at the bottom and "work up in the American way" seemed to him to offer more chance of success than agitation or protest. Thus, when Washington insisted that Tuskegee students learn such practical subjects as blacksmithing, caning, brickmaking, basketry, and wheelwrighting, he believed graduates would appear attractive to benevolent white employers. Although manual training often proved irrelevant in an industrializing South, Washington's lessons in "orderliness, cleanliness, discipline, and a 'cooperative spirit' had relevance for the new era."[15]

To Ellis Island and America

In 1901, Washington told the world his story in *Up from Slavery*. By then, the war with Spain, which began idealistically in 1898 to liberate Cuba, had led to the acquisition of the Philippines and to the brutal suppression of the Philippine independence movement. Thirty-six years after the Constitution ended slavery, white supremacy had "become the American Way" in the South, the North, and in the nation's new colony across the Pacific.[16] In this context and at a time when municipalities were making large investments in city cleansing, it was not simply coincidental that white, middle-class Americans—and those like Washington who wished to win their favor—placed such strong emphasis on personal cleanliness. In 1896 Edward Bok, the didactic editor of the *Ladies' Home Journal* and a Danish immigrant himself, noted with pride the advances the United States had been made in plumbing and hygiene. "The bath," he reported, was "becoming a national institution." In a vein strikingly similar to Washington's, he opined that

> The man who makes a point of keeping himself clean, and whose clothes look neat, no matter how moderate of cost they may be, works better, feels better, and is in every sense a better business man than his fellow worker who is disregardful of both his body and dress, or either. He works at a distinct advantage. The external man unquestionably influences the internal man.

Bok directly connected "the cleanliness of a people" and their moral superiority.[17]

Late nineteenth-century Americans were certainly not the first to view their superiority in terms of a physical characteristic such as whiteness or even cleanliness. At least a century earlier they, like their English relatives, had often associated the color black with dirt. Hence people who had darker skins than Anglo-Saxons—always African-Americans and frequently Jews and southern Italians—usually suffered a stamp of inferiority. Seen by some as "vast masses of filth" who were "foul and stagnant," southern and eastern European immigrants made nativist Americans uneasy and anxious. They argued that it was not the size of the immigration pool that concerned them but its "character"; they maintained that the personal habits of these newcomers (occasionally referred to as "mudsills") were "repugnant" to the "inherited tastes" of Americans and would weaken the nation's wealth and power.[18]

Of course, not everyone viewed the new immigrants as a threat to the country's greatness. Yet few were unconcerned about how these foreigners would adjust to American life. Even those who welcomed them (their own relatives included) encouraged them to discard their old ways as quickly as possible and become Americans. Thus those who intended to stay in the United States "dressed from head to foot in American clothing" almost immediately. Others, who wanted to return to Europe with enough cash to better their lives back home, went in search of the most lucrative jobs. Over time, though, more and more immigrants put down roots and began raising families in America.[19]

The immigrants who remained needed little prodding to adopt American ways that they believed would help them succeed. For, contrary to popular opinion at the turn of the century, those who chose to emigrate with their families (or with plans for them to follow) were not "the dregs" or "the scum" of the Old World; instead they tended to be venturesome and ambitious people, eager for opportunity. They sought success in "the incredible land." Despite the variety of motives and circumstances that caused them to leave their homeland, the several million immigrants who came to the United States were drawn by hopes and visions of achievement.[20]

The majority arrived in New York City, following two weeks of uncomfortable and congested steamship travel. Although steerage provisions had improved from those endured by the Irish following the Great Famine of the late 1840s, they remained less than adequate for passengers concerned about cleanliness. There was no fresh air on the lower decks, where travelers kept their bedding and baggage. There were lavatories with toilets and some basins of porcelain or coarse metal; but bathtubs and showers were only occasionally provided, and then fees were charged for their use. Water was available primarily for drinking or cooking, so clothes could be washed only on deck and in salt water. Under these conditions, it is little wonder that a last-minute scrubbing and change of clothes before setting foot on Ellis Island was "the best that could be hoped for."[21]

Ship companies were largely responsible for the lack of sanitation on their vessels, but immigrants also contributed to the unsavory atmosphere. Although washing and bathing facilities were in short supply, passengers frequently failed to use those that were provided. Many did not bother to clean their eating utensils or assist one another in keeping their quarters in order. Some were probably too seasick to care. Others, who found the food plentiful but poorly prepared, took little interest or initiative in cleaning up before or after meals. Finally, the Old World habits of many immigrants, who came from Europe's peasant farmlands, did not serve them well on crowded ships that were inadequately equipped and staffed. Thus, despite periodic attempts by stewards to wash down and disinfect steerage passage-ways and cabins, they were usually filthy.[22]

Immigrants approaching the coast of America for the first time remembered how happy they were to see land, view the Statue of Liberty, and leave their "dank and dreary" ship compartments. Ellis Island offered them a reception that stood in stark contrast to the treatment they had received on board ship. In the dining room, a young man from Romania recalled eating "the best dinner . . . in my entire life." He wondered, "What kind of a country is this, receiving me, a lowly immigrant, with a great dinner . . . ?" A Russian Jew was "startled by the tremendous whiteness" of the dormitories above the Great Hall. He had never seen so much white in one place—"the tile was white, the bed was white, the sheets were white, the light was bright and white."[23]

Besides dining rooms and dormitories, Ellis Island had enough showers for 8000 immigrants each day. All newcomers could bathe, but many were not accustomed to such facilities and chose only to rinse their feet. Women who had never washed their hair were not eager to begin at Ellis Island. Others, who had already tidied up and changed into their best clothes aboard ship, wanted the physical examinations to begin. Although most of the migrants had been vaccinated, disinfected, and inspected before sailing (beginning in 1891 American immigration law demanded this of steamship companies), they were required to undergo similar procedures upon arrival. Within a few hours or a couple of days at most, 98 percent were admitted to the United States; yet, years later, most remembered this short period of time with enormous dread. They vividly recalled their trepidation as they came before uniformed physicians and immigration officials as well as their panicky fear that they or family members would fail the examinations.[24]

First impressions of living conditions in America were at once varied and similar. The experiences of individual families differed, but most were both surprised and disappointed at what they found. Instead of avenues paved with gold, they saw in New York City "narrow streets of squeezed-in stores and houses, ragged clothes, dirty bedding oozing out of the windows, ash-cans and garbage-cans cluttering the side-walks."[25] Writer Mary Antin described the Boston alleyway where she first lived as a box in which "two rows of three-story tenements [were] its sides, a stingy strip of sky . . . its lid, a littered pavement . . . its floor, and a narrow mouth its exit." A Polish woman in Chicago remembered 44th Street and Ashland Avenue, where her family boarded, as "the stinkiest place in the world." Like so many others, she was shocked by urban America. Their neighborhoods, filled with "the stinking smells of crowded poverty," lacked the open spaces, forests, and streams that many of the first generation would always associate with their European villages. "Where," they wondered, was "the golden country of [their] dreams?"[26]

If their streets and neighborhoods were found lacking, so too were their dwellings. Women especially found them disappointing. One southern Italian, confined to a congested tenement in New York City, missed the warm weather that allowed so much outdoor living; thoughts of the public fountain, where she had gone for water and visited with neighbors, made her sad. In the New York flat, her family shared "a sink in the hall" and "one bathroom in the yard where garbage was thrown" with four families who were strangers. She confessed that every time she used the privy she "died a little." Another Italian woman who accompanied her husband to a wooden shack in a coal-mining community in Wayne County, Iowa, around 1900 said she "cried her heart out for the first year." These experiences led them and many others like them to conclude that "America, America, it's no good."[27]

Although numerous immigrant families worked in mines or on farms in the Midwest and West, the majority lived their lives in an urban environment. The frontier of settlement had moved so far from the Atlantic and the cost of starting up a competitive farm had risen so much that most "greenhorns" remained in seaboard and Great Lakes cities. And, following the agricultural depression of the 1870s, they were joined by American farmers who left the countryside for industrial jobs. From the 1880s onward, Chicago proved to be a major destination for both native-born farmers and immigrants. Its attractiveness stemmed from the employment opportunities it offered. Located on Lake Michigan, Chicago was a port city and railroad hub as well as "a center for the grain and lumber trades, livestock processing, and meat packing, and the home of breweries and iron and steel mills and the Midwestern garment and financial center;" it always needed laborers.[28] For that reason, its population doubled from half a million to a million between 1880 and 1890.

This urban population explosion explains in large part the monumental health problems that followed in its wake. Cities were unprepared for the massive influx of newcomers. Public works infrastructure, housing, and health facilities could not handle the critical demands of a burgeoning population, let alone one so unfamiliar with the ways of the metropolis. Most of these people, who were rural in orientation, had few skills and little capital. As a result, they worked the longest hours for the lowest wages in the dirtiest surroundings. These "mudsills" of northern cities (shrewd enough to know, however, that they had more opportunities there than in the South) took jobs digging sewers, mining coal, excavating tunnels, puddling iron, building railroads, collecting garbage, washing dishes, and shining shoes. In short, they eked out a living in pestilential slums located near the industries that gave them work.[29]

In Chicago's stockyard neighborhood, known as Back of the Yards, swarms of flies literally blackened the air. They seemed to come from everywhere—massive slaughterhouses, open trucks from local fertilizer plants, four city garbage dumps, alleys piled high with uncollected refuse, and a stinking sewer called Bubbly Creek. Besides the flies, heavy clouds of smoke, "thick, oily, and black as night" carried a sickening, rancid odor. To this blighted region, the location of the well-known Union Stock Yards, went 45,000 immigrants—Irish, then German, and finally Slavic—in search of a better life.[30]

Sickness, especially tuberculosis, was commonplace in this exceptionally filthy place. In 1901 sanitary conditions in Back of the Yards were "as bad as any in the world." Ten years later, when Poles and Lithuanians predominated (but lived apart on separate blocks), the area had definitely improved. Chicago had extended its sewers as well as enlarged and treated Bubbly Creek, making it a good deal less offensive; most cellar apartments had been abandoned, and many streets had been paved. But sanitary arrangements remained primitive. Too many immigrant families still used outdoor privies, while most shared hall or basement water closets with several households. In one case, a single closet served forty-seven people, an overcrowding reminiscent of steerage, except it was permanent.[31]

The four city dumps that distinguished this Chicago community also remained. These large, landmark holes, from which clay had been taken for nearby brickyards, were regularly filled with refuse of every kind by municipal garbage collectors, private scavengers, and local packers. Since material of some value was mixed in with worthless items, women and children took their turn (following commercial pickers who paid $15 a week for the privilege), hunting through the wastes for kindling wood, old mattresses, used clothing, pieces of food, and the occasional silver utensil or toy. Ignorant of the hazards such as flies and rodents, especially from the decaying organic matter, as many as twenty women and sixty children might ordinarily be found looking for goods they could not afford to buy.[32]

Would these women have discontinued their visits to the dump had they realized the danger? To assume that they would have stopped, had they known, fails to recognize how desperate many of them were. By 1910, when a family of five needed $900 a year to maintain a modest standard of living, only one immigrant in seven earned that much. Wives—and often children—worked for a pittance at home or found low-paying jobs in neighborhood industries. Struggling to keep their families fed and alive, many also toiled as domestics, laundresses, and janitresses in private residences, commercial establishments, and public buildings. One Russian woman summed up what so many believed about their future—it was little more than "long and hard work in the unsanitary buildings."[33]

Almost all immigrant women had "two irons in the fire." Besides working outside the home, they also carried out their home-making responsibilities in temporary shacks on the outskirts of towns or in makeshift tenements situated in the oldest and least desirable sections of cities. These dwellings were often built before the advent of modern sanitary facilities or codes, and absentee landlords generally refused or were unable to remodel or repair them. Many families—frequently with several children under six and a few boarders—crowded into small, dark shanties or apartments that lacked adequate water and toilet facilities.[34]

A 1911 Senate investigation of immigrant living conditions in New York, Philadelphia, Chicago, Boston, Cleveland, Buffalo, and Milwaukee found home plumbing facilities in a deplorable state. In nearly all instances "the water supply was found to be either a faucet within the house or a yard hydrant." Where there was a faucet, it was almost always located in the kitchen. Only 30 percent of the households studied had separate, indoor toilet accommodations; about half shared toilets with a second household. A minority still depended on dry toilets in yard privies. In Cleveland, where many of the streets remained unsewered, the majority of immigrant households had nothing else.[35]

Housing in Chicago's ethnic neighborhoods also had its peculiarities. Compared with New York City's tenements, which were usually five to seven stories high, Chicago's were not tall. There were seldom more than three stories above the basement, and many apartments had more closet and pantry space than did flats in New York and elsewhere. But Chicago had by far the largest number of basement apartments and toilets located under the sidewalks of raised streets. Both features proved particularly troublesome and unhealthy. Not only was there little light and ventilation in cellar dwellings and underground privies, but they were also damp and fetid since the wastewater and sewage from adjacent yards "drained under the floors and around the walls." In these places, not surprisingly, it was "practically impossible to keep any degree of cleanliness."[36]

In Chicago and elsewhere cleanliness was definitely a luxury for immigrant families, and they paid a high price for it. Writer Anzia Yezierska, a Jewish immigrant from Russian Poland, showed in story after story that soap and water were not cheap and that the poor could not easily keep clean. Despite what contemporaries may have believed, her point of view was officially borne out in the final reports of the Senate's Immigration Commission. It concluded its study of immigrant living conditions by stating

that "in general the proportion of well-kept homes [was] high." Where it
was not so, the commission blamed "circumstances over which the inhabi-
tants [had] little direct control, such as a poor water supply or unsanitary
drainage. . . ." Another 1911 survey, by the federal Bureau of Labor, reported that the majority of immigrant kitchens and bathrooms rated "good"
or "fair" as to cleanliness, and that Italian women, for example, who had
been in New York for several years and had "moved uptown" were indeed
fastidious homemakers.[37] Like Yezierska's fictional characters, many foreigners were "slaving" to keep clean.

The burden of cleanliness fell primarily on wives and mothers. Although
they came to America from a variety of places and brought different customs with them, immigrant women from southern and eastern Europe were
chiefly responsible for the care of their homes and children. In the villages
and towns of the Old World, they maintained simple and orderly dwellings,
where even their earthen floors suggested cleanliness. In one village in
Sicily, for example, housework usually began before sunrise when women
went out to draw their families' water from nearby fountains. During the
day housewives took care of children and small animals, while they did
many chores; besides sewing and preparing meals, they made beds, swept
straw and feces from corners into the streets, and carried "night pots" to
dumping areas outside the village. If they happened to have brick or tile
floors, they washed them and threw the used water into the street, following
local practice. When they did laundry, poorer women carried their clothes
(lighter than water) to public fountains or open springs. Others, lucky
enough to own washtubs or to hire help, washed clothes at home.[38]

On Elizabeth Street in New York City, where many Sicilian women lived
after arriving in the United States, they found flats that were small and dark,
not unlike the dwellings they had left behind. They probably would have
been surprised and perplexed had their new apartments had large windows,
running water, or flush toilets. Strangers to American ways, they did not
know how to adapt the customs of their old homes to their new ones. Most
immigrant women found housework in America more difficult "with the
cleaning of woodwork, washing windows, care of curtains, carpets, and
dishes, and more elaborate cooking." Scrubbing floors, changing bedding,
and doing laundry proved especially arduous for those accustomed to
earthen floors, feather beds, and clothes rinsed alongside their neighbors' in
the open air. An Italian woman who emigrated to Chicago in August 1900
and subsequently had four children, remembered that "everything was
wash, wash, wash. . . ."[39]

Although "everything was pretty hard to keep clean" for Polish and
Lithuanian women who lived in Chicago's Back of the Yards, they did not

ordinarily shirk their housekeeping duties. In fact, many of them were meticulous housekeepers who acquired a reputation for the scrupulous care they gave their floors and laundry as well as the sidewalks and streets in front of where they lived. They brought high standards from the old country; in their case, settlement workers would preach to the converted. Soap and water actually helped them master their environment. A spotless house and front walk demonstrated that they could rise above their harsh new surroundings. In the end, cleanliness enhanced their self-esteem and made them proud of the little they had.[40]

The daily battle against dirt meant more than keeping homes and clothing clean. It also included personal hygiene, and bathing posed special problems. Many, who considered the practice useless and possibly dangerous, were accustomed to bathing only occasionally, usually during the summer months in local rivers or streams. Others, who recognized the importance of taking frequent baths, lacked the plumbing and privacy necessary to achieve "the spick-and-span cleanliness" of so many Americans. Yet everyone seemed to recall standing in line on a Saturday evening or before the holidays to take a turn in the hot showers at a public bath or a large washtub at home. One Polish woman explained what was known in her family as the "Russian bath." It was the one taken by the last in line—it had "the coldest and the dirtiest water."[41]

As immigrants struggled to keep clean in an almost impossible environment, middle-class Americans became more aware of the germ theory and grew more anxious about the spread of contagious diseases. By the 1890s street cars, paper money, and library books were thought to be threatening carriers of deadly microbes. But nothing caused more alarm than unwashed immigrants in neighboring slums. Eleanor Roosevelt's "Cousin Susie" begged the nineteen-year-old Eleanor, for example, "to quit all her settlement work and join her in Newport; she feared that Eleanor would bring home an immigrant's disease." Sanitarians and physicians also expressed concern:

A man may live on the splendid "avenue," in a mansion plumbed in the latest and costliest style, but if, half a mile away, in range with his open window, there is a "slum," or even a neglected tenement-house, the zephyr will come along and pick up the disease-germs and bear them onward, distributing them to whomsoever it meets, whether he be a millionaire or a shillingaire, with a perfectly leveling and democratic impartiality.[42]

In rural societies, where land served as a buffer, cleanliness had few of the imperatives it took on in a nation of cities. By the late nineteenth century, however, middle-class city dwellers believed in the importance of cleanliness to health, civility, and morality. They had been convinced by the coming together of a large immigrant population, stunning (although not easily understood) public health discoveries, and major public works investments. In 1899, when Mayor Josiah Quincy of Boston declared that "an unclean man could not feel the same sense of self-respect as a clean man" and that "a man was less likely to fall into moral evil if he kept himself physically clean," he expressed sentiments popular among the new urban middle class.[43] Cleanliness was no longer valued solely by an elite; it was accepted by a broad public.

For the most part, immigrants from southern and eastern Europe had little knowledge of the germ theory and did not understand American habits of personal hygiene. Only Jews, who brought with them specific religious rules and rituals that emphasized cleanliness, agreed with native-born Americans on this critical matter. Yet even immigrant Jews expressed astonishment at American plumbing. One man remembered how he reacted when his father, who had been to the United States, first described a faucet with running water: "How is that possible, you open a valve, and water, water, all you want?"[44]

Good Neighbors, Good Teachers: The Settlement Workers

Bewildered by modern city life and discriminated against because they were foreigners, immigrants had few places to go for advice or protection. Many, however, found "good neighbors" in the settlement workers. Jane Addams, the most celebrated of those who dedicated their lives to serving the immigrant poor at the turn of the century, opened the door of Hull-House in Chicago in 1889. To her and others like her, no concern was too insignificant and no task too menial in their attempt to improve the newcomers' lot. Living in slums, they understood as few Americans did the hardships that arose out of poverty, squalor, and disorientation.[45]

Settlement houses, which frequently had a neighborhood's "cleanest windows and shiniest doorknob," did not hide the middle-class backgrounds of their residents. At Hull-House, for example, they planned their work around the availability of servants hired to do the cooking and cleaning. In New York City, Lillian Wald, founder of the Henry Street Settlement, recalled how difficult it had been for her and Mary Brewster to locate quarters on the East Side simply because they "clung to the civilization of a bathroom." After a long and careful search, they chose an apartment with a tiny closet and a small bathroom in the hall. When they moved in, they brought good furniture, a Baltimore heater, and lovely dinnerware with them. Here Wald and Brewster lived for two years—in space the same size as that occupied by the large families below them.[46]

As paradoxical and artificial as these living arrangements may have appeared, they enabled settlement workers to become effective mediators between immigrant neighborhoods and the surrounding communities of which they were a part. And, in matters of cleanliness, working-class families received an array of services from settlement folks. They established nurseries and staffed dispensaries where they taught mothers how to bathe and feed their infants; they inspected streets and alleys to force landlords to clean up their properties and prod city officials to remove garbage. They also sponsored evening classes and informal gatherings where adults learned the hazards of slaughtering sheep in their basements, drinking water from horse troughs, and sorting rags culled from dumps.[47] Settlement workers believed that many of the newcomers' troubles arose from their unfamiliarity with city living; in time, they would also know that their neighbors' most serious difficulties stemmed from social and environmental problems beyond their control.

That knowledge came directly from the settlement folks' experience of living beside the immigrants they tried to help. "Good neighbors"—like Addams in Chicago or Wald in New York City—were not casual, friendly visitors like the charity organization people of the 1870s. Instead of living in working-class neighborhoods, those charity volunteers (often older upper- or middle-class women who had actively assisted the Sanitary Commission or the Freedmen's Bureau during the Civil War) periodically visited the poor to investigate their needs, establish cordial relations, and encourage such provident habits as industry, thrift, and cleanliness.[48] Settlement workers and charity volunteers shared a desire to improve immigrant life and eliminate divisions between classes and ethnic groups, but they differed significantly in their approaches.

Josephine Shaw Lowell, director of the New York Charity Organization Society, believed that immigrants were personally responsible for the impoverished conditions in which they lived. Their poverty and squalor had roots in their character—people whom she described as "idlers." At various times she ruefully described the unfortunate circumstances of slum life, but she always seemed to be searching for "the moral flaws that underlay such conditions." She counseled charity volunteers when visiting the unemployed to "find some sort of means of letting the head . . . earn a dollar to provide for their immediate necessities." She even suggested such jobs as chopping wood, scrubbing floors, washing clothes—"anything to avoid teaching the dreadful lesson that it is easy to get a day's living without working for it."[49]

In contrast to Lowell, Addams did not think the immigrant families she knew on Chicago's West Side were lazy or irresponsible. In fact, she sometimes seemed surprised at how hard they worked. In her autobiography she remarked that the poorest immigrant women kept on "with the hard night scrubbing or the long days of washing" for the sake of their children. These people were poor, she contended, not because of individual weaknesses but rather because of the harsh environments in which they lived and worked. Defects in character were more the consequence than the cause of their poverty. The 1893 depression provided these reformers with the first tangible indication that their immigrant neighbors suffered from forces beyond their control.[50]

Living in a slum during the winter of 1893–94 gave Hull-House residents an opportunity to witness at firsthand the appalling misery that afflicted communities when hundreds of thousands of people were out of work. It was, for settlement folk everywhere, "an ordeal by fire." In Chicago, where unemployed visitors to the World's Fair saw no reason to return home, the situation was especially wrenching. The newly formed Civic Federation established relief stations and temporary lodging houses; Hull-House sheltered homeless women and children. Addams, who had been appointed to a fumbling committee of the Civic Federation to assist the masses of unemployed, resigned in disgust. She asked in dismay: "When has a committee ever dealt satisfactorily with the unemployed?" She subsequently began "the most serious economic reading" she had ever done and commenced "a decade of economic discussion" to identify the broader causes of such distress.[51]

Addams and other settlement workers discovered that the misery of the urban poor stemmed primarily from low wages, bad housing, polluted water, and inadequate health care. They knew that, despite their good intentions and their eagerness to respond to their neighbors' suffering, "public motherhood" would not solve the monumental problems of the poor. As they shifted their attention from private charity to social justice and from remedy to prevention, they looked beyond themselves to the state, viewing government as the "active, positive agency of community welfare." Addams, for one, came to believe that government fostered the good life; municipal housekeepers everywhere soon agreed with her. Not only would they initiate such operations as milk stations or kindergartens, and later give them to city hall, they would also demand more health-related services and better protection.[52]

Because they grew up in an age alert to the dangers of sewer gas and germs, settlement workers could not ignore rotting garbage and faulty drains. They lived in houses located in some of the poorest quarters of

America's cities, and they shared with working-class families filthy streets and alleys, impure water supplies, and defective (or non-existent) sewerage. They also experienced the smoke, soot, and foul odors of nearby factories and stables. Unlike the majority of their immigrant neighbors, however, settlement folks knew the perils of pollution. And to some extent they realized how difficult it would be to remove, or effectively reduce, health hazards that were "multiple and interconnected."[53]

Besides attacking the environmental threats that surrounded all of them, settlement workers wanted the urban poor to understand how cleanliness could improve and lengthen their lives. In other words, the reformers wanted their neighbors to see what they saw—the links between unsanitary conditions, repeated illnesses, and high rates of mortality. Products of their time, they shared the assumption held by many sanitary experts that uncollected garbage and poor drainage caused disease. In fact, Lillian Wald's successful Visiting Nurse Service, begun in 1893 on New York's Lower East Side, drew inspiration from the most famous sanitarian of the late nineteenth century, Florence Nightingale.[54]

Still committed to the principles that had fueled her highly publicized work during the Crimean War, Nightingale took a particular interest in district nursing during the 1890s. She liked its focus on prevention. Believing that nurses should do more than simply attend to the sick, she wanted them to teach hygiene and preventive medicine as well. She encouraged them to become "health missioners" and take their knowledge of prevention and cleanliness "to uneducated women in their own houses." Unconvinced of the merits of bacteriology, Nightingale cautioned against it. "Looking into the drains," this anti-contagionist believed, was more important.[55]

Jane Addams and the Hull-House Women's Club took this advice to heart in the summer of 1894. In an attempt to lower the death rate in Chicago's Nineteenth Ward, they investigated the work of the city's garbage collectors. But, instead of looking into drains, they checked backyards, alleys, and the huge wooden garbage boxes that were fastened to street pavements. For three nights each week during August and September, after a full day's labor, these immigrant women carried out their inspection assignments. Besides learning how to clean up their neighborhood, they found out why it was so important. As wives, mothers, and municipal housekeepers, they acted "to prevent the breeding of so-called 'filth diseases'" that endangered their families' health and lives.[56]

As a result of this two-month project, three city garbage inspectors were transferred in succession out of the ward. But that was only the beginning. After continued protests to City Hall about the inadequate collection service provided by a local contractor, Addams submitted a bid (with the support of two well-known businessmen) for the garbage removal contract of the Nineteenth Ward. The bid was thrown out on a technicality, but the mayor decided to appoint her garbage inspector for the ward at a salary of $1000 a year. She and her deputy, Amanda Johnson, stayed on the job for three years. They supervised the work of the contractor and his men, took landlords to court for not providing suitable garbage receptacles, kept their neighbors involved in a series of clean-up campaigns, and even built several small incinerators at Hull-House.[57]

Addams received a good deal of local and national attention for what she accomplished as garbage inspector. The *Chicago Times-Herald* described the radically improved appearance of specific streets and alleys, after emergency teams removed thousands of cubic yards of dirt and rubbish that the contractor had refused to handle. The *Omaha Bee* reflected on the real purpose of Addams's experiment. It was not to make life more difficult for garbage collectors, as some contractors had complained; rather it was to raise the standards of cleanliness and health for people "greatly in need of both." And in giving special attention to the sanitary conditions of the Nineteenth Ward, Addams had "rallied to her assistance every mother in it."[58]

When health department figures showed that the death rate of the Nineteenth Ward dropped from third to seventh among Chicago's wards, these mothers cheered. Their dirt-chasing had paid off.[59] The irony of their perception lay in the fact that the filth theory of disease, while scientifically out-of-date, continued to motivate clean-up efforts that *did* ameliorate some health problems. Thus, seven years later, in 1902, when the Nineteenth Ward suffered disproportionately from a typhoid epidemic, Hull-House residents undertook another investigation. This time they looked into the drains for the cause of the disaster.

From Miasmas to Microbes

The woman who headed the second Hull-House investigation looked into the drains with eyes trained from a decade's work in bacteriology and pathology. Alice Hamilton undoubtedly shared Nightingale's dedication to sanitary reform, but Hamilton's commitment to creating a healthy environment incorporated late nineteenth-century discoveries in microbiology and immunology. She earned a degree in medicine from the University of Michigan in 1893 and interned that summer at the Northwestern Hospital for Women and Children in Minneapolis. Shortly after arriving Hamilton complained to her sister that the hospital lacked a laboratory, and its microscope was not as good as her own. Even before she began advanced studies at the German universities of Leipzig and Munich and at the Johns Hopkins

Medical School in Baltimore, she prized "careful, elaborate work" over "off-hand diagnoses" of infectious diseases.[60]

Hamilton came to Chicago from Johns Hopkins in 1897 as a professor of pathology at the Woman's Medical School of Northwestern University. It was her first job. Instead of living alone or with another woman doctor, she moved into Hull-House. Life there, she later recalled, "satisfied every long-ing, for companionship, for the excitement of new experiences, for constant intellectual stimulation, and for the sense of being caught up in a big move-ment which enlisted [my] enthusiastic loyalty."[61]

Known as a "woman-of-all-work," Hamilton involved herself in a number of Hull-House activities. She visited sick children at home, taught English to Greeks and Russian Jews, and instructed Italian women in basket weav-ing. In addition to investigating the 1902 typhoid epidemic, Hamilton was especially remembered by Addams and others for the well-baby clinic she ran in the shower room of the basement gymnasium. Several mornings each week, she presided over baths and gave classes in hygiene. Here she learned that she could ease "the Italian mothers' dread of water" by anointing their babies with olive oil.[62]

In the fall of 1902 Hamilton returned from a vacation on Mackinac Island to find Chicago in the grip of another outbreak of typhoid fever. Particularly troublesome to the Hull-House neighborhood was that, with less than 3 percent of the city's population, it suffered more than 14 percent of the ca-sualties. Addams wanted to know why. "A bacteriologist ought to be able to discover the reason," she declared.[63] Hamilton figured that some local con-dition was responsible since the entire West Side drew its water from the same source. To discover the cause, two Hull-House residents made a care-ful examination of 2000 dwellings and found that only 48 percent had mod-ern plumbing, even though open privies and undrained vaults were against the law.

Hamilton suspected that flies were the culprits. Putting her theory to the test, she and her two assistants collected and tested quantities of them in the laboratory of the Memorial Institute for Infectious Diseases where she worked. Hamilton found the typhoid bacillus and believed she had discov-ered "why the slums had so much more typhoid than the well-screened and decently drained homes of the well-to-do." In January 1903 she presented her findings to the Chicago Medical Society, and a month later they were published in the *Journal of the American Medical Association*. Looking back on her career, Hamilton said she "gained more kudos from [her] paper on flies and typhoid than from any other piece of work."[64]

Her research had a very real impact on the Nineteenth Ward. With the evidence Hamilton provided, Hull-House residents lambasted the Chicago

Board of Health for failing to enforce municipal sanitary regulations. A Civil Service inquiry supported their charge, and a number of city inspectors were dismissed; five were also indicted for bribery. The mayor refused, however, to replace the health commissioner. Still, with the appointment of a new chief sanitary inspector, who forced compliance with the law, conditions around Hull-House improved.[65]

Once the hullabaloo died down, Hamilton learned to her surprise that flies "had little or nothing to do with the cases of typhoid in the Nineteenth Ward." A broken water main at the local pumping station had allowed sewage to escape into the drinking water. Contaminated water, therefore, was the real cause (although flies do carry typhoid bacteria) of the severity of the typhoid epidemic. For three days after it had begun and before the leak was detected, people living in the neighborhood drank and cooked with polluted water. Since the truth was more shocking than Hamilton's fly theory, the Board of Health did not admit it to the public. Yet 402 people in the Nineteenth Ward died of typhoid during July, August, and September 1902. And more might have done so if housewives were not fairly accustomed to boiling their water.[66]

If Jane Addams and her coworkers had any doubts that they had entered a new age as well as a new century, this incident must certainly have removed them. Although middle-class Americans had been exposed to popular versions of the germ theory since the 1880s, many of them would remain confused well into the 1920s about the best ways to prevent infectious disease. The "Age of Plumbing" had brought with it the threat of sewer gas and then germs. It had also demonstrated that lives could not be protected simply by removing dirt and debris; uncollected garbage and faulty drains were not the only health hazards. For in Chicago's Nineteenth Ward in the summer of 1902 water that had appeared clean was, in fact, unclean. Had all housewives boiled their families' water (and cooked their vegetables), there would have been fewer deaths. But even the most diligent housekeeping could not alone ensure safety against disease.[67] Thus turn-of-the-century reformers linked themselves and their health causes ever more closely to city hall *and* continued to stress the need for personal cleanliness.

When settlement workers and nurses began visiting working-class homes in the 1880s and 1890s, they had no idea that the discovery of germs would increase the value of their work. Although local governments were spending enormous sums to build and expand their public works, they gave little money to promote instruction in hygiene. In 1902, Charles V. Chapin, health commissioner of Providence, Rhode Island, said most Americans believed the filth theory of disease—that "everything decaying and offensive to the sense of smell was dangerous"; they made no distinctions "between dangerous dirt and dirt not dangerous." Early sanitarians like Nightingale or George Waring had given short shrift to personal cleanliness, preoccupied as they were with ventilation, drainage, sewer gas, and garbage. The shift from the miasma theory (and anti-contagionism) to the germ theory was not sudden or complete, but it began in the United States during the 1880s. Of that time, William Sedgwick, public-health bacteriologist of Lawrence, Massachusetts, later wrote, " 'Before 1880 we knew nothing; after 1890 we knew it all; it was a glorious ten years.' "[68]

Buoyed up by this new knowledge, Chapin sought to reverse the old anti-contagionist emphasis with a "smashing attack on the conventional theories of sanitation," first in an article in *Popular Science Monthly* and then in an address before the American Public Health Association. In both instances, he stated that the germ theory of disease enabled a new generation of sanitarians to "discriminate between filth that is dangerous and that which is not." Because germs are parasites that live in the bodies of people (or animals) and die quickly when exposed in the environment, Chapin urged municipalities to end their almost exclusive preoccupation with cleaning up the physical environment. He admitted the need for protecting water supplies since many infectious diseases were transmitted through fecal matter, but he contended that it would make "no demonstrable difference in a city's mortality whether its streets are clean or not, whether the garbage is removed promptly or allowed to accumulate, or whether it has a plumbing law."[69]

Instead Chapin encouraged Americans, especially health officials, to pay closer attention to personal cleanliness. Contagious diseases, he maintained, "spread more among filthy people just because such persons use very little soap and water and allow their faces, hands, belongings and dwellings to become and remain smeared with mucus, saliva, pus and other infectious material." Chapin also pointed out that personal cleanliness was a great deal cheaper than public cleanliness. It "cost nothing," he insisted, "to wash the hands before eating and after the toilet," while purifying water and building sewers required millions of dollars.[70]

Not all sanitarians agreed with Chapin's distinction between safe and dangerous dirt, but advocates of what came to be called the "new public health" did. And while immigrant women would probably have laughed at the assertion that it "cost nothing" to keep clean, they undoubtedly would have attested to some of its benefits. Personal cleanliness, in fact, became the new rallying cry in the twentieth century. The scientific claims of Chapin and the "new public health" converged with domestic hygiene practices of middle-class women, and together they had a profound effect on immigrant lives. Health departments and settlement houses, in particular, carried out a major assault on contagious diseases and infant mortality through formal and informal instruction in personal hygiene. Immigrant mothers, all agreed, were the key.[71]

Public health was well on its way to becoming private health. Public works services and municipal housekeeping efforts continued, of course, but a new consensus developed among sanitarians and reformers on the need for inculcating standards of germ-free cleanliness among working-class families. Immigrant women saw little value in dirt; yet they often were too poor or ignorant to protect themselves from its dangers. Unclean milk, which caused the deaths of so many of their children, was an enigma. An Italian mother in Chicago, for example, thought the babies in Italy were healthy because they drank goat's milk whereas babies in her neighborhood were sick because they drank cow's milk. She did not understand that the milk she had given her baby in Italy was "clean," but the milk she purchased at a grocery store in Chicago was "dirty." In this instance, Chapin was correct. Many cities had done "much to improve the milk supply" but had done "nothing to show the people [that is, mothers] where to get the good milk." Hence, although Chicago was the first city in the world to legislate the use of pasteurized milk in 1909, babies still died there from drinking infected milk.[72]

Advocates of the new public health never appeared as extreme as Chapin. They knew that the purification of public water and the pasteurization of urban milk were major factors in controlling epidemic diseases. Yet their focus on education in personal hygiene and on medical examination of school children and workers also produced significant results in changing popular attitudes toward disease and death early in the twentieth century. They were no longer seen as inevitable. Americans began to believe that most illnesses could be prevented or cured and that nearly all newborn babies would live.[73] Many of these modern expectations actually started with lessons in cleanliness.

But in crowded immigrant quarters, where the importance of personal hygiene was only vaguely understood, instructions in cleanliness were few and far between. This was especially true in families where mothers found New World child-rearing and housekeeping practices both perplexing and frustrating. In the view of one editorialist, most Polish mothers in Chicago did not "know how to take care of children, what to give them to eat, how and when to bathe them, and how to dress them." Yet, when shown how good hygiene habits could affect their children's welfare, immigrant women offered little resistance. Thus the challenge for those who knew that cleanliness could save lives was to carry the "findings of the scientists and laboratories to the people" in a way they could be understood.[74]

Slavic women living in American cities had a good chance of losing one baby in three. In 1910, in states that registered births and deaths, 124 infants died for every 1000 live births; and children under five accounted for a fourth of all deaths. Until 1915 the most important cause of these deaths was diarrhea and dehydration, the direct result of impure water, unclean milk, and inadequate personal hygiene. As sanitarians and settlement workers knew, a direct correlation existed between infant mortality and poverty, especially among urban immigrants. In 1913 investigators from the Children's Bureau, a federal agency created the previous year, discovered that infant deaths in Johnstown, Pennsylvania, increased by 40 percent when homes lacked running water and that a child whose father earned less than $521 annually was almost twice as likely to die as one whose father earned over $1200.[75]

Poverty was the major culprit, and its devastating effects were found everywhere. Settlement workers had first glimpsed the extent of this reality during the 1893 depression, and they saw much more in the two decades that followed. As they gathered evidence, it became clear that they needed the aid of government agencies and labor organizations to raise the standard of living of the immigrant poor. A decent living wage and improved housing could "Americanize" immigrants more quickly than any combination of outreach services and special classes. In 1909, a study of working-class families in New York City, funded by the Russell Sage Foundation, made this very point—an annual income of $1100 changed bathtubs and toilets from luxuries to necessities.[76]

This is not to say, however, that immigrant mothers did not need instruction in infant hygiene to prevent their babies from dying. The conquest of disease required the education of mothers as much as it demanded the treatment of water and sewage by public works engineers. C.-E. A. Winslow, Yale's preeminent public health educator, explained the challenge:

> Typhoid fever and malaria can often be routed on a large scale by the engineer; but infant mortality must be met and conquered in the home. The intelligence of the individual mother is the only ultimate safeguard against the perils of infancy; and it is much harder to bring education to the mothers of a community than to lead pure water into its house.

It was notoriously difficult when mothers knew little or no English and hardly ever ventured far from their homes or neighborhoods.[77]

In New York City's tenements, where infant deaths were grimly frequent in the summers between 1904 and 1908, immigrant women received advice

on home sanitation and child care—at times in the languages they spoke—
from a phalanx of local activists concerned about milk.[78] They knew that a
good supply, if improperly stored, was useless. In 1907, when the New York
City Milk Committee opened milk stations in seven immigrant neighborhoods, it not only dispensed clean milk but also provided instruction on its
care. Besides learning the dietary value of milk, mothers were shown how to
boil it, if they had any doubts about the milk's cleanliness, and how to keep
it cold and covered. Do not allow the "typhoid fly" to bathe in it, they were
warned, while taught to wash empty containers with soap and hot water.[79]

Between classes nurses visited their "students" at home to answer more
personal questions and show them practical ways to improve the care of
their children. In some instances, infants who had been fed the best milk
died because their mothers had given them indigestible foods such as pick-
les or had clothed them improperly. But under the nurses' direct supervision, most mothers and babies did exceedingly well. By 1910 New York
City's health department, through its Division of Child Hygiene, had begun
operating milk stations that also instructed mothers in personal hygiene.
The New York Milk Committee, which had demonstrated on a large scale
the need to educate immigrant mothers near and in their homes, assisted
the health department in establishing its stations and also coordinated the
work of another seventy-nine milk stations located in various Manhattan
and Brooklyn neighborhoods.[80]

Metropolitan's Health Messengers

Lillian Wald's Visiting Nurse Service, begun at the Henry Street Settlement
House on New York's Lower East Side before the shift in orientation from
public to personal cleanliness, continued to expand its health work in new
ways. As early as 1903 the settlement had started an infant welfare station,
where immigrant mothers received clean milk and lessons in hygiene. It was
still in operation and caring for over 500 babies in 1914, five years after
Wald signed an unusual contract with the Metropolitan Life Insurance
Company. In this unique partnership, Wald agreed that nurses from Henry
Street would provide home care and health instruction to Metropolitan
Life's policyholders on the West Side of New York City. In return the
nurses would receive fifty cents for each visit.[81]

The public health nurse, as a kind of community mother and health
teacher, soon became a "central figure in the modern public health campaign." Over 500 visiting-nurse organizations promoted her as "a messenger
of care, cleanliness, and character" to America's working-class population.
Wald's Henry Street nurses had certainly fostered this image as they minis-

tered to the immigrants in their neighborhood. In fact, it was through their involvement with Lower East Side Jews that Wald met Lee K. Frankel, director of United Hebrew Charities until 1909 when he became manager of Metropolitan Life's Welfare Division. He accepted this position because he was convinced that the insurance company had "joined in the battle against disease" and "hoped to lead the world in preserving lives."[82]

This was a tall but very real order for a world that had become, in Frankel's words, "health mad." Yet it was the natural result of the "startling and revolutionary" scientific discoveries of the previous twenty-five years that still remained inscrutable to many people. Nearly every American institution—the press, states and municipalities through their health departments, settlement houses and welfare organizations, schools, and even insurance companies—had been forced into the modern health campaign, "educating the great masses of the population in human life extension." Frankel believed Metropolitan agents should act more as social workers than businessmen when they entered the homes of working men and women. After all, he pointed out, Metropolitan had encouraged "long life and right living" from its beginning in 1868; and its agents and medical examiners now had scientific reasons for instructing families in "the doctrines of sanitation and hygiene."[83]

Frankel hired a young Lithuanian Jew, Louis Israel Dublin, who as a child had lived in the tenements on the Lower East Side, to help him make Metropolitan a socially responsible institution. Both men shared the concerns of New York City's settlement workers and the goals of the nation's progressives. In this context, the visiting-nurse agreement reached between Frankel and Wald appears less unusual. So too do the other phases of the major educational campaigns crafted by the Frankel-Dublin team and sponsored by Metropolitan to improve the public's health. Nevertheless, the size and impact of these joint efforts were phenomenal. What is particularly striking is the message that was delivered time and again, in old ways and new, in printed matter, and in person:

> We must learn the simple fundamental laws of health and hygiene. Foremost, WE MUST BREATHE CLEAN AIR! EAT CLEAN FOOD! DRINK CLEAN WATER! HAVE CLEAN HOMES! HAVE CLEAN BODIES! LIVE CLEAN LIVES![84]

Metropolitan looked upon its policyholders as children in need of instruction and protection. Beginning in 1909 with the creation of its Welfare Division, "Mother Met," as its employees affectionately called the company, stood ready to use either tried-and-true methods or innovative strategies against such killers as typhoid fever, infant diarrhea, and tuberculosis. Its motives were not, of course, completely unselfish; it knew that in reducing mortality rates it could also increase profits and enhance its image. Thus, when the Henry Street nurses successfully "demonstrated in a practical, visible way the responsibility which Mother Met feels toward her children," the company extended the nursing service throughout Manhattan and to other major cities.[85]

Frankel's Welfare Division launched its premier educational campaign in 1909 with *A War Upon Consumption*, an illustrated pamphlet explaining the causes of tuberculosis and how it might be prevented. Since the "white plague" was responsible for 17 percent of the deaths of the company's policyholders, the pamphlet showed its readers exactly how "the germs of consumption" were carried from the sick to the well. It singled out the germs' allies—dirt, dampness, and darkness—as enemies to be fought with cleanliness, pure air, and sunshine. Within a few years, company agents, visiting nurses, physicians, branches of the Young Men's Christian Association, and public and private health organizations had distributed twelve million copies in twelve languages. In 1913 and 1914, as a continuation of its crusade to educate policyholders in disease prevention and personal hygiene, Metropolitan placed twenty million disposable drinking cups on the cars of several railroad lines. The following year it gave away thousands of fly swatters to promote "Clean Homes, Pure Food, Clean Milk, No Flies, and No Mosquitos."[86]

Since so many of Metropolitan's policyholders were foreign born or of foreign parentage, the company approached them "along special lines." It was one of the first to recognize the value of selling products—whether insurance or cleanliness—through the potential buyers' language. Most of its health publications, especially those on the care of infants, were printed in German, Italian, French, Spanish, Polish, and Yiddish. As early as 1910 it placed ads in *Yiddishes Tageblatt*, explaining its interest in helping working families. The Borden Milk Company, which had a Baby Welfare Department in the 1920s, also approached immigrants about life-and-death matters in this way. Both knew from the experiences of settlement workers and visiting nurses the importance of involving foreign-language speakers in their cause.[87]

Metropolitan's health pamphlets and its innovative advertising were unusually successful, but company agents—or "health messengers," as Frankel liked to call them—deserved the greatest credit for carrying personal hygiene education into the home. Not surprisingly, a good many of these agents spoke foreign languages, coming as they often did from the same immigrant communities they targeted. In the 1890s, only a third of the agents canvassing households were born in the United States, and some of them were from immigrant families. Of the total, 24 percent came from Germany and 12 percent from England; the remainder were from English Canada, French Canada, Ireland, Italy, Bohemia, Russia, Austria, and Hungary. They were carefully selected, but none had any formal education beyond grade school. Most of them had previously been employed as skilled artisans, sales clerks, or industrial workers.[88]

It is not easy to know how families received these agents when they came calling. They represented, at one and the same time, many of the progressive reform groups of the early twentieth century as well as the new ethnic middle class. Since large numbers of immigrants invested in insurance premiums (chiefly death benefits because few could afford more) and believed in buying from their own, it seems safe to assume that Metropolitan agents were welcomed on their weekly rounds. As regular daytime visitors, they usually dealt with housewives and mothers who took responsibility for making the payments and who placed great value on their investment. The relationship between these health messengers and immigrant women was close, according to Frankel, since they met "not only when joy is in the home, but when sorrow and death enter there." For this reason he always believed Metropolitan agents provided "a knowledge of the laws and rules of sanitation and hygiene which [could] not be obtained in any other way."[89]

Americanizing the Immigrant Home

There were other ways, besides Metropolitan's way, to help immigrant women understand American standards of cleanliness and make the difficult adjustment to city life. Basic housekeeping classes offered in homes or neighborhood centers proved popular among housewives weak in English. Settlement workers and nurses, functioning as educators rather than inspectors, offered the most successful programs; they, unlike many representatives of women's clubs, tended to appreciate the difficulties under which immigrants labored and to know the kind of changes they would accept. For instance, most settlement folks saw no reason for concern about "the use of black bread instead of white, or in the wearing of a shawl instead of a hat." But in matters of personal and domestic hygiene, particularly when a family's health seemed in jeopardy, they gave straightforward advice, often in the form of demonstrations.[90]

Annie L. Hansen worked in Buffalo as a public health nurse and "domestic educator" for the North American Civic League for Immigrants. Beginning in 1911, for a two-year period, she visited Polish, Italian, and Hungarian homes to teach housewives the rudiments of household sanitation and personal cleanliness. She soon discovered that, since most of the women had come from rural villages, they found "modern methods of sanitation" as foreign as the English language. Day after day, Hansen showed them, among other things, how to bathe and feed their infants, what to do with potato peelings, where to dispose of floor sweepings, and when to wash their children's hair. She found her work onerous only when faced with the attitude, held by a few of different nationalities, that "cleanliness is a condition only for the rich."[91]

In 1915, after the California legislature passed a law permitting local boards of education to employ "domestic educators," immigrant mothers throughout the state began learning "the rules of health, sanitation, and hygiene" at home. They also received advice on buying food and clothing, becoming citizens, and understanding American customs and laws. "Home teachers," as their instructors came to be called, exerted "a direct Americanizing influence" not only by raising cleanliness standards but also by speaking English whenever possible, observing public holidays with patriotic souvenirs and songs, explaining school regulations and traditions, and involving mothers in their children's activities. From the prewar years through the 1920s, Americanizers encouraged immigrant mothers "to maintain the new American standard of living in diet, hygiene, and infant and child care" by promising them they would make their children *true* Americans.[92]

Settlement workers frequently established housekeeping centers, giving immigrants "a home to copy." They transformed ordinary flats into "model" tenements and taught groups of mothers (and often daughters) how to live as Americans. In Boston the Women's Municipal League paid the rent on a three-room flat where workers from the South End House gave advice, for example, on how to deal with landlords in securing adequate garbage receptacles, more light, and better plumbing. While these lessons did not always yield results, tenants learned they had rights. Esther G. Barrows, who lived more than twenty years at South End House, recalled that four months after their center opened property owners in the neighborhood began repair or remodeling work in five apartment buildings.[93]

In New York City Wald and her close friend Mabel Hyde Kittredge wanted their Lower East Side neighbors to know "the art of healthful housekeeping." To make tuberculosis less threatening and American ways less intimidating, they opened "The Flat" at the Henry Street Settlement. There they taught women and girls how "to make tenement life more healthy and . . . cleaner and prettier." Like their colleagues in Boston, Wald and Kittredge explained to those who came for instruction that they need not accept leaks in ceilings, falling plaster, and dirty toilets that did not work.[94]

Because "The Flat" succeeded, Kittredge started other model tenements, organized the Association of Practical Housekeeping Centers, and published a textbook in 1911. In it she described in detail "how to furnish and keep house in a tenement flat." She recommended painted (not papered) walls in light colors, uncluttered surfaces, floors without carpets, shelves and window seats for storage, un-upholstered chairs, iron bed frames, and only a few pictures on parlor walls. Kittredge and her followers believed this simplicity would lead to cleanliness. In case it did not, she gave explicit directions on how each room (and the objects in it) should be cleaned. She also included recipes for cleaning solutions.[95]

How much of this advice immigrant women took to heart is difficult to know. If beauty is in the eye of the beholder, American middle-class reformers and newcomers from southern and eastern Europe probably had very different opinions about what was beautiful. Recent arrivals generally measured their success in America against an old-country standard of gentility and nobility. When they purchased clothes or furnishings for their homes, Italians, Slavs, Poles, and others alike had their native lands in mind. Once they had a parlor, for instance, they often filled it with a piano. For Jews from Germany and Austria, where parlors of only the bourgeoisie had pianos, it signified their realized aspirations.[96]

Kittredge and her friends would probably not have advised placing a large piano in a small parlor. Nor, for that matter, did they approve of the vivid blue walls and red carpets found in many tenement flats; and they especially disliked the dust-gathering stuffed furniture, feather beds, heavy carpets, long lace curtains, and draped mantles that distinguished immigrant homes (and, for that matter, many Victorian American ones). Simple, mission-style or early American furniture seemed so much more appropriate to them, and certainly more conducive to cleanliness. But, to European immigrants who wanted their couches and sideboards to have "heft, color, and strong lines," that kind of furniture lacked substance and status. After all, as Mary Antin observed, her family had "achieved" a red carpet in their parlor! Bright colors on the floors and walls indicated a new level of prosperity and offered some relief to the monotony of their daily lives.[97]

The bric-a-brac and wall hangings of new immigrants, most of whom were either Catholic or Jewish, also reflected their European backgrounds and tastes. Catholics especially displayed religious objects—statues, crucifixes, blessed candles, and holy cards—throughout their homes; they often hung small holy water fonts near doorways and wrapped palms distributed on Palm Sunday around crucifixes. Well into the twentieth century, there could be found a representation of the Sacred Heart of Jesus in the best room of almost every Catholic house. Multi-color calendars with pictures of the Pope and St. Peter's in Rome that listed feast and fast days along with Holy Days of Obligation also graced the walls of immigrant flats. In observant Jewish quarters, parents sometimes displayed prints of rabbinical figures; far more common were photographs of loved ones left behind in the Old World and brightly colored *yahrzeit* (birthday) plaques. Richly illustrated calendars from local merchants and clippings from Sunday newspapers also found their place on tenement walls.[98]

These foreign ways prompted expert housekeepers to insist that the furniture and ornamentation cherished by immigrants made cleanliness nearly impossible. "A place for everything, and everything in its place" had been a shibboleth of domestic educators since before the Civil War when Catharine Beecher first began giving household advice. But, as Anzia Yezierska countered in one of her novels, the rule was "no good" for immigrants because "there weren't enough places." Nor were there enough sinks, bathrooms, running water, or electricity. Only after 1900, when new tenement house laws started to require a separate water closet in every new apartment, did American reformers see genuine improvement in the cleanliness of immigrant homes and belongings. Builders began installing bathtubs as well as toilets and gave newcomers their first real chance to "convert" to the gospel of cleanliness.[99]

In most cities, however, years passed before immigrant communities benefited from adequately plumbed housing. Although new dwellings had been critically needed since the 1880s, contractors and realtors responded first to the suburban demands of the more prosperous middle class. And landlords, who profited from overcrowding in poorly maintained apartments and cottages, resisted initiating any major household improvements until forced to do so. In the meantime, immigrants did the best they could. They shared privies and hall toilets, carried water from the closest supply, tried to keep a healthy and orderly home, and from time to time protested the filthy conditions under which they had to live. Some took advantage of public baths built in America's largest cities at the turn of the century; but southern and eastern Europeans, who were unaccustomed to bathing year-round, showed no great enthusiasm for them, except on hot summer days. A few reformers had believed that these baths would ensure cleanliness among the urban poor, but private bathrooms eventually made them obsolete.[100]

America's immigrants—regardless of nationality, gender, or generation—longed to escape miserable housing and live in places with running water, electricity, and private bathrooms. Yezierska, who knew the disabling and degrading effects of "deadening dirt," explained the delight that accompanied a bathroom of one's own:

Bathtub, washbowl, and toilet. My own. . . . How could I desecrate the cleanliness of that tub with my dirty body? I thought of the hours I had to stand in line at the public bathhouse before Passover and the New Year—and the greasy tub smelling of the sweat of the crowd. The iron sink in the hall on Hester Street. One faucet for eight families. Here were two faucets. Hot water, cold water, all the water in the world. I turned on both faucets and let them run for the sheer joy of it.[101]

In search of better plumbing, first-generation immigrants were often nomads, willing to move from one apartment to another for the sake of stationary tubs. It was not unusual, in fact, for a family to begin in a cold-water flat, then move to one with running hot water; from there, the same family might soon move again to an apartment that had a toilet exclusively for its use, followed by a third one that had a bathtub and a toilet. In the end, they generally settled in new neighborhoods where they bought homes of their own, equipped with modern conveniences.[102]

African-Americans, Cleanliness, and the Great Migration

Ironically, the "American way" of cleanliness was also pressed upon a group of Americans whose ancestors had almost all arrived here before 1808, when the international slave trade officially ended. African-Americans are the oldest Americans except for Indians and the descendants of a handful of Europeans. But seniority counted for nothing where poverty ruled. Rural blacks moving to northern cities got the soap-and-water message not only from white society but also from the small African-American middle class, who preached Washington's "gospel of the toothbrush" and related admonitions.

From black slums, where housing conditions were deplorable, there were few opportunities to escape. Immigrants may have been poor, but they were white; better jobs with better pay enabled them to move to better neighborhoods. For immigrants, the slums became bearable with the knowledge that they could improve their lives if they worked hard. But African-Americans, also burdened by extreme poverty, knew their skin color prohibited their mobility and restricted them to ghettos. In Chicago, to which over 50,000 black Southerners migrated between 1916 and 1919, their ghetto was known as the Black Belt, virtually "a city within a city."[103]

Chicago's black ghetto did not result from the Great Migration during and after World War I. The color line had been drawn a good deal earlier. By 1900 several colonies of residential areas had already become linked to form a long, narrow Black Belt that housed 30,000 people on the city's

South Side. In 1930, when the African-American population increased to about 250,000, the ghetto was still intact, only five times larger. Yet African-American families had even less chance of living outside it. No eastern and southern European immigrant group experienced anything comparable to the racial segregation and discrimination that plagued all blacks.[104]

Chicago's settlement workers recognized this fact. Jane Addams and her Hull-House associates were especially sympathetic; others were not. All, however, accepted the color line. Even reformers like Addams, who admitted that the slavery and subsequent segregation experienced by African-Americans were far worse than the dislocations and exploitation suffered by immigrants, failed to treat poor southern blacks as they did other migrant groups. But Addams and her friends were often as realistic as they were idealistic; their goal was racial tolerance, not equality. As a result black settlement houses, often with white as well as black sponsors, opened their doors to those in need. Poorly financed and equipped, these separate but hardly equal settlements could only make a stab at ameliorating the horrendous living and working conditions of the thousands of African-Americans who poured into the city in search of jobs following the outbreak of World War I.[105]

Although southern blacks moved in great numbers to New York and Detroit, their mecca was Chicago. The Illinois Central Railroad made it easy for anyone in the Deep South to reach what appeared to be the promised land. And the Chicago *Defender*, the most popular newspaper among southern blacks, invited its readers to hop a train by telling them about job opportunities and showing them how prosperous and influential Chicago's African-American community had become. Pullman porters and dining-car waiters, individuals held in especially high esteem, confirmed these images of Chicago as they traveled through the South; they not only spoke proudly of their home town, but they also faithfully distributed copies of the *Defender* to their southern friends and relatives. Without doubt, they bore some responsibility for creating the momentum of the Great Migration and for making the *Defender* the largest-selling African-American newspaper in the United States by World War I.[106]

The individual most responsible for these events was Robert S. Abbott. A graduate of Hampton Institute and friend of Booker T. Washington, Abbott founded the Chicago *Defender* in 1905. He believed in Washington's philosophy of individual achievement, but Abbott was not an accommodationist. He knew the minds of his readers and catered to them by publishing news they could understand and appreciate. His outspokenness against discrimination, his virulent anti-South attitudes, and the bold coverage he gave lynchings and other violent racial incidents accounted for the newspaper's amazing success.[107] Yet the *Defender* reflected Washington's notions of self-

help too. Frequent editorials on manners and morals accompanied by Dr.
A. Wilberforce Williams's weekly columns on health and hygiene were rem-
iniscent of advice given to African-Americans in the pages of the *Southern
Workman*.

Williams, a physician at Provident Hospital, began his "Keep Healthy"
column in 1913 before the wartime arrival of black migrants. But his regular
and oftentimes repetitious exhortations on cleanliness, bathing, tuberculosis, sanitary homes, spring cleaning, and summer hygiene took on additional
significance as these newcomers struggled to make homes for themselves in
Chicago's black neighborhoods.[108] On the South and West sides, long neglected by the city, they found filthy, dilapidated apartments and shacks.
Most of them were crowded on lots surrounded by unpaved streets and alleys clogged with heaps of rubbish and rotting garbage; toilet facilities were
scarce or in need of repair. And, despite these frightful conditions, rents
were notoriously high. In fact, in some cases, rents doubled after African-
American families moved into buildings previously occupied by whites.[109]

Like the immigrants before them, black Southerners were innocent of
city ways. They knew very little about "sanitation, ventilation, filtered water,
the effects of overcrowding, or the use of the bath tub." Thus it is hardly
surprising that tuberculosis, a disease of poor people, fell particularly hard
on them; from 1914 to 1926 Chicago's African-Americans died from tuberculosis at a rate six times greater than that of whites. In his columns
Williams, an active member of the National Association for the Study and
Prevention of Tuberculosis, hammered away at the importance of cleanliness in combating this disease. The Chicago Urban League initiated health
campaigns and funded an array of social services, hoping to halt its spread.
The exclusion of African-American tuberculars from sanitoriums (the best
treatment then known) shamefully perpetuated the higher rates among this
group. In 1926, when Chicago boasted that it had the lowest death rate of
any city of a million or more people, black mortality was still more than
twice that of whites. Confined to their ghettos, where they remained ill-
housed and ill-fed, they continued to suffer and die at disproportionate
rates a decade later.[110]

As living conditions worsened, the African-American middle-class, the
Urban League, and the Chicago *Defender* placed the burden of improvement on the migrants' backs. In the spirit of Washington and "the gospel of
the toothbrush," middle-class African-Americans advised these poor Southerners to become industrious, thrifty, disciplined, and clean. Embarrassed
by their backward ways and afraid that "the Race" would be discredited by
their slovenliness, established blacks told newcomers "to emulate the 'Gold
Dust Twins' and make the dirt fly." Urban League volunteers passed out

leaflets and made door-to-door visits, counseling migrants on their duties as American citizens—"cleanliness, sobriety, thrift, efficiency, and respectable, restrained behavior in public places." The *Defender*, which had promoted migration, now expected the newcomers to adopt "modern methods of sanitation"; to prevent unnecessary illness and hostile comments against "members of the Race," the newspaper urged them to use water freely.[111]

The message was the same in other cities where southern African-Americans moved in great numbers. The St. Louis Urban League instructed them to "use the toothbrush, the hairbrush and comb, and soap and water freely." "Habits of dress and behavior," which may have been appropriate in small towns, were "perniciously conspicuous in a community like Detroit," according to its Urban League. As in Chicago, Detroit's migrants were advised not to "crowd inside of a street car filled with people in your dirty, greasy overalls"; instead they were encouraged to follow the lead of the much admired Pullman porter. His face may have been "as black as ebony" but his soul and body were "as white as snow."[112] Immaculate, disciplined, and deferential, he epitomized what Washington and the black middle-class hoped their southern brothers and sisters might become.

The attitudes of middle-class African-Americans mirrored those of many prosperous German Jews in New York City in the late nineteenth century. They had viewed the influx of eastern European Jews as a threat to their "hard-won respectability" and shunned them until they were "civilized" by reformers like Minnie Louis, founder of the Louis Downtown Sabbath School in 1880. Its purpose was none other than "to inculcate habits of cleanliness" among Lower East Side Jewish immigrants who, Louis believed, were ignorant of "the cleansing properties of water."[113] For immigrants and blacks alike, cleanliness had deep cultural and social significance; it signaled an early step in the process of assimilation and acceptance. For African-Americans, however, integration proved to be only a mirage. Once they removed their dirt, whites found it nearly impossible to forgive them their color.

Until the recent resurgence of tuberculosis, Americans have had little reason to fear contagious diseases and have largely forgotten that cleanliness is necessary for survival in urban areas. Before the turn of the twentieth century, Booker T. Washington had admonished African-Americans that cleanliness was necessary for their acceptance, and in the 1910s the Chicago *Defender* and branches of the National Urban League carried this message to thousands of African-American migrants. Settlement workers and sanitarians "Americanized" European immigrants in similar fashion, inculcating middle-class values as well as trying to improve living conditions—all of this taking place between Booker's boyhood during Reconstruction and the early years of the Great Migration, and from the enormous influx of immigrants in the 1880s through the pioneering days of the settlement houses. By 1910, Americanizers, one and all, had succeeded in making cleanliness a hallmark of being American.

Behind all of this work, in what now appears to have been "a golden age for public health," were varying degrees of knowledge that, without cleanliness, rural folk moving to cities became the easy victims of disease and death.[114] For this reason, more than any other, health and hygiene programs were introduced into schools and workplaces nationwide. State and local health departments, already committed to promulgating habits of personal cleanliness, would guide them and witness incomparable advances. Settlement-house and other private initiatives with immigrants and African-Americans continued. But the new story after 1910 was that efforts to promote cleanliness were no longer limited to the personal, not to say amateur, but became institutionalized and bureaucratized.

CHAPTER FIVE

Persuading the Masses

Our job is bringing cleanliness into a dirty world.
—LEVER BROTHERS EXECUTIVE, 1940[1]

Education and Business Team Up

After 1910 reformers did not stop chasing dirt, nor did public health threats
become mere memories. In this pre-sulfa, pre-antibiotic age, when tuberculosis, diphtheria, typhoid, and polio remained real killers, campaigns to
destroy deadly germs did not simply replace efforts to do away with stinking
dirt; instead they supplemented them. In the 1910s and 1920s, the critical
arenas of public health and cleanliness activity centered in *education*—not
only by schools but also by organized philanthropy and boards of health—
and in *business*—both in the workplace and through advertising. By the
early 1930s, the twin arms of education and business had used their mighty
influence to turn cleanliness into a cultural value. Keeping clean was not
only healthy; it was patriotic, success-driven, and very American. And it had
the overwhelming support of physicians and sanitarians, school teachers and
nurses, parents, state and local officialdom, philanthropists, and, most pow-
erfully of all, corporate America.

From Settlement House to School

Throughout the nineteenth century Americans continued to believe that
mothers played the most important role in teaching national ideals to their
children. But a question arose concerning mothers who were foreign and
unfamiliar with American standards and customs. In the eyes of many middle-class reformers, educators, and employers, immigrant mothers made up

"a reactionary force" of Old World ways, which threatened the nation's physical and moral health. As a result the public schools took on new significance, and by 1920 "if you ask[ed] ten immigrants who [had] been in America long enough to rear families what American institution is most effective in making the immigrant part and parcel of American life, nine [would] reply 'the public school.' "[2]

In school as well as at home, child training remained largely in women's hands. In one-room schoolhouses and in large city buildings, teachers tended to be young, single, native-born women, who were respectable representatives of the communities in which they worked. They instructed their pupils in the three Rs, disciplined them, and built character; in fact, with the massive immigration of southern and eastern Europeans in the 1880s and 1890s, teachers and superintendents (who were usually men) began to place more emphasis on "character." Educating for citizenship in a new industrial America became equally as important as teaching the rudiments.[3]

Settlement workers, who recognized their own limitations in meeting the social needs of their immigrant neighbors, encouraged the public school to enlarge its function and develop the "whole child." Learning English was only the beginning. Immigrant children needed so much more, often more than their homes could give them: daily, practical instruction on how to keep clean and stay healthy; manual training to learn skills and help them find jobs; and group recreation where they could meet friends for dancing, swimming, and competitive sports. Neighborhood organizations and immigrant-run societies occasionally sponsored these kinds of activities, but settlement folks believed the public school should lead the way. It belonged to everybody as nothing else did or could. "The common school is common ground . . . ," according to Graham Taylor of the Chicago Commons Settlement, "that little patch of Mother Earth which belongs to all of us."[4]

The persuasion and pressure exerted by settlement houses changed many schools into neighborhood centers. Julia Richman, the district superintendent of New York City's Lower East Side schools from 1903 to 1912, admitted that when she was a principal her school was different because it was "inspired by settlement work." Schools that were "different" opened kindergartens for slum children, introduced courses in domestic science and mechanical arts, offered free medical examinations, built public baths, and invited adults to evening English and citizenship classes. Jane Addams praised such schools for their effectiveness as "Americanizing agencies"—for connecting entire households to American habits and customs.[5]

Immigrant children *and* their mothers learned a good deal about cleanliness in kindergartens. They provided the "earliest opportunity to catch the little Russian, the little Italian, the little German, Pole, Syrian and the rest and begin to make good American citizens of them." Often the children were "mere babies" and had "everything to learn," but usually they were youngsters who had previously played in the streets, since they were too young to go to school or work. While they attended kindergarten, their mothers sometimes went to classes on child care and housekeeping; more frequently they received "home visits" and learned how to bathe their babies and dispose of troublesome garbage, where to get clean milk and underwear, and the dangers of flies and mosquitoes, broken glass, and rusty nails. Sons and daughters also brought home instructions in cleanliness. One German mother in Chicago, for example, reported good-naturedly that her four-year-old son made her "wipe up kvick anything what I shpill!"[6]

Pupils took their cleanliness lessons to heart. They did not always understand their hygienic value, but they wanted to avoid embarrassing or humiliating incidents. Two Jewish girls, who had used rags for handkerchiefs, immediately got rid of them when a teacher said they were disgusting. They feared being called to her desk, given a clean handkerchief, and forced to blow their noses in front of their classmates. A Polish student in the Bronx was mortified the day she was called to her brother's classroom. There, for all to see, the teacher pulled at her brother's collar and showed her "a broad band of dirt that began at a sharp edge just below his clean jaws." Promptly dismissed with "See that he washes better," she left ashamed and angry at her brother.[7]

One immigrant, reflecting on his school days, remembered the routine clearly. Early in the day, the teacher would "inspect our hair, turn our hands around, look at our ears, examine my neck to see if it was dirty"; later on, the school nurse would "come and look at [our] hair, with two little wooden sticks" and examine throats with wooden tongue depressors. She referred students with symptoms of diphtheria to the medical inspector, and she sent those with lice home for a delousing—a responsibility that school administrators and medical inspectors generally believed belonged to mothers. In some places, health centers regularly sponsored demonstrations "in head cleaning" for mothers and their oldest daughters.[8]

School nurses almost always found other health problems while checking for the most prevalent contagious diseases. Decayed teeth proved an especially conspicuous and serious one. Most immigrant children had never used a toothbrush. They did not know why their teeth—or their siblings' teeth—were discolored or loose; nor did they understand why their teeth sometimes ached or how they contributed to nose, throat, and ear disorders. Yet these children never failed to notice when their "dirty, ugly" teeth set them apart from classmates with "shining white ones."[9]

Americans, young and old, would in time be recognized worldwide for teeth that "always seem to have been furiously brushed not more than an hour ago." Although they had not yet achieved this distinction at the turn of the century, middle-class Americans and their children had begun to appropriate the details of personal cleanliness. For reasons of "standing" as well as health, it was considered as "inexcusable" to ignore one's teeth as it was "to go with uncut and dirty finger-nails, or to appear in public with facial and manual blemishes of dirt and neglect." As schoolchildren learned the basics of oral hygiene through school programs or ones sponsored by dental societies, children's aid organizations, and local clinics, entire families began using toothbrushes and toothpowders as readily as they had substituted handkerchiefs and towels for rags. A few people even went so far as to have all of their decayed or crooked teeth pulled and replaced with "a set of good false teeth."[10]

The unsanitary conditions of school buildings disturbed school and health officials as much as the sight of unclean children. This concern, while not new, was exacerbated by the burgeoning foreign population and its eagerness for free education. Nearly all the schools in immigrant neighborhoods were crowded, filthy, and poorly ventilated—perfectly suited for the spread of contagious diseases. Indeed too many of these old buildings, all in need of better classroom furniture and toilet facilities, remained in use far too long. Pre-1900 schools, which were often without bathrooms or lunchrooms, remained the lot of African-American children in Chicago well into the 1920s. But the schools they left behind in the rural South were worse.[11]

By 1900 a national movement to improve school buildings, started in large cities, resulted in the passage of basic sanitary codes in most states, including southern ones. In urban schools water closets and urinals gradually replaced privies; and, since most tenement homes lacked showers or bathtubs, public facilities (usually showers) were often installed. Jane Addams reported in 1892 that the whole Italian neighborhood adjacent to Hull-House possessed only three bathtubs. Not surprisingly, she and her associates supported Chicago's Municipal Order League in establishing a system of public baths. They also encouraged Lucy Flower, their friend on the Chicago Board of Education from 1891 to 1894, in her successful attempt to introduce showers into local schools. Cleanliness, which they believed *preceded* godliness, also promoted health, decency, and self-respect.[12]

In parochial schools cleanliness tended to occupy a place *next* to godliness. The schools themselves, which frequently began in the basements of Catholic churches, were as ill-equipped and crowded as public schools. But the religious women who staffed parochial schools were "free to create a discipline and an order unknown in most nineteenth century schools" because they had dedicated their lives to service and were willing to work for subsistence wages. Nuns used textbooks that emphasized the same social values taught in public schools—obedience, diligence, thrift, patriotism, piety, honesty, and cleanliness. They also gave students explicit instructions on how to wash their hands and clean their nails; those who refused to comply were sent to bathrooms "where there [was] no heat and the water [was] cold." Nuns (often Irish themselves), who provided a "wide range of services for Irish women in the large Catholic cities," helped poor mothers "to have the children regular in their attendance at school, neatly dressed, with their clothes mended and all marks of degrading poverty removed."[13]

The rising nationalism of the 1890s encouraged farm communities to give some much-needed attention to the appearance of their schools too. Besides cleaning up yards and purchasing flags and flagpoles, they began supplying toiletries since few families could afford such niceties, or enough of them. In 1893 a Kansas girl wrote that at her school, "We have a mirror, comb, towels, and a washbasin." And for good reason. There was "scarcely a sounder principle of pedagogy," according to a committee studying rural education in Wisconsin, "than that care begets care; order, order; cleanliness, cleanliness; and beauty, beauty."[14]

Teachers, who inherited the problem of how to promote cleanliness, devised their own techniques or tried ones recently learned in the new normal schools. A Kansas teacher made her pupils aware of one of their deficiencies by writing "dirty hands" on the blackboard, while another simply washed her hands and cleaned her nails in front of a class. In Delaware County, Iowa, Sarah Gillespie Huftalen was more direct with her students—she "compelled them to be clean at the price of eternal vigilance"; she also made boys who soiled toilet seats wash them. Farther west, in Mitchell, South Dakota, the Presentation Sisters at Holy Family School sent home children who were not clean.[15]

Most rural schools were little more than frame or log structures that occasionally had a privy or, in rare cases, two at the corner of the school yard. The single-room building, which housed the educational activities of farm children of all ages, ordinarily had several windows on each side, a door at the back, and a wood- or coal-burning stove. Before rural schools began consolidating after World War II, teachers generally did the housekeeping chores and repair work that were later assigned to janitors. But responsibility for the upkeep of outhouses rested with those who used them. Thus they usually appeared uninviting and once in a while even seemed dangerous. In some parts of the country, mud wasps nested in their corners, and, almost everywhere, pranksters threatened to tip them over or secure their doors.[16]

Nonetheless, despite all of these shortcomings, education became "the keystone of the modern campaign for public health" in the twentieth century. Its proponents—many of whom were classroom teachers—stressed that schoolchildren had power over their health, without denying the hazards of untreated sewage, stagnant water, or unsanitary privies. They merely shifted the balance from public cleanliness to personal hygiene. Laboratory tests had clearly demonstrated that communicable infections resulted more or less directly from "the passage of fresh germs from person to person." Consequently, scientific medicine in the 1910s and 1920s concerned itself as much with changing behavior as with epidemiology, while school and health officials conducted the actual campaigns. The crusade against tuberculosis, with its focus on personal hygiene, would reflect the emphasis on strengthening individuals to ward off contagious diseases.[17]

This "new public health" was a change in accent then, not an abrupt reversal. Laggard cities continued to install sewerage and water purification plants, for instance. But as society increasingly demanded a work force with white-collar skills, the public schools became the principal and most accepted agency for educating, socializing, and sanitizing the young. Elementary-school texts in hygiene and biology shifted in content from 65 percent anatomy and physiology in the 1890s to 5 percent in 1925, while discussions of sanitation and health rules rose from 4 percent to 40 percent. High-school biology courses in New York City taught "upwardly mobile, immigrant Manhattan boys between the ages of thirteen and sixteen . . . what to consider clean and precious or dirty and dispensable"; students learned from their textbooks how sewer and water systems got built and why clean tableware and thorough disposal of manure and garbage were important. Enrollments in home economics rose from under 4 percent of public high-school students in 1910 to 17 percent in 1928, and in physical education (inevitably including aspects of personal hygiene) from nothing before 1922 to over 50 percent in 1934.[18]

School and health reformers went to great lengths to keep the children in their custody well, especially youngsters whose lives were threatened daily by poverty and contagion. However, educators also felt obligated to socialize and integrate millions of poor, immigrant children into American society. The majority of native-born principals and teachers were proud of their middle-class values (as were most second-generation teachers) and convinced that education could convert foreigners into American citizens; therefore, their rhetoric mixed elements of hope and fear as they sought equality of opportunity as well as conformity for their students. Teachers tended to believe—and probably correctly—that "in an opportunity structure dominated by WASPS the immigrant youth would find success easier with an Anglicized name, 'correct' speech, a scrubbed face, and well-starched collar." In 1922 an Italian eighth-grader in Chicago said he intended to go on to high school because he wanted "an office job" where he could be "clean and not digging in the dirt and building sewers." He knew, as did others, that an education and cleanliness brought white-collar status.[19]

Philanthropy Changes the South

School conditions in the rural South created health problems that inhibited learning. In fact, a health official remarked that "hardly one" of the school-houses built in the nineteenth century was "so constructed as not to seriously impair the physical constitution of the children" who attended them. African-American youngsters, often prohibited from going to even these miserable schools, stayed home where they played unsupervised or helped their parents. But this situation began to change in 1904, when Anna T. Jeanes, a Quaker philanthropist from Philadelphia, made the first of several sizable contributions to improve black schools. In 1907 she created the Negro Rural School Fund, also known as the Anna T. Jeanes Foundation, with a million-dollar donation.[20]

The predominantly rural South, which was nearly one-third black in 1910, trailed behind the public health and school reform movements of the rest of the country. Although African-American communities existed in the North, 90 percent of the nation's blacks still lived in the South before World War I. They had emerged from slavery with a desire to become literate and had welcomed assistance from the Freedmen's Bureau, northern missionaries, and graduates from Hampton and Tuskegee. Despite their training programs and good intentions, however, African-Americans continued to suffer disenfranchisement and discrimination. Southern whites opposed universal public education and regularly distributed local funds more generously to white schools than to black ones.[21]

As a result of the Jeanes Fund (and money from the Julius Rosenwald Fund, established in 1914), African-Americans and their country schools benefited from the supervision and dedication of a long line of "Jeanes teachers." Perhaps the most notable of these was Virginia Estelle Randolph, a black teacher in Henrico County, Virginia, who transformed a dilapidated, "little wayside school" into a "model progressive rural school." In so doing, she caught the attention of the county schools' superintendent, who appointed her the first Jeanes teacher supervisor of the rural African-American schools of Henrico County.[22]

Randolph and other Jeanes teachers, almost all of whom were African-American women, succeeded because they responded to the urgent needs of their elementary school pupils. Besides fund-raising campaigns and attempts at modernizing school facilities, they emphasized the importance of hygiene. "It must be impressed upon the minds of the pupils," Randolph wrote in her first annual report in 1909, "that 'Cleanliness is next to Godliness,' and when this law of Hygiene is obeyed, they have conquered a great giant." Jeanes teachers taught Henrico County's youngsters how to make their environs "neat and clean" and explained again and again why they had to know the contents of "a book on the 'Laws of Health' " that hung in their classrooms.[23]

The Jeanes teachers had considerable influence in African-American communities during the early twentieth century. Besides improving school attendance and instruction, they also "fostered habits of personal cleanliness" mainly through demonstrations on health and hygiene.[24] Their notable efforts to change the sanitary practices of African-American Southerners were complemented by another million-dollar philanthropic undertaking aimed largely at poor whites. In 1909 the Rockefeller Foundation announced the formation of the Sanitary Commission for the Eradication of Hookworm.

During the following year, nine states invited the new commission to the South to support their educational work against hookworm, or, as it was commonly known, the "germ of laziness." Hookworm was a riveting target; a problem of both physical and mental health, of both private and public sanitary practice, it required education as well as treatment. And the fight against it succeeded, becoming a model for later public health campaigns. Contracted in many cases by walking barefooted over ground contaminated by animal or human wastes, hookworm's victims, physically underdeveloped and mentally dull, were "despised by others as lazy, shiftless, indolent, untrustworthy good-for-nothings." However, state health officials and the Sanitary Commissioners regarded these poor folks as primarily *unsanitary* and, besides medical treatment, prescribed what they judged even more important—instruction in hygiene and sanitation. In short, they placed their faith in the "gospel of the sanitary privy" to halt the spread of hookworm and other contagious diseases such as typhoid and malaria. Privies, at least, could confine waterborne infections.[25]

The name "Sanitary Commission" had historical significance for these Progressive-era health reformers. They knew the legendary "cleansing" successes of Florence Nightingale and the British Sanitary Commission during the Crimean War; they also held in high regard the achievements of the United States Sanitary Commission, which had emphasized prevention over cure during the Civil War. Drawing on this illustrious past, the Rockefeller Sanitary Commission envisioned its work as largely educational and preventive. Thus it called on public health officials, school teachers, physicians, church leaders, businessmen, and journalists to join hands in a crusade against hookworm.[26]

Public school teachers initially proved more receptive to the campaign than any other group, even physicians. The Sanitary Commission and its inspectors wisely targeted the schools, seeing them as "the most ready form of access to the general public." Besides distributing leaflets and brochures that pupils could take home, they examined children who appeared infected and gave them instruction on habits of hygiene. In the summer months commission field workers also attended teacher institutes, where they explained what caused the disease. Before long students and teachers alike noticed positive improvements. One Georgia schoolteacher, astonished at the transformation of his class, thanked a field worker for changing his "peevish and stupid" pupils into "cheerful and studious" ones.[27]

As the hookworm campaign progressed through the southern states, it began to resemble a religious revival. Large, poor families journeyed long distances to hear how they could be saved from the ravages of disease. In 1911 in Pike County, Alabama, the Stevens family—a woman and her seven children, all with advanced cases of hookworm—walked and rode carts fourteen miles to attend the opening day of the Free Hookworm Clinic. "Anxious to do all she could to save her children from further trouble," Mrs. Stevens listened carefully to the advice she received and "took home with her a ten cent pail to store in the corner of the barn" until she could afford to build a sanitary privy. Convinced by the "almost miraculous results of a single treatment," she returned with her children the following week.[28]

Cleanliness did, indeed, seem close to godliness in the churches, schoolhouses, and make-shift dispensaries that welcomed serious country folk who gathered together to learn "the value of personal sanitation." In Alamance County, North Carolina, where 90 percent of the homes had inadequate privies and 50 percent of the schools had no privies at all, an estimated 9000 people received treatment for hookworm, viewed exhibits on the sanitary privy, and heard health presentations during a six-week period from August 8 to September 20, 1913. While not all were immediately converted, "quite a number of people" built sanitary privies at their homes. In coastal North Carolina, at about the same time, a field worker for the commission bragged: "We woke up the natives," who were ready "to erect sanitary privies just as soon as we tell them what kind to build."[29]

The school campaign in North Carolina had greater success because the Sanitary Commission collaborated with the Woman's Association for the Betterment of Public School Houses. This organization, which had existed since 1902, was committed to making rural schools into "models of cleanliness." Not unlike health and school reformers in the North, this southern group of middle-class white women believed that environment shaped character. Thus, early in the hookworm crusade, their association endorsed the construction of sanitary privies and pressured school boards to build them. By joining with local organizations and strengthening them, the Sanitary Commission's influence endured long after its official work ended in 1914. What had begun as a narrowly focused program to eradicate hookworm finally developed into "a program of mass education."[30]

Although the Sanitary Commission did not completely eradicate hookworm from the eleven southern states in which it worked, it brought "health to thousands" by improving "countless dwellings and schools." Twenty-five years later, Dr. Francis Arthur Bell said that in South Carolina many of the adults who were children during the hookworm campaign still remembered the pertinent points of his lectures and continued "putting them to practical use in regards to health matters and sanitation." Equally important was the commission's impact on state and local health departments. From 1910 through 1914 they became better funded, better staffed, and better able to implement their responsibilities.[31]

Once the Sanitary Commission left the South, progressive Southerners depended on their public health agencies to involve them in national developments. For example, by 1914 the regular examination of schoolchildren and school buildings had become fairly commonplace in the North, especially in cities heavily populated by European immigrants. In the South such activities became routine only during the ensuing ten years, when state medical inspectors carried forward the Sanitary Commission's baton and became health educators and boosters. While some areas were more receptive than others to state intervention in local health matters, nearly all Southerners participated to some degree in nationwide sanitary efforts to swat the fly and avoid spitting on sidewalks.[32]

Although slow to join the anti-fly and anti-spitting crusades that began at the turn of the century, southern health and school reformers eventually became a part of the chorus of voices that transformed annoying, pesky houseflies into dangerous "dealers in deaths" or "germs with legs." In 1921, the Winston-Salem Department of Health distributed leaflets encouraging North Carolinians of all ages to "Swat the Fly . . . Kill Him." A decade earlier in Kansas, the Boy Scouts "carried on war" against flies:

> they divided [Weir] township into districts and assigned each district to a corps. . . . Then they constructed fly-traps, distributed them among the citizens, covered manure piles, screened the privies, and before the end of the season they boasted that Weir was the cleanest district in the United States.[33]

The spectacular "swat the fly" drives that remained in vogue for years in Kansas and elsewhere demonstrate the extent to which early twentieth-century health reformers—in both the North and South—relied on popular education to change attitudes about disease. Not unlike the struggle against hookworm, the war against deadly flies became "a campaign for general cleanliness," especially following the 1916 polio epidemic, when flies were blamed for its spread.[34] Flies had nothing to do with polio, but they did carry germs. Hence "swatting the fly" was a useful slogan in the cause of public health education.

Soap and Water for Modern Health Crusaders

Cleanliness also seemed part of the answer to tuberculosis, or consumption as most people called it, a common cause of death at the turn of the century. The "White Plague," a disease of the poor and the working class, flourished in crowded, poorly ventilated, and unsanitary dwellings where hygiene was inadequate. As "a disease of the masses"—one that was particularly devastating to immigrants, African-Americans, and Native Americans—advice for its cure and prevention was frequently laced with middle-class prescriptions for acceptable behavior.[35] And because tuberculosis was transmitted through close contact, personal cleanliness ranked first among the exhortations of those who joined the fight against it.

Although these activists were inclined to accept the germ theory, they still thought that disease among the poor was largely the result of "filthy habits." As a result, the National Association for the Study and Prevention of Tuberculosis, along with local health agencies, developed innovative educational techniques to alter what it saw as dirty and harmful practices. Exhibitions, posters, streetcar tickets, and films warned of the dangers of spitting—an especially common and vulgar habit shared by many Americans until they gave up chewing tobacco in favor of "cleaner" cigarettes—and drinking from the common cup found in trains, office buildings, and schools. However, with the growing belief that tuberculosis was often acquired in childhood, the anti-tuberculosis crusade directed a considerable amount of its energy and funds to teaching "health chores" to schoolchildren. They were not only more malleable, but they almost unfailingly brought the health message home to less approachable parents and older siblings.[36]

Only a small number of tubercular children attended open-air schools, but few young people (tubercular or not) remained untouched by the campaign against juvenile tuberculosis. For example, by 1914, Harriet Fulmer of the Visiting Nurse Association had organized 9000 children in southern

Illinois and Chicago as "Open Air Crusaders"; in 1915, under the aegis of the National Tuberculosis Association, 100,000 children became "Modern Health Crusaders." Bathing regularly, washing hands before meals, and brushing teeth twice each day were among the eight health chores that, when completed and charted, enabled participants to qualify as "pages," "squires," or "knights." A very popular program, the "Crusade" enlisted three million children in 1919 and became established in every state and in many public school curricula by 1930. The Metropolitan Life Insurance Company, a pioneer in the fight against tuberculosis, organized a "Health and Happiness League." Its members pledged not to use a public drinking cup, to spit in public places, or to throw rubbish in streets, and they promised to bathe, wash, brush teeth, and "destroy every house-fly [they] possibly [could]."[37]

Schools, which were unaffected by the ebbing of patriotic furor after World War I, continued to civilize and socialize the young. Indeed, throughout the 1920s, the public school remained a forceful agent in inculcating American, middle-class habits of cleanliness—showing children just how much fun keeping clean could be. A renewed sense of purpose and excitement resulted from the ideas of a new breed of health educators who formed the Child Health Organization (CHO) in 1918. Committed to a curriculum that focused on teaching health habits through active participation, these educators hoped to change how schoolchildren behaved and create in them a "sanitary conscience." World War I catalyzed school health efforts further, since almost one-third of the potential draftees (731,000 of 2,511,000) were rejected as physically unfit:

> We won the war, but when the smoke of battle had cleared away, we realized, as never before, the pathetic weakness of our citizens . . . A large proportion of these physical defects might have been corrected or prevented if the schools had been doing their part.[38]

Inspired by the shocking rate of draftee rejections and evidence of widespread malnutrition among schoolchildren, Sally Lucas Jean, a school nurse trained in education, developed the CHO into "a tremendous force in the promotion of health in the schools of the United States." Physicians, educators, public health officials, and others backed CHO's attempts to place "health education"—a term they preferred to "hygiene"—in school curricula. From 1919 to 1923 Jean and her associates led CHO along these lines and then merged it into the American Child Health Association. Jean thereupon became a freelance consultant on health education, working with corporations that sold processed food and dairy products, insurance, and finally soap; in the mid-1920s she served as "School Health Consultant" for Lee Frankel's Health and Welfare Division of Metropolitan Life. In Sally Lucas Jean, the connections between professional public health work and business enterprise were close. Appealing to corporate self-interest, she helped make it enlightened.[39]

To bring about the behavioral changes they desired, the CHO encouraged teachers to adopt techniques reminiscent of those used earlier by the National Tuberculosis Association. Instead of the "Modern Health Crusade," in which children were promoted from pages to knights upon completion of their "health chores," Jean and her staff of six women organized youngsters into toothbrush brigades and introduced them to a health clown named "CHO-CHO." His performances were so popular that in 1919 Jean hired a "CHO-CHO the Second," who could "draw clever cartoons." Children themselves were urged to become health educators, by drawing posters and composing health slogans. One child wrote, "A good American is clean."[40]

In the early 1920s Grace T. Hallock, a CHO staff member and prominent author of storybooks about hygiene, invented the imaginative "Healthland," which was the "vacation ground of millions of boys and girls." Four trains (one called the "Red Cheek Local"), all desperately in need of young passengers, traveled each day to this unusual vacation spot. En route children could choose to stop at various points of interest: *Milky Way*, the capital of Healthland and the battleground on which "the Coffee King was defeated"; *Bathtubville*, "known and visited by every man of eminence"; or *East Toothbrush*, famous because of "the efficiency of its housewives, who were the first to adopt the modern method of sweeping up and down, instead of from side to side." There were other places too—such as "Play Meadows," "Ice Cream Mountain," and "Dreamtown"—that, it seems safe to say, travelers found more enticing and probably chose to stop at more frequently.[41]

During the 1920s health educators sought to improve the hygiene habits of all school-age children, not just immigrants. By bringing clowns and trains into classrooms, telling soap-and-water tales, and organizing health plays and toothbrush brigades, they effectively changed the behavior of many children and also influenced their parents, who heard about these educational activities at home. Such success did not go unnoticed. In fact, several of these educators (including Jean and later Hallock) took on new assignments in 1927, when a group of soap manufacturers contributed $500,000 to create the Cleanliness Institute (discussed below).[42]

School programs—and eventually industrial ones—to Americanize adults also existed. But immigrants who worked had little time, energy, or desire to attend night classes, even those initiated especially for them. With the

onset of World War I, however, programs multiplied in response to a growing consensus that "the adult foreigner must be prepared for citizenship no
less than his children." Although women taught in or directed nearly all
adult Americanization operations, most of their efforts were aimed at working men who, as potential voters or possible subversives, needed "a stake in
America—a home to fight for." The links connecting cleanliness, health,
good citizenship, and success were made ever clearer.[43]

In 1915 California's Home-Teacher Act empowered public schools in
Los Angeles and other areas to instruct immigrant mothers in English and
"Americanism." Classes took place in schools, factories, boarding houses,
hospitals, and elsewhere. By 1916 at least 500 communities offered special
public school programs to Americanize foreign-born adults. A minimum of
120,000 individuals annually enrolled in these classes, although a good deal
fewer completed them. Still, between 1916 and 1925 hundreds of thousands of immigrants, almost all of them adult males, completed courses in
English and civics. The subject matter varied widely, but in those considered the most successful teachers learned how to adapt their material and
methods to adults. Peter Roberts, immigration secretary of the Young
Men's Christian Association, actively promoted a "new scheme" for teaching English to adult foreigners that became quite popular. It drew on "the
daily experiences of an ordinary man" and encouraged the repetition of
short sentences—such as "I wash myself; I comb my hair; I put on my collar
and necktie"—that could be used in everyday conversation.[44]

Americanizers, who thought that "right living" led to good citizenship,
generally believed that foreign-speaking workers were not clean. Thus they
emphasized personal cleanliness to the point of obsession, as did their textbooks. In *English for Foreigners*, for example, there were separate lessons
on the care of the hands, hair, and teeth in addition to those on "Taking a
Bath," "How to Dress," and "Good Health." All of them stressed the value
of keeping clean, while many lessons here and elsewhere implied that their
readers knew little or nothing about soap and water. The author of *First
Lessons in English for Foreigners in Evening Schools*, who was also principal of a Buffalo public school, instructed:

> What is this? That is soap. What can you do with soap and water? I wash my
> hands and face with soap and water. What do you use the basin for? I put the
> water into the basin.

The insensitivity and tediousness of such readings, coupled with the long
hours that immigrants worked each day, suggest why so many of them
dropped out of school.[45]

Americanizing the Workplace

It hardly mattered that schools attracted few foreign-born men because, unlike their children, most were Americanized in the workplace. Their new identities, as writer Philip Roth observed, were "forged on the job" rather than "by schools, teachers, and textbooks." Employers introduced "welfare" programs out of a fear of labor unrest and in the hope of undercutting union appeals. These programs operated so well, particularly in raising sympathy and understanding between employers and employees, that by 1914 a National Civic Federation survey showed that 2500 employers had begun them. The intense nationalism surrounding World War I further encouraged them to eliminate divided allegiances and create English-speaking citizens who would be loyal to their country and their company.[46]

The war effort brought Americanizers to factories, where they created or helped shape employee welfare programs. International Harvester, for example, adopted Peter Roberts's method for teaching English, the same one used in many public school classes for adult foreigners. But at the workplace the repeated, short sentences stressed industrial discipline, safety, and sanitation: "I work until the whistle blows to quit. I leave my place nice and clean. I put all my clothes in my locker." The Ford Motor Company, which instituted English classes also designed by Roberts, tied its hiring, firing, and promotion practices to its educational program. Once again only those committed to "right living" would succeed—"the man and his home had to come up to certain standards of cleanliness and citizenship."[47]

Ford employees became indoctrinated with middle-class standards of hygiene in Americanization classes at company plants. Besides English, they learned how to eat, what to wear, and when to bathe. White-collar company investigators also visited auto workers' homes, looking for signs of uncleanliness, drunkenness, gambling, or poorly cared-for children. Ford did not want his employees living "like cattle" and using "their bath tubs for coalbins"; instead they were to spend their unusually high ($5 a day) wages in ways that would exemplify his ideals. Since he believed that "the most advanced people are the cleanest," he demanded that his workers live "in clean, well conducted homes" and use "plenty of soap and water" on themselves and their children.[48]

These Americanization efforts served as models for others. Detroit, for one, built its "Americans First" campaign in 1915 on Ford's apparent success. In the interest of nationalism, defense, and industrial peace, the Detroit Board of Commerce struck a deal with the Board of Education and the city's major manufacturers. The schools promised to offer well-organized and widely publicized evening courses in citizenship and English (again employing "the Roberts Method") to the thousands of foreigners who were looking for work. In return, manufacturers agreed to give preference to job applicants who completed the course-work and earned certificates.[49]

Detroit was not alone in drawing inspiration from Henry Ford. In 1916 the Kohler Manufacturing Company, located four miles west of Sheboygan, Wisconsin, decided to award "positions of trust and responsibility to only those men who are native born or naturalized citizens of the United States or those of foreign birth who have filed their first papers for citizenship." The president, Walter J. Kohler, was the third son of an Austrian immigrant who founded the company during the Panic of 1873. It succeeded and eventually prospered by offering a wide range of products. In the beginning, it made and sold farm plows, railroad frogs, and castings for local furniture factories. By the 1890s the company had added windmills, haybalers, urns and settees, cemetery crosses, railings for stairs and porches, and a cast-iron, enameled water trough and hog scalder that doubled "as a bathtub when fitted with legs." This enameled tub—when produced in 1911 as a single, *"sanitary"* piece, without crevices, joints, or seams—turned the Kohler Company into a nationally recognized producer of plumbing fixtures.[50]

Kohler relied on immigrant labor from the start. By 1914, with its products in demand, the company required at least a thousand workers to turn out its white, enamel bathroom and kitchen fixtures. Kohler then began hiring large numbers of foreigners in need of jobs, mostly single men from central and southern Europe, who initially found living quarters in Sheboygan until Walter Kohler developed Kohler Village, an industrial community adjacent to the plant. In 1918 his "American Club," the first building of the village, opened its doors. It was designed specifically, Kohler announced, to provide hygienic housing for single men of foreign birth. And at its dedication on Sunday, June 23, Kohler stated that "the name American Club was decided upon as it was thought that with high standards of living and clean, healthful recreation it would be a factor in inculcating in the men of foreign antecedents, a love for their adopted country."[51]

American flags, large clocks, and photographs of George Washington and Abraham Lincoln graced the walls of this two-story, red-brick Gothic building that is today a luxury hotel. Until a second wing was added in 1924, it held eighty-two "clean, cozy, and comfortable" single rooms that rented at $27.50 a month and included board and "plain washing." In the American Club dining room, which accommodated about 300 (and is currently the site of the Immigrant Restaurant and Winery), Kohler employees could take "a warm, well-cooked noon meal at a very nominal cost." And they, like the boarders, were free to use the lounge and reading room as well as the billiard and pool tables. Also available to them were four large, well-lighted, white-tiled bathrooms, fitted with Kohler's distinctive plumbing ware.[52]

Kohler's paternalism was far-reaching. Not only did the company build modern homes, free of "insanitary plumbing and foul air," but it also supported a medical and dental department with two full-time physicians, a dentist, and three visiting nurses. They devoted themselves to the workers and their families, while crews of inspectors and janitors from the safety and sanitation department looked after the workplace. Enameling plumbing fixtures was always a "dangerous trade," according to Alice Hamilton, the public health physician and expert in urban and industrial diseases. In 1912 she worked as a special investigator for the United States Bureau of Labor and later remembered Walter Kohler as "the only employer . . . who was seriously concerned with the problems of lead poisoning and of dust" at that time. By 1929 Hamilton said he "stood at the head" for making his plant's sandblast chambers "dust-proof."[53]

Walter Kohler, like Henry Ford, brought heavy pressure to bear on immigrant employees to become American citizens. Through his "Americans only" promotion policy, he prodded newcomers into attending night classes to learn "our language, our manners, our customs, our government." Beginning in October and then again in March, Sheboygan and Kohler schools offered free courses in English, civics, and hygiene. Workers enrolled in them at the company's Employment Department or through shop foremen.[54]

In classes they learned English and the basics of personal cleanliness from *First Lessons in English for Foreigners*. There is no direct record of what was taught in the hygiene classes, but the company newsletter offers many clues. "Teeth Tell Tales," for example, advised its readers that "a clean well-kept set of teeth is an asset to health and good looks and tells the story of cleanliness and careful attention." Notices in the "Health and Safety" column continually listed cleanliness as important, particularly in preventing tuberculosis. Spitting on streets or sidewalks, while endangering the community's health, also offended its pride.[55]

The company believed that its cleanliness, patriotism, and worthy purpose made it a "beacon" for other industries. Each year on April 7, which became "Americanization Day" at Kohler, company representatives drove workers who wished to take out citizenship papers to the Sheboygan County Court House in automobiles decorated with American flags. In 1926, a decade after the tradition began and with flags still flying, a Kohler bus transported seventy-five men of ten different nationalities to the courthouse. Their names appeared on the Kohler's Americanization Day Honor Roll, and newly naturalized citizens celebrated at a company-sponsored banquet.[56]

So many immigrants worked at Kohler that local citizens thought "you almost had to be a foreigner" to get a job. Some also speculated that the company recruited greenhorns because they would work for less than Americans. These conjectures were probably true since profits were small in the early years. Only during World War I, when the company obtained munitions contracts, and during the prosperous 1920s, when markets for their plumbing products expanded, did Kohler show large profits. During these years, it operated at full capacity, employing nearly 4000 people and paying better wages than most factories in Sheboygan. By 1934, however, some workers—joining the first union at Kohler—complained that they labored harder at more hazardous jobs and were unfairly penalized for defective work.[57]

But during the 1920s, when prosperity seemed endless, few employees at Kohler or anywhere else voiced much dissatisfaction. Corporate Americanization programs offered opportunity and security to immigrant workers in pursuit of both. Yet by the end of the decade most of these educational efforts had been terminated. The superpatriotism and nationalism that had fueled them waned as the 1920s rolled on. Programs that managed to survive at all finally ended in the early years of the Depression as a result of the major financial losses suffered by large companies. By then Kohler had long since become a leading manufacturer of the standard American bathroom, or what it called "the shrine of cleanliness."[58]

Advertising campaigns replaced Americanization efforts in showing immigrants and other middle-class aspirants "how to cleanse themselves." In ad after ad, throughout the 1920s, "Kohler of Kohler" promoted the "small and simple" modern bathroom with its standard three fixtures of "immaculately white enamel." In 1925, Kohler's most extensive advertising year, it ran large, four-color ads touting "the fun of being clean" and the "magic" of cleanliness to middle-class subscribers of fifteen national periodicals. Two years later, the company created new demands for its products by illustrating the inconveniences and troubles that arose when there were "not enough bathrooms to go around."[59]

The Business of Cleanliness

There remained one final impulse to complete the magnet-like force that was pulling Americans and their culture toward a modern version of cleanliness. Up to the 1910s, the energy to persuade the masses of the benefits of keeping clean flowed largely from private individuals and public servants—people with charitable, philanthropic, or simply public-spirited motives. Education (in several forms, not just the public school) had become a great engine of value reinforcement. But, during the 1920s, a second great dynamic—the profit motive—added such power as to drive the train of cleanliness irresistibly. Harnessing both public spirit and the hope of private gain, the business of cleanliness made personal hygiene an obsession as well as a virtue.

American society was increasingly "corporatizing" in the early twentieth century, and companies almost inevitably carried out campaigns for cleanliness in their own way. In this venture, as in others, not all segments of corporate America contributed positively. The first truly large businesses, the railroads, had to be brought kicking and screaming through the courts to acknowledge responsibility for injured workers. For a long time, mining and steel companies were immune to pleas for the safety and health of workers and their families, and meatpackers' procedures remained notoriously unsanitary until state and federal regulation forced improvements. But in cases where corporate well-being connected directly with cleanliness, surprising linkages resulted. Henry Ford and Walter Kohler believed that a clean work force made for a more efficient one; and Kohler tried to make his bathroom fixtures a necessity in every home. Thus for their own purposes, which were by no means nefarious or always the same, they promoted cleanliness.

Cleanliness, however, enjoyed other corporate connections. An early example, beginning in 1909, led Lillian Wald, the settlement-house pioneer, to the Metropolitan Life Insurance Company (described in the preceding chapter). Another case linking health educators with corporate America began in 1927, when Sally Lucas Jean and Grace Hallock of the Child Health Organization became involved with the Cleanliness Institute. Although the soap manufacturers who founded it may have been genuinely concerned about America's "slovenly folk," the Association of American Soap and Glycerine Producers was undoubtedly worried that the nation did not use enough soap. The cosmetics industry, whose product sales tripled between 1919 and 1929 as more women began wearing makeup, had begun taking customers away.[60]

Even more troubling was the fact that Americans had actually become cleaner. Paved streets and closed cars were the major elements in eliminating the layers of dirt and dust that had permeated so much of everyday life. Filthy, unsanitary working conditions also improved as machines took over back-breaking, sweaty jobs. Tractor-pulled graders and conveyors, instead of wheelbarrows and muscle, moved heavy loads; mechanical sweepers and bulldozers gradually replaced brooms, picks, and shovels. Thousands of jobs, which had for decades been grimy and hard, were sufficiently transformed to make soap producers anxious. And there was reason for concern inside the home, where electric lights and gas stoves began replacing kerosene lamps and coal stoves. So, although many Americans had *incidentally* become cleaner, the Cleanliness Institute told them they had not become clean enough.[61]

The institute's birth on June 23, 1927, at a dinner at the Park Lane Hotel in New York City, marked "the formal inauguration of a nationwide cleanliness movement." Sidney M. Colgate, president of the Association of American Soap and Glycerine Producers, pledged "large-scale cooperation" between soap manufacturers and their guests—health officials, educators, publicists, heads of social service organizations, and representatives of women's clubs. Reminding them of the "more than one billion dollars" expended annually by Americans to keep clean, Colgate made the point that cleanliness had become good business. Important to the country's standard of living, health, and social welfare, it was also a potential source of mega-profits.[62]

During the 1920s, "the business of cleanliness" was to produce an abundant supply of soap that both the rich and poor would buy. To sell it all, the manufacturers decided to educate as well as advertise. Soap advertisements were hardly new. Sapolio and Ivory had become widely known at the turn of the century through innovative advertising that used memorable slogans, photographs, and trademarks. Sapolio's nationalistic ads in the 1890s, for example, preached that "a clean nation has ever been a strong nation." Slogans such as "It floats" and "99 and 44/100% pure" sold millions of Ivory cakes during the same decade, pushing its maker's profits to $1.5 million by 1904. Twenty-five years later, when soap manufacturers desperately wanted to boost sales and guarantee a future for their products, they put aside their rivalries (as they had during World War I) and made children the main targets of their cleanliness campaign.[63]

"Shake Hands *Often* with Soap" typified the kind of advice the Cleanliness Institute gave America's schoolchildren once it discovered how few of them were truly clean. In a survey of "handwashing" at 145 schools in fifteen states, only 31 percent provided pupils with hot and cold water, soap, and towels; in one school alone did students obey the primary rule of "the health game"—"hands must be thoroughly washed before meals and after toilet." Since children were "not born with a 'sanitary sense,'" they had to be taught cleanliness. With this as its purpose, the institute initiated an all-out drive against dirt. It began by inundating schools with thousands of pamphlets, posters, flyers, and textbooks, all emphasizing in one way or another "common sense applications of cleanliness principles to everyday life." It prepared outlines for "Cleanliness Teaching" that showed educators how to inculcate bathing and grooming habits in children from kindergarten to high school. The institute also distributed bibliographies on cleanliness to hundreds of libraries and sent its *Cleanliness Journal* free to health officials, civic leaders, school teachers, and others who were partners in its sanitary crusade.[64]

All of these publications and activities concentrated on a few simple, clear messages. Cleanliness as "the basis of all good health" was the one most frequently stated. But there were others, many of which highlighted the new properties cleanliness acquired as the United States became more industrial, urban, and ethnically diverse. Of course, cleanliness continued to be used as an indicator that some individuals were morally superior, of better character, or more civilized than others. While certainly not novel, these qualities now served to differentiate larger numbers of Americans, especially as society became more middle-class and white-collar. Those with "clean collars," according to the Cleanliness Institute, not only got the best jobs but were more successful in them. Why? Because clean people had more self-respect and were also more confident, efficient, and affable.[65]

Articles in the *Cleanliness Journal* reflected values that had become popular in the early twentieth century.[66] Those who defined success as largely the consequence of appearance and sociability shared the mentality of the business world, where good grooming and personal congeniality transformed the "culture of character" into the "culture of personality." Middle-class youths and their parents, for example, looked upon the ability to please others through dress and manners as more important than discipline, earnestness, and diligence. Sociologists Robert and Helen Lynd found that in "Middletown" (Muncie, Indiana), where education was "a faith" in the 1920s, parents seemed uninterested in the subjects taught in local schools. They were far more concerned that their children learn "habits of industry" and form friendships for the purpose of "getting on . . . in the world."[67]

In classrooms as well as in advertising copy, manufacturers of soap and other cleansing products taught young adults some hard, real-world lessons. To neglect cleanliness, without doubt, was to court disaster. Failure to bathe and shave, as described in a Cleanliness Institute ad, explained why one salesmen could not close a deal or, in 1920s' terms, "put it over." In Listerine's "Don't Fool Yourself" ads, readers were graphically reminded of the kind of people "employers like to have around" and the ones that make the best "life partners." No one with halitosis—"a deliberate offense"—would endure.[68]

Prosperity touched a large segment of the population during the 1920s. But prosperity had its perils. Besides undermining a reliance on character, it "encouraged an anxious concern for social approbation." The emphasis on a clean, genial personality fed a striving for acceptance, approval, and popularity. Advertisements for soaps, mouth washes, toothpastes, and deodorants in mass-circulation magazines showed working men and women how to cleanse themselves and become part of the increasingly sweatless, odorless, and successful business class. Ad men, who benefited from instructions in behaviorist psychology and trade journal reports indicating that "more people still took a bath only on Saturday night than bathed daily," made the cleansing process seem so easy and so rewarding. And, in the end, advertising "made us cleaner." According to an Eastman Kodak publicist:

> It [advertising] has plumbed us from Maine to California. A generation ago the joke about the Saturday night bath had not yet been sprung. Today a new hotel has nearly as many bathrooms as sleeping rooms or it's a failure. A new house without one or more bathrooms can't be rented. In another generation there will be nobody who can see the point to that Saturday night bath joke, for we who used to lug the tub up from the cellar every week-end will be gone. And it's advertising that has done this—the irresistible appeal of pages upon pages of pictures of tile bathrooms and porcelain tubs and clean linen, and of soap that floats has made us want better things.[69]

Between June 1930 and November 1931, the Cleanliness Institute undertook a major advertising campaign of its own, one underwritten entirely by the Association of American Soap and Glycerine Producers. Consumers who returned coupons cut from ads or soap packages got answers about grooming and cleaning practices. This experiment promoted the highly touted notions that cleanliness was within everyone's reach—it was easy—and that it paid large dividends—it was rewarding. The institute spent $500,000 on three advertising appeals—on loveliness, bathing, and housecleaning—and received 685,154 requests from ordinary "folks" for over a million free booklets that offered help on "cleanliness problems." A qualmy adolescent in California who asked for *The Thirty Day Loveliness Test* commented on the margin of the coupon: "If you only knew how I *need* that book." The promise of more beautiful complexions for those willing to commit themselves to a month-long, "soap-scrub" regimen proved the most popular of seven "loveliness" ads that appeared in seventeen women's magazines. The second most compelling one, which pictured a woman alone versus a woman surrounded by six attentive men, simply asked: "Will YOU be a lovelier person by Dec. 15th?" With daily doses of soap and water, every woman could become a lovelier *and* "more likable, happier person." The reward for such attention and diligence was not simply cleanliness, but also popularity and self-esteem at a time when life had become "more intimate."[70]

The Cleanliness Institute's advertisements, like so many others in the

1920s and 1930s, exploited women's worst fears of giving offense, while manipulating their hidden desires to be sought-after and liked. A Listerine ad that asked "What's Wrong with Me, Mother?" gave a more straightforward, and unnerving, explanation of how to be popular than did the Cleanliness Institute's copy on loveliness. "Good looks, personality, and stylish clothes" did not always ensure "a good time"; for one "insidious thing"—unpleasant breath, or halitosis—could make "the most beautiful girl in the world unpopular." But Listerine guaranteed to wash it away and place every young women "on the acceptable side." Early Kotex ads discreetly shared the secret of "better-class women" who found "peace-of-mind, comfort, and immaculacy" from a product that *"thoroughly deodorizes."*[71]

Since women were considered more vulnerable than men to emotional appeals, advertisements heralding the benefits of cleanliness were directed largely at women who lived in cities and had money to spend. It would be mistaken, however, to assume that poorer women were not exposed to these entreaties. The Cleanliness Institute, for instance, ran almost all of its coupon ads in *True Story*, a magazine aimed at young, working-class women. By 1926 its circulation approached two million, and two years later it carried an impressive roster of national advertisers that included Pepsodent, Kotex, and Lux along with the Cleanliness Institute.[72]

Immigrant women did not escape ads with an emotional bite, even though advertisers generally believed their incomes were too low to warrant much attention. The makers of Fels-Naptha, the "golden bar with the clean naptha odor," placed a series of ads in *Survey*, the magazine for professional social workers, during the 1920s and 1930s. Rather than appealing directly to immigrant women, Fels-Naptha decided to reach them through social workers—using blatant ethnic stereotypes. Foreign women were portrayed as sub-standard, but eager to learn the American way of cleanliness. "Mrs. Rizzuto," said one ad, wanted "to live up to our standards of cleanliness," but she found that difficult because "her methods are so primitive, so ineffective." The solution? "Coaching on American ways of keeping house . . . [and] when you're teaching her, suggest Fels-Naptha Soap." Other ads in the series aimed the same message at "Mrs. Orozco," "Mrs. Kowalski," and other ethnics including a woman who would be "summering on her fire escape," or another whose daughter would get a "black star" for coming to school dirty—unless Fels-Naptha saved the day.[73]

At times advertisers spoke directly to immigrants (and African-Americans) through their own newspapers. One publicist, who claimed, "I have never seen a better purchasing agent than the foreign-born mother, trained in the hard school of experience and necessity," urged advertisers to use the foreign-language press, especially those that "preach the gospel of law and order, counseling good American citizenship." T. Coleman Du Pont, who believed that "advertising is the biggest Americanizer in America today," also encouraged more direct use of foreign-language papers. They would sell more American goods, "dispel this Bolshevism cloud," and "interest immigrants to like America and stay here and buy homes here and help us build this big country."[74]

Lever Brothers ran large ads with photographs in Milwaukee's Polish newspaper, *Kuryer Polski*. One explained the plight of a young woman whom men avoided because of underarm odor after only a few dances. Deeply embarrassed, the woman stopped going until she discovered Lifebuoy soap; it gave her the "immaculate cleanliness" and "pleasant freshness" that rescued her from distress. Readers of the Chicago *Defender* who "never understood the secret of Maizie Turner's charm" finally learned through a Lever Brothers' ad how Lifebuoy soap helped her become "popular." Another African-American woman who brushed with Colgate toothpaste won "a leading position in Chicago's upper society set," became "queen of the Delta Sigs," and married a happy man who proclaimed "Yes Sir . . . She's My Baby . . . Now!"[75]

Young men, presumably less fastidious than their wives and sisters, were seldom the targets of ad men's pitches. When they were, words such as "popular" or "charming" did not appear very often. The Cleanliness Institute's poster of a man showering, for example, simply said: "Swim for exercise; bathe for cleanness. Both for Health." Another poster, designed with men in mind, stated: "A Clean Machine Runs Better—Your Body is a Machine—KEEP IT CLEAN." On occasion, especially when soap ads concentrated on body odor, men could be subjected to the same insensitive treatment as women. In one Lifebuoy series entitled "Behind His Back," a man with "b.o." finally figured out, before losing his friends and a promotion, "what they're saying behind my back!" But in contrast to the legions of anxious and confused women who starred in thousands of advertising tableaux promoting personal hygiene products, only a scattering of uneasy, white-collared men found their way into these ads.[76]

In fact, when men appeared as consumers, they were almost always clean-shaven businessmen—never factory workers, builders, firemen, or engineers. Safety razors and disposable blades had removed their turn-of-the-century beards and mustaches and given them "quicker, cleaner, more lasting" shaves. Williams Shaving Cream promised its users a "face that's fit," one that could "get orders or give orders" with confidence and calm. These well-groomed, clean-cut businessmen generally sat behind large desks or, when pictured with women, stood off-center and in the background. From there they looked approvingly on their wives or disapprovingly on women at the office who were "despised" because they suffered from bad breath or perspiration odors.[77]

Married women, as wives and mothers, shouldered the heavy obligation for their family's success. This is probably best demonstrated in the ways they carried out their household responsibilities, which began to include purchasing an ever-growing assortment of dirt chasers. Indeed, when it came to personal hygiene, the makers of Williams Shaving Cream knew they could "count on her to keep him on the road to success," for wives realized that "tomorrows are brightest for the man who is face-fit today." According to the B.V.D. Company, women sensed "even better than *he* does" that the smartest purchases were the ingredients for advancement and popularity. That, at least, is the answer the company gave when its ad men asked: "Why Do We Advertise Men's Underwear in a Woman's Magazine?"[78]

By 1929, when national periodicals carried over $300 million in advertising copy, the majority included photographs. They were cheaper than drawings and paintings and more effective in showing emotions; three years later, a single issue of the *Ladies' Home Journal* used photographs in half of its ads. This change is noteworthy, since as late as the mid-1920s most advertisers still believed color and modern art attracted more attention. What is more remarkable—and extremely telling in regard to the nation's increasing preoccupation with cleanliness in the years after World War I—was the $20 million that businesses spent in advertising soaps, toilet goods, and cleansers in 1935, when all but the very rich felt the severe hardships of a depressed economy.[79]

Lever Brothers, the makers of Rinso, Lifebuoy, and Lux soap, revised its advertising copy over the years to reflect the changing cultural meanings of soap itself. In 1902, Lifebuoy was "the Friend of Health—the soap that cleans and disinfects, purifies—at one operation." It was still called "health soap" in 1926, but an ad notified consumers that Lifebuoy could also stop body odor and ensure social acceptability. In 1916, Lux was "a wonderful new product" for "laundering fine fabrics"; by the mid-twenties it could also preserve "soft, youthful, lovely feminine hands" and, by the early thirties, prevent "undie odor" as well—"She never omits her Daily Bath, yet she wears underthings a SECOND DAY." Francis Countway, the president of Lever Brothers and the individual most responsible for the "discovery" of body odors and the "stop smelling" ad pitch, was inspired by Listerine's successful advertising campaign against the previously unknown halitosis. Countway and his associates admitted, while Lever Brothers' business boomed, that they cared little "about the opinions of softies who think that the Body and Undie Odor copy is disgusting." They were simply doing their job, "bringing cleanliness into a dirty world."[80]

Americans may have become cleaner as a result of these incessant and irresistible appeals, but radio advertising could also claim some credit. By 1930 almost twelve million homes (about 40 percent of the total) had radios, and the number continued to rise as more low-income families acquired them and came to prefer the radio to magazines or books as a source of information on "how to run their homes and how to improve themselves." Listening to the radio became the nation's favorite pastime during the Depression, and financially hard-pressed advertisers overcame their initial wariness about how listeners would react to "hard-sell" interruptions of their music. In fact, advertisers soon discovered that the most intrusive commercials often worked best. The continual "Lucky Strike means fine tobacco" and the eerie Lifebuoy "B.O." foghorn were two of many.[81]

Radio advertisements began supplementing the print media from the late 1920s on. Sales of another Lever Brothers' product, Pepsodent toothpaste, skyrocketed in 1929, when it became the sponsor of *Amos 'n' Andy*, a national radio sensation. Even before the National Broadcasting Company purchased the series, Freeman F. Gosden (Amos) and Charles J. Correll (Andy) had created a "chainless chain" of broadcasts that made the adventures of Amos and Andy available to select stations from East Coast to West six nights a week. But the NBC Blue network enlarged their audience, made Gosden and Correll Depression celebrities, and quadrupled Pepsodent's sales. Interestingly, the *Amos 'n' Andy* show won approval from the press, as well as from ministers and mothers, for its " 'clean,' wholesome character."[82]

The advertising successes of Lucky Strike and Pepsodent encouraged competitors of every stripe to use the personal contact that radio provided. Before hard times forced the Cleanliness Institute to shut down in December 1932, it also went on the air in a series of broadcasts—"A Tale of Soap and Water," "A Doctor Looks at Cleanliness and Health," "Summer Camps and Cleanliness," and "The Search for Beauty," to name only a few—that highlighted the benefits of cleanliness. For housewives, the special target of an array of daytime programs, the institute created the "Homeville Country Club" and offered what it hoped were powerful suggestions on "Houseworking Your Way to Good Looks" through "Kitchen Calisthenics," "A Boat Ride in the Bedroom," and "Dance of the Mop and Duster."[83] Like schoolchildren, whom the Cleanliness Institute and health educators had long considered a wedge into the home, the radio too broke through the privacy of the family circle with persuasive entreaties that reached even those who bought only a few magazines or knew only a little English.

Persuading the masses to keep clean united soap producers and their ad men along with educators, health officials, and industrialists in a unique cultural enterprise. Although their reasons for trying to convince the upwardly mobile to rid themselves of working-class or hick ways were not always exactly congruent, they all equated cleanliness with success and the American way of life. The wife and mother who wanted her husband and children to succeed, therefore, found "a way to send them out in freshly laundered and ironed white shirts each day." And the father who came to America in search of opportunity shared his experience about clean clothes and good grooming with his son: "It was better to buy some nice clothes and have them on because people look at your appearance . . . even if you have to let your stomach go for a day."[84]

As the nation slid into the Depression of the 1930s, workplace Americanization and philanthropy ebbed, but other powerful messengers of personal cleanliness continued to reach the public's ear. At school children still heard how they should keep clean and avoid germs. In 1942, the health magazine *Hygeia* once again made the distinction between "visible dirt" and "contagion," and told its readers how "essential" it was to wash hands, avoid common drinking cups, and use only clean towels.[85] Radios too blared what almost everyone seemed to know, catchy advertisements for soaps, mouthwashes, and toothpastes. Like so much else in American society, the culture of cleanliness had become institutionalized. The *mix* of public and private value-reinforcers, both pointing in the same direction, made its triumph virtually inevitable. Only rural Americans remained outside what had become a mass movement. But, before cleanliness peaked in the 1950s, they too would adopt the ways of their city cousins.

CHAPTER SIX

Whiter Than White—
and a Glimmer of Green

The average American home is among the cleanest and most hygienic in the world. But there are many American cities the
cleanliness of whose streets set a municipal standard which
would make a European blush.

—P.B., 1952[1]

Cleanliness Peaks

The American pursuit of cleanliness, which began in earnest during the
mid-nineteenth century, reached its peak in the years following World War
II. Almost everyone had become convinced of its value by the 1930s, yet the
quest continued slowly and deliberately during the Depression decade.
Home economics became part and parcel of high-school and college curricula, and rural electrification began to make cleanliness possible on remote
farms. In the early 1940s, despite the horrors of World War II, full employment returned and catapulted the American economy into "the wild blue
yonder of skyhigh prosperity." At the war's end and through the 1950s, advertising expenditures doubled and electricity use nearly tripled as millions
of suburban homeowners bought household appliances and hygiene products in such quantities as to create a "culture of cleanliness"—a people that
used more water and had more bathrooms per family than any other nation
on earth. "Whiter than white," which for so long could be the goal of only a
few, had finally become the national norm, seemingly possible for all.[2]

The culture of cleanliness took root in the "modern" American home during the 1920s and 1930s, when the economy lurched, then sped, away from

blue-collar manufacturing and toward white- and pink-collar service jobs. As a result, the whole family, from breadwinner to teenager, demanded a "cleaner clean" to win acceptance and success. Women took up the challenge at home by purchasing more appliances and cleansers but employing fewer domestic servants—even though large postwar families meant, in historian Ruth Schwartz Cowan's telling phrase, "more work for mother." Another postwar paradox characterized the situation of farmers. Just as rural electrification began to close the gap in life style between them and their city cousins, the number of farm families started falling. Up to the late 1930s, nearly a third of American families lived on farms; but only about 4 percent remained there by the late 1960s. Suburbs gradually replaced farms as the living-space norm. After World War II a consumer-goods revolution also occurred, providing a plethora of soap, deodorants, detergents, and bathroom fixtures to those who had the will and the wherewithal to buy them. Since minorities were ordinarily paid less for their work and excluded from modern homes in suburbia, they found it almost impossible to keep up with the expanding white middle-class.

These themes defined the culture of cleanliness from the 1930s to the 1960s. The "normal" middle-class home was mostly a coveted idea, an advertiser's dream, in the 1920s. Only in the future, some thirty years away, would women—the majority of whom by then lived in homes with central heating, indoor plumbing, running hot and cold water, and electricity—search, often without respite, for "the cleanest clean possible."[3] The live-in maid or twice-a-week cleaning lady were in part casualties of the Depression but continued to become scarcer as the quality of appliances improved. Housewives readily replaced servants with machines endowed with the "greatest cleaning power." The Model 10 Eureka vacuum cleaner, for example, was advertised as "so revolutionary" and powerful that it " 'eats up' dust, sand, grit, lint—any kind of dirt" and "solves every cleaning problem." Something few servants could do! For good reason, then, the generation of middle-class women who became housewives *after* 1930 depended more on machines than maids to maintain a decent standard of living for their families.[4]

At no time did the nation's poor women (and more than half of them still lived on farms) face the maid-or-machine dilemma. Indeed, many of them were themselves domestics, while others worked in factories, laundries, fields, or canneries just to make ends meet. They lived with their families (and sometimes boarders) in crowded, poorly equipped housing in urban neighborhoods or small towns, or along country roads. Central heat, indoor plumbing, running hot and cold water, electric light and power had yet to reach their tenement flats and isolated farmhouses. Working as they did in the dirtiest jobs and living in the most undesirable places, they hardly ever had clean homes and belongings.[5]

In such circumstances, doing laundry or taking baths remained difficult and time-consuming. Without a nearby water supply, both chores meant carrying heavy buckets of water some distance, heating them on a stove, and again transporting them to washing or bathing tubs. Keeping a home was as labor-intensive in the 1930s as it had been in the 1840s. It is hardly surprising that

> underclothing might be changed only once a week, or even once a season; sheets likewise (if they were used at all, since featherbeds did not require them); outerclothes might do with just a brushing; shirts or shirtwaists might go for weeks without benefit of soap; faces and hands might get splashed with water once a day; full body bathing might occur only on Saturday nights (and then with a sponge and a wooden tub and water that was used and reused) or only when underwear was changed—or never at all.[6]

Housewives as Targets

The rapid spread of home economics in high schools and colleges in the 1930s and later, coupled with the increasing availability of modern conveniences, appeared novel and liberating, but proved to be a new way of tying most women to a very old job. Whether struggling to get ahead or striving to keep up with the times, few women doubted that their place was in the home; almost all, especially the more prosperous, became targets of home economists and manufacturers of appliances and cleansers. Poor women, who knew that cleanliness was important, anticipated the possibility of living in a home with central heating, running water, and a toilet—a decent home they could call their own.[7] Middle-class women, who watched their husbands' work-worlds transformed by efficiency experts, channeled much of their energy into becoming competent household managers.

Home economists had been seeking ready pupils since early in the century, back in the days when cleanliness was still primarily sought as insurance against disease. Well before the advent of electric-powered home appliances, Ellen Swallow Richards, the renowned home-economics pioneer, encouraged progressive methods. "The twentieth-century housewife," she said in 1900, "must bestir herself and bring her ideas [and tools] up to date." When a "pin-point of dust" could yield "three thousand living organisms, not all malignant, but all enemies of health," cleanliness was, as Richards insisted, "a sanitary necessity of the Twentieth Century whatever it may cost."[8]

Cleanliness standards rose quickly as a result of explicit warnings from home economists and graphic descriptions of germs from manufacturers of cleansing products. They regularly reminded housewives that microbes multiplied "a thousandfold in an exceedingly short space of time." Since no one could be too careful, discriminating wives and mothers were urged to buy cleansers that chased "both the seen and unseen dirt" from every nook and cranny. Only "the highest degree of cleanliness" brought "real satisfaction" and, presumably, peace of mind in what had become a daily battle against a hidden enemy.[9]

"Domestic scientists," as home economists were sometimes known, had called on the findings of laboratory scientists to energize homemaking. Since middle-class women no longer needed to make soap, candles, bread, cloth, and other domestic necessities, a commonly asked question was, "What were women to *do*?" Housework, it appeared, had been "robbed by the removal of *creative* work." A few critics of American domesticity believed with Charlotte Perkins Gilman that housewives had a perfect opportunity to free themselves from their homes and "the tyranny of bric-a-brac," a tyranny which had forced them "to wait upon . . . things, and keep them clean."[10]

But with the home at stake, housewives refused to leave. They chose instead to become part of a major domestic reform movement that promised to save the home through efficiency and more exacting standards. In 1909 home economics became a full-fledged profession with the founding of a national association and quickly won the support of education, government, and industry. In 1917 the federal Smith-Hughes Act subsidized programs to train girls and women as homemakers, and by 1920 over thirty states had initiated home economics courses in their public schools. The advertising industry welcomed these women who could be counted on "to promote the splendors of domesticity—and the necessity to buy new products in order to realize those splendors."[11]

In the late 1920s, power and light companies employed home economists to explain the new washing machines, vacuum cleaners, and refrigerators to potential consumers. These women were so successful that by 1930 there were 400 "home service departments" operating in public utilities across the country. The home economists who conducted these how-to demonstrations gave a whole range of household advice, mixing "the technics of products with middle-class values of domesticity." More than simply salespersons, they "played a dynamic translating role" that helped customers understand how electric appliances could make them healthier, cleaner, and more efficient.[12]

Christine Frederick, another home economist turned saleswoman, also became a mediator between companies and consumers. An educated mother of four, she began her career testing household products in the Applecroft Home Experiment Station that she set up in her Long Island home. In 1912 she became household editor for *Ladies' Home Journal* and subsequently published *The New Housekeeping* (1913) and *Household Engineering: Scientific Management in the Home* (1915). Hoping to liberate women from the dirt, drudgery, and despair of never-ending housework, she promoted "efficiency" measures that all too frequently resulted in more work or "make work."[13]

Frederick's "new housekeeping" promised to elevate housework to a profession and turn housewives into managers. She believed she could help women remove their feelings of inadequacy, make it possible for them to spend more time with their children, and allow them "to rest, to play, to stay young—to widen the circle of pleasant social contact." No longer would they have to place "good tools" in the hands of bad servants. And, finally, in servantless homes *"exact standards"* could be followed and "greater perfection" achieved.[14]

Frederick contended that the "business" of homemaking in the twentieth century relied upon machines. She and other home economists convinced American women, who held in their hands "enormous purchasing power," that household appliances were not "luxury" items but "productive machinery" as essential to the well-equipped home as to the well-equipped factory or office. And she advised manufacturers of these products, usually men, on how to sell their wares to women. She discovered that one of the greatest appeals was cleanliness, for Americans "do not like dirt or anything that suggests it." Although most homemakers did not yet understand the germ theory, Frederick reported, "they meticulously act upon the assumption that germs must be outwitted."[15]

Frederick also encouraged manufacturers to appeal to women's emotions and to show "Mrs. Consumer" in cities and on farms what electric appliances could do for themselves and their families. As a result, in advertising copy, dishwashing, laundering, and bathroom cleaning ceased to be time-consuming, dreaded chores; they became instead efficient expressions of affection and concern or embarrassing signs of carelessness. During the interwar years, housewives who were already concerned about cleanliness read over and over again heart-warming testimonials to modern conveniences. Thanks to a General Electric dishwasher—rather than to "Mother and the girls"—in "millions of kitchens, the warm soapy smell of fresh-washed china and sparkling glassware mingled with the lingering fragrance of Sunday-dinners-done." Housewives also learned that Rinso soap and electric washing machines got one smart woman's wash "at least 4 or 5 shades whiter" without scrubbing or boiling; while Sani-Flush warned them that "a dirty dingy toilet" could bring "whispered comments" from guests who "go upstairs."[16]

Perfect cleanliness, women were led to believe, could not be achieved outside the privacy of their own homes. Commercial laundries were too expensive and could not be trusted, according to promoters of the electric washing machine. Frederick, for one, insisted that clothes done commercially were too often lost, damaged, or improperly cleaned, touched as they were by strangers. The fact went unnoticed that, for years, African-American women had cleaned white women's clothes, houses, and babies (and continued to do so in many southern and wealthy homes). Advertisers of Automatic Electric Washers simply reiterated the experts' warnings: "Only in your home can you . . . know that nothing is lost, nothing mishandled, and everything washed perfectly clean." During the 1930s, the electric washer entered many homes when its price dropped and when "energetic advertising" by soap companies "accelerated the trend of the previous one hundred years of increasing standards of cleanliness."[17]

Advertising of this kind had several consequences: the consumption of electricity rose rapidly; middle-class, urban households acquired a hodge-podge of electrical appliances; and women became trapped during the 1920s in a "feminine mystique" usually associated with the 1950s. Even before the Depression, advertisers and domestic reformers had idealized the wife and mother who did not work outside the home, who systematically and happily did her own housework, and who found sole satisfaction in caring responsibly and creatively for her house and family. Admittedly, not all home economists intended to glorify housework and keep women at home. Some had actually hoped to free them from their time-consuming chores so they might give their energies to charitable, cultural, or social causes. Hardly anyone suggested, however, that contented or sane women pursue careers—or that men share in homemaking. Only in an emergency, Frederick counseled, should "the smooth running of the house" be placed "on the man's shoulders."[18]

Ideal husbands were to make their wives' work easier and their homes cleaner by providing them with up-to-date equipment and conveniences. Few families could afford to purchase everything at once. But during the 1920s many began by buying houses of their own—encouraged as they were by the Better Homes movement and offers from building and loan associations. By 1930, 48 percent of American families owned their houses; in some of them, thanks to tinted fixtures, the bathroom was "a show place." Smaller than Victorian residences and frequently located in suburbs, outside dirty, dense cities, most (certainly the newer ones) had gas, electricity, and indoor plumbing.[19]

Yet not all houses did. In towns of 10,000 people or less, for example, 49 percent had no bathtubs in 1925. In Muncie, Indiana, where 30,000 people lived in 1920, it was quite common "to observe 1890 and 1924 habits jostling along side by side in a family with primitive back-yard water or sewage habits, yet using an automobile, electric washer, electric iron, and vacuum cleaner." Still, it was only a matter of time. In large cities like Chicago, about 92 percent of all houses had electricity in 1925, and 82 percent of those owned by the poorest families had private bathrooms in 1932. Only farms remained untouched by modern conveniences before World War II.[20]

Bathrooms in the Country

Farm women barely felt the effects of the revolution that transformed housework in middle-class, city homes in the early twentieth century. Girls like Rose Landsown, who lived in Chicago, dreaded visits to their grandmothers' houses in the country where everybody took baths in a portable tub and "in the same water." Farm women, for their part, knew how city folks lived from reading the Sears catalogue or from visits to town to see relatives or to do business. Hazel Clawson of Benton County, Indiana, remembered the first bathtub she ever bathed in; it was at her sister-in-law's in Homewood, Illinois, just outside Chicago. She also recalled how much she enjoyed attending teachers' meetings in Evansville, Indiana, because the hotel where she stayed had a private bathroom.[21]

Through the 1920s and most of the 1930s, farm life changed little from what it had been during the nineteenth century. Although housekeeping had never been easy for women who did their own work, it proved particularly difficult for women who lived on farms. Not only were they more isolated than housewives who lived in towns and cities, but they also were more overworked. Besides the usual household labor, farm women had to look after cows and chickens, and on many farms they worked in the fields between preparing meals for any number of hard-working and hungry hired hands. For these women there was not a moment to relax. One southern housewife complained that her only break from a sweltering, hot kitchen on a summer day was a "walk to the well for a fresh bucket of water, or to the chicken lot to care for the little biddies."[22]

Houses were almost impossible to clean and, when cleanliness was achieved, it lasted only a very short time. An Indiana farm woman remarked that "people who kept their houses nice and clean . . . really had to work." The culprits were many: roaming animals that smelled bad and attracted flies, wood- and coal-burning stoves that left smoke stains on the walls and ceilings, and dirt roads that easily turned to mud but, when dry, always gave off dust—so much dust that "you could write your name any place."[23]

The time spent cleaning varied greatly. By not being too fastidious, housewives could lessen their frustration as well as the number of house-keeping chores performed every day or every week. Yet a farmhouse full of people demanded endless attention. At least once a year, usually in the spring and sometimes again after the harvest, farm women would "start from scratch" and give their houses a thorough cleaning. Taking one room at a time, they cleaned—and often painted or wallpapered—each room. Many houses had rag carpets that housewives and their daughters had woven themselves. These floor coverings were taken outside, hung on a clothes line, and beaten until the dust was gone. An eighty-four-year-old woman from Scott County, Indiana, remembered in the early 1980s how her mother ripped their carpets apart during the 1920s and 1930s, washed them on a zinc-covered washboard, sewed the rags back together, and re-turned the rugs to the floors.[24]

Nothing proved as burdensome to farm women as the annual spring cleaning, save washing and ironing. Doing the laundry was their most back-breaking and time-consuming chore, especially since it took at least two days every week. An Indiana farmer noticed that his wife "washed one day and ironed the rest of the week." But, even more than time, it was the lack of water and the sheer bulk of farm dirt in clothes that made the job so onerous.[25]

Washing had to be done outside, in good and bad weather alike. All the water used for rinsing as well as for washing—about eight gallons for each washtub, and there were usually two or three tubs—had to be carried in buckets from a spring or well. Water was boiled in huge, iron kettles over open fires and then was transferred to washtubs, to be mixed with buckets of cold water. In the Texas Hill Country, women usually did about four loads (sheets, shirts and other white clothing, colored clothes, and dish tow-els) in a week's wash, and the water had to be changed for each load. More buckets of water, holding about three or four gallons and weighing about twenty-five pounds, were again hauled from the spring or well to the fire. On hot days, "you felt like you were being roasted alive."[26]

Dirty, greasy farm overalls demanded vigorous scrubbing with home-made lye soap or, quite often, a bar of Fels-Naptha and rapid "punching" with a wooden broomstick or paddle to make them clean. Lifting wet over-alls from a washtub and placing them in another tub for rinsing also re-quired strong arms. Each washed item was "swished" through the rinse water and occasionally transferred to a third tub for blueing to make it white. After the bending, punching, and lifting, came the wringing, which was done before anything was hung on a line to dry, winter or summer. "By the time you got done washing, your back was broke," said Ava Cox, who lived and washed in the Hill Country during the 1930s.[27]

Women with babies washed diapers by hand nearly every day. When there were many babies—or sick ones—"it was just wash, wash, wash." Diapers, boiled clean, were also hung in the sun to dry. In fact, they were frequently the first announcement to neighbors that a new baby had arrived. But, whether it was diapers or sheets, a clean wash hung properly on the line gave many tired farm women a sense of satisfaction. One woman said she made a "picture" out of her clothesline, where "everything was separated and hung together." Another boasted that her wash "was the whitest and was on the line first."[28]

Yet even women who took pride in a white wash became distressed as they saw modern equipment change their husbands' farm work along with the housework of friends and relatives who lived in the city. In 1907 a southern woman who identified herself in the *Progressive Farmer* as "Nellie of Magnolia" explained that farm women were "not complaining about the task that is ours, though we do sometimes feel in our weary, worn-out hours that the good things in this world are not equally divided." Over a decade later, a woman in Greene, New York, who seemed more embarrassed than angry that her farmhouse lacked modern conveniences, echoed what had become a familiar lament—that farm women "haven't had their just share of things—material things." She said she was a grandmother who did not want to die until she had "fitted up a farm house—one with hot and cold water, with a bath, with good lighting and heating systems, with a power washer, etc. etc." Without electricity, she could have none of these "material things."[29]

Farm women wanted indoor plumbing and electric washing machines, first of all, to reduce their workload. They valued health and hygiene, but they also "longed for life, more life and still more life." They wanted "some means of lessening the continual grind" because it was exactly that, along with isolation, crushed ambition, and lack of time for improvement that made them feel like drudges. And their discontent grew larger as their awareness increased that they had been left behind and were living in "the Dark Ages." They also saw many of their sons and daughters drawn off the land, attracted by city lights and modern amenities.[30]

Women who thought living conditions on their farms resembled those of the Middle Ages were not greatly mistaken, for they remained strikingly primitive. In 1919 a survey conducted by the Department of Agriculture indicated that, while 96 percent of those interviewed did have screens on their windows, 90 percent still had outdoor toilets and, of necessity, "walked the path" in sickness and in health, in cold weather as in warm. Anticipating the arrival of electricity, a few better-off farm families built bathrooms—but *without* fixtures. Electric pumps were useless without current; farm people still had to haul water from the outside. In fact, in 1919, farmers (primarily women) spent over ten hours each week pumping water and carrying it from outdoor sources to kitchens.[31]

The "Dirty Thirties," characterized by dust storms, droughts, and the Great Depression, made life on America's farms—particularly in the Midwest, Great Plains, and South—exceedingly difficult. Distressed and desperate women gave less attention to cleaning (although many saved money by making their own soap) as they increased the size of their gardens, canned nearly everything they produced, and sold whatever they could—hooked rugs, baby ducks, cottage cheese, yeast cakes, canned fruits and vegetables. Some, especially farm daughters, took jobs outside the home (often as teachers) to help their families survive. But farm women were anxious and impatient; they wanted "an American standard of living upon the farm." One woman in rural Stickney, South Dakota, even asked Eleanor Roosevelt to come to their aid:

[E]verything which we have to buy has gone up and the things we have to sell are going down in price. . . . I haven't had [a new dress] for almost a year and a half and there are women right in this community who are much worse off than I am. If the men cannot think of helping the women of the Country then surely we must intercede for ourselves.[32]

Early in the twentieth century, as farmers acquired gas-powered tractors and corn shredders, their wives began to speak openly about the unequal distribution of power within rural families. They were often angry that so much was spent on farm equipment and so little on household appliances. In 1908 an unidentified "Farmer's Wife" wrote a "Word to Husbands":

A farmer spends freely for this and for that if it lessens his toil a bit.
The reaper, the mower, the new fangled sower, have each made with
    him, quite a hit.
But while he is riding at ease in his field 'neath skies that are calm
    and serene,
His spouse has to rub all day at the tub for lack of a washing machine.[33]

Women's unhappiness with this indifference and lack of regard intensified as electricity began to reach more farms through the Rural Electrification Administration (REA), a New Deal program established in 1935. Less than 10 percent of American farm families had high-line electric service prior to the establishment of the REA. Some in isolated areas tried to make do with home generators powered by gasoline engines or windmills, but they were only sporadically reliable. Utility companies refused to serve areas with only a few families, citing the high costs of stringing lines through the countryside.[34]

Rural electrification was concentrated mostly in the Far West and Northeast. Well watered and densely populated, farms in the Northeast were typically intensive poultry-raising and dairying enterprises. There, the closeness of farms persuaded the utility companies that it was worthwhile serving them. In the Far West, with its hydroelectric dams and advanced methods of irrigation, half the farms had electricity by 1935; in California, which produced enormous amounts of fruits and vegetables, 63 percent of the farms were electrified. But small "dirt farms" in the Midwest and South had almost no electricity; fewer than 5 percent of the sprawling, sparsely settled ranches of Montana, Wyoming, the Dakotas, Oklahoma, and west Texas had electricity, much of that self-generated.[35]

Electrification, even without the involvement of profit-oriented power companies, was not cheap. Construction of a mile-long REA electrical line cost $1000 (instead of the utilities' $2000), and at least three families along this mile had to agree to pay for the line and use it. This agreement implied that farmers would wire their houses and farm buildings and then purchase electrical appliances and equipment. As eager as many may have been to have electricity, a large number of small, poor farm folk were scared—of not being able to pay their electric bills, of falling into debt, of losing the only land they possessed. In the Texas Hill Country, they were also afraid of the wires that ran across their land and the official papers they had to sign. Could the wires, like lightning, hurt their cows or possibly their children? And in signing an easement, were they giving up control of their farmland?[36]

Because of such fears, the REA launched a vigorous campaign to educate prospective clients as well as offer them loans for wiring and equipment. Not unlike the agents sent out by the Agricultural Extension Service during the 1920s and 1930s, REA representatives (male and female) explained, in very practical terms, how electricity could benefit farm life and make it more like city living. The REA, copying the initiatives of private power and light companies, also employed home economists to persuade farm families to buy and use electric appliances. They argued convincingly that "electricity would create less work for the farm woman." However, as with city women, the workload shifted rather than diminished.[37]

In 1938 an REA traveling "circus," or Farm Demonstration Tour, took to the road. A procession of large trucks carrying tents, washing machines, stoves, refrigerators, hay dryers, and other kinds of electric machinery made its way through the Midwest and South. County newspapers and extension agents trumpeted their arrival. Under tents set up in open fields, big crowds—occasionally 5000 people in a single day—witnessed the magic of electricity.[38]

They also learned how "electricity pays its way in the rural home" from home electrification specialists like Louisan Mamer. A home-economics graduate of the University of Illinois, Mamer began working for the REA in 1935 and three years later became responsible for developing its Farm Tour publicity. After that she traveled around the country offering "study courses"—her elaborate, self-prepared curriculum—to female members of REA-financed cooperatives and 4-H clubs.

Mamer emphasized the housewife's partnership role in the family farm and business, and then demonstrated how electricity could help her "produce, provide, and prosper" in her "big job." Clothes cleaned quickly and easily in electric washers and hot meals cooked on electric stoves (and tasted by the audience) removed some doubts. More important were the testimonials from women who were using electricity. They reported that "it saves my food, my time, my energy, my money and, most of all, my disposition."[39]

By 1940 the REA had built 200,000 electrical lines and was serving over half a million consumers. The transformation was so remarkable that a grateful Tennessee farmer testified in church that "the greatest thing on earth is to have the love of God in your heart, and the next greatest thing is to have electricity in your house." An Iowa farm woman, within the reach of a transmission line and also blessed with several major appliances, described electricity as a "good fairy . . . [who] waved her magic wand across my path." However, not all farm women were so fortunate. Some would have to wait until after World War II for REA lines to reach them, while others had yet to "be given a square deal in the matter of home improvement."[40]

Farm women's magazines and agricultural agents continued to comment that, while most good farmers had the power equipment they needed in their barns and fields, their wives and daughters "still carr[ied] water into the house as women did a hundred years ago." Wives usually encouraged the purchase of a tractor or harvesting machine because it was good business and generally reduced the number of hired hands they had to feed. But they complained that the modern conveniences they desired had to wait for those "extra funds" that were always so hard to come by. What farm women wanted most was indoor plumbing; more than any other improvement, it would remove much of the physical drudgery from their lives.[41]

Running water would also help make their homes cleaner and healthier. Before electric lights revealed every corner cobweb, some women said they had no idea that their houses were "so dirty!" But lights, like irons and radios, were relatively inexpensive and easy to install. A ready supply of water for kitchen sinks, washing machines, and bathtubs was not. In 1939 self-installed plumbing equipment in a typical Iowa farmhouse cost about as much as a small tractor (approximately $500); plumbers could install the equipment, but they were frequently reluctant to accept jobs outside town and would charge more. That, however, was only the beginning. Once the pumps and pipes were in place, housewives eagerly anticipated—and occasionally fought for—the *next* new purchase that would bring them up to the level of city life. In Scott County, Indiana, Margaret Dean went "on a strike" against her husband until she acquired her first washing machine.[42]

In time, most rural women acquired the modern conveniences they had longed for. World War II brought high incomes to farm people and, eventually, cooperation between the private utilities and REA. In 1936, after its first year, REA served 8000 consumers; by 1940, over half a million; and by 1950, over three million. Only families living in the most remote areas of the country did not have service. Some farm folk even claimed that war was "the miracle" that "changed everything." In 1974 the mother of writer Alice Walker reminisced that in 1952 her sharefarmer shack outside Milledgeville, Georgia, gave her "one good thing"—"my first washing machine!"[43]

But these "good things" caused housekeeping standards and germ consciousness to escalate for rural women just as they had for urban women. More conveniences, ironically, made for more work, even though they could do it in less time and more easily. Jobs that housewives previously performed only once a week had by 1953 become a part of most daily routines. Helen Musselman of Hamilton County, Indiana, recalled her grandmother's amazement at the amount of time she spent cleaning the bathroom every day "in spite of all the convenience." The grandmother had done her washing on Monday, taken the used wash water to the privy, and scrubbed it out. "It was done once a week, and that was the chore." A less old-fashioned woman argued, however, that one of "the charms" of the electric washer was that "half a dozen extra sheets and towels . . . mean very little extra work."[44]

The War Changed Everything

In 1940, 72.9 percent of Americans surveyed by *Fortune* magazine considered themselves "middle-class." But it was not until the postwar years (1946–60) that these "middle-class" men and women could afford enough amenities and conveniences to live up to their aspirations and gain a piece of the Good Life. During the 1950s, for the first time in American history, white-collar workers verged on making up more than half of the labor force, and by 1960 the great majority of families described themselves as "middle-class," with more material reason than ever before. Thus most people could (and did) acquire what had formerly been *luxuries* only dreamed of. In the process, they achieved standards—even obsessions—of cleanliness that continue to mark American society.[45]

People's lives seemed to change almost overnight after the bombing of Pearl Harbor on December 7, 1941. As men left their jobs for the armed services, government recruitment campaigns promising good wages lured women into work places that previously had been off-limits. By 1944, 1.7 million women—married as well as single, black as well as white—were employed in steel, machinery, shipbuilding, aircraft, and auto factories. Five years earlier, only 230,000 women had these kinds of heavy-duty jobs. Rosie the Riveter had so won the public's patriotic support that the *Ladies' Home Journal* featured a fictional woman combat pilot on its cover.[46]

All in all, nineteen million women worked for wages at some time during the war years. However, the majority were not Rosie the Riveters. White women filled clerical or sales positions, while African-Americans once again had to be satisfied with blue-collar factory jobs that few whites would consider. Women worked largely because they needed to—not because they felt overly patriotic or desired a career. Once on the job they shied away from "dirty work" and were "much more concerned than [were] men about the general neatness and cleanliness of their surroundings, especially of the washrooms." Women fixed up dingy, old restrooms by adding wallpaper, curtains, or plants. And in factories where there were no restrooms for anybody, employers frequently installed new ones to improve morale.[47]

Unlike peacetime when most white women who had jobs were young and single, during the war older, married women worked in much larger numbers. By the spring of 1945, three million of the five million women with jobs were over thirty-five, and most of them were married with children. They hated leaving home, especially if they had youngsters or sick husbands and little help with the shopping, laundry, and housecleaning; many of them returned home quickly when the war ended. Their memories of the Depression, however, motivated them "to get what they could while they could."[48]

Fears of economic insecurity would influence the behavior of Americans for decades. One might think that the turn-around began in the 1940s since so many Americans earned better wages, opened savings accounts, and purchased war bonds. Yet few who experienced wartime inflation, shortages, and rationing became fully persuaded that their economic situation had permanently improved. For housewives, everyday life was tough even if they made good money. They became annoyed with the shortages of house-keeping goods (washing machines, vacuum cleaners, and irons), to say nothing of their frustration as they stood in line to exchange government coupons for sugar, meat, and soap. Adequate housing was so scarce, even well after V-J Day, that by 1947 six million families had doubled up with friends or relatives, while others set up housekeeping in the most unlikely and unacceptable places—tents, used trolley cars, chicken coops, and tool sheds.[49]

Mobile homes and trailers provided some relief but few comforts. Living in cramped quarters, with too few bathrooms and questionable water supplies, meant that hygiene was generally bad. Even families who had decent housing often took in less fortunate relatives or friends, and thus missed their privacy and found it hard to keep themselves and their houses clean. With adults and children living on top of one another, housekeeping became nearly impossible; with soap and washing machines so hard to find, housewives in cities adopted tried-and-true farm methods to do their laundry. The demand for good commercial laundries increased, but they were expensive for families to use; coin-operated machines were also a costly, and inconvenient, answer to household needs.[50]

African-American women, many of whom left the rural South for better-paying industrial jobs in the North, had a great deal more difficulty in finding places to live and ways to keep clean. And, on the job, they were sometimes shunned for being "dirty and diseased." But they never seemed too filthy or too sick to qualify as scrubwomen and janitors. If they were lucky enough to land a munitions job, they usually found themselves in locations where the work was dangerous or exceedingly unpleasant. In airplane assembly plants, for instance, they got hired in "dope rooms," where glue fumes were overpowering and often nauseating; they also found jobs among the blast furnaces of the sintering shops. Later, the Women's Bureau of the Department of Labor credited them with "moving as much dirt and material as men." It may have been because they worked around the clock. African-Americans regularly received night-shift assignments, which added more burdens on them as mothers and homemakers.[51]

Whatever the hours, conditions, or wages, American men and women at war anticipated and planned for peace. What did they hope for and desperately want? "Significant improvements in living," according to a national insurance company that advertised its "packaged mortgage" in late 1945. William Levitt, who would bring Henry Ford's mass production techniques to housing, recalled that he and his Navy buddies spent endless nights during the war talking about what they would do when it was over. It boiled down to this: if they weren't married, they were going to get married; and if they didn't have kids, they were going to have kids. But they worried most about where they would live. Probably with their parents, at least for a couple of years, since they had no other options.[52]

Women wanted much the same, which explains in good part "the rush to the altar and the delivery room." Raising a family and managing a home became the twin goals of most American women. The baby boom began in 1942, with full employment; after the war ended in 1945 young adults married in unprecedented numbers and gave birth to more children at shorter intervals. As wartime strains faded, men and women alike began to believe that they had been given another chance to get on with their lives. They sometimes acted quickly and seemed impatient with delays, but they generally made "life decisions on the basis of safety and security." Reacting to years of loneliness, deprivations, and postponements, they wanted to return to "normal" living—remembered nostalgically from the twenties. Not surprisingly, they longed for family togetherness and more prosperous times.[53]

Postwar life would be better, as Americans hoped, but it would never be quite the same. Of the millions of married women whom the war brought into the labor force, many were laid off or simply quit when war production ended; but others took sales, clerical, or service jobs. These did not pay as well and were sex-segregated, yet because of them society would gradually come to accept the idea of married women working outside the home. In 1950, 21 percent of all married white women held jobs. But most 1950s' women preferred "the family over work" and found more fulfillment in homemaking tasks than clerical ones. Having grown up during hard times, they associated economic insecurity and hardship with their mothers' employment. Thus, without a positive image of work and with few good jobs available, they chose domesticity.[54]

Strong cultural forces also came into play. Even during the war popular images of Rosie the Riveter did not seriously alter the age-old notion that a woman's place was in the home. And after the war good, well-adjusted moms like Harriet Nelson of *Ozzie and Harriet* and June Cleaver of *Leave It to Beaver* hardly ever left home for paying jobs. Femininity prohibited them from doing so, from competing with men. Instead they found happiness as wives and mothers. In marriage and motherhood, they discovered romance, a sense of purpose, and plenty of enjoyment. No one made mention of "the problem that has no name," the one Betty Friedan came upon in 1957 and revealed six years later in *The Feminine Mystique*. Perhaps everyone was too busy making up for lost time and chasing after their dreams.[55]

Looking for a "Cleaner Clean"

Owning a house represented, above all else, the quintessential American dream. By 1960 that dream had come true for 31 million of the nation's 44 million families, according to President Eisenhower in his State of the Union message. And most of these homes had modern kitchens, washing-machines, and at least one bathroom. Companies like Kohler had promised that "fine-quality plumbing fixtures and fittings," so limited during the war, would be available once victory was won, and they were. Until then Americans waited patiently, saved what they could, and even picked out a plot for a house with "more living space, greater utility with increased cleanliness and comfort."[56]

But their dream remained just that in 1945 and 1946. World War II veterans returned to find that the housing shortage they remembered all too well had not improved. Clamoring for places to live, they complained: "If this country can build an $80 billion war industry, make the atomic bomb and win the war, why can't it build enough houses?" In the end, it could and did, but not without healthy assistance from the federal government and a revolution in the construction industry. The single-family, mass-produced tract houses built in the late 1940s for young veterans and their families depended on mortgages underwritten by the Federal Housing Administration (FHA) and the GI bill.[57]

Many economists feared that the country would sink back into depression after the war. Had they gone out to suburban Long Island, where William Levitt was building new houses in an unusual way, they would have been greatly reassured. Short-story writer W. D. Wetherell later described the activity:

> Down the street is a Quonset hut with a long line of men waiting out in front, half of them still in uniform. Waiting for jobs I figure, like in the Depression . . . here we go again. But here's what happens. A truck comes along, stops in front of the house, half a dozen men pile out . . . in fifteen minutes they put in a bathroom. Pop! Off they go to the next house, just in time, too, because here comes another truck with the kitchen. Pop! In goes the kitchen. They move on one house, here comes the electricians. Pop! Pop! Pop! the house goes up. . . . And then it finally dawns on me. What these men are lined up for isn't work, it's homes![58]

Long Island's Levittown houses, built on concrete slabs in twenty-seven steps, were small and unimaginative, but well-built and reasonably priced. Ordinary citizens—principally war veterans and blue-collar workers—stood in line in October 1947 to buy their first houses: Cape Cod-like boxes with living room, kitchen, two bedrooms, and a bathroom. They cost $7,990 and required no down payment; nor were there closing costs or "hidden extras." "All yours for $58" a month, according to a *New York Times* ad. "Mr. Veteran" was indeed "a lucky fellow," for Levittown was the American dream reduced "to a practical and affordable reality."[59]

Levittown and many other communities like it succeeded, despite an avalanche of criticism. Architectural critics insisted that the homogenized houses were backward, bland, and lacking in dignity; local residents feared that mass-produced housing and low-income, first-time buyers would turn Levittown into a shanty town. They failed to understand, however, that these young Americans hungered for stability, normality, and "a piece of the American Dream." Cele Roberts, who bought a ranch model with her husband in 1949, recalled:

> The house was surrounded by a lake of mud. But I was thrilled—it was a very exciting thing to have a house of your own. And everything you dreamed about was there, everything was working, brand-new, no cockroaches. You got a beautiful stainless steel sink with two drains, cabinets, drawers, a three-burner General Electric stove with oven, a Bendix washing machine. The only thing I had to buy for the house when we moved in was a fluorescent tube over the kitchen sink.[60]

Well-constructed, inexpensive suburban housing with modern conveniences attracted young people who wanted to raise their children outside crowded and unsafe city neighborhoods. African-American veterans, who dreamed the same dreams and also hoped for an opportunity to get ahead, were denied the chance. In 1949 Gene Burnett read advertisements for Levittown in several newspapers, but, when he and his fiancée arrived there from East Harlem, a salesman refused to give them an application form. New suburban developments used restrictive covenants in sales or rental contracts (at first legally, then informally after 1948) that excluded primarily African-Americans but sometimes other minorities as well. Not until the late 1960s could they buy a house in Levittown or developments modeled after it. William Levitt's attitude was brutally frank: "We can solve a housing problem, or we can try to solve a racial problem. But we cannot combine the two." That injustice kept African-Americans from the dream for another twenty years.[61]

People who lived in white Levittown (eventually there were three of them)—or in Park Forest, Illinois, or Panorama City, California, for that matter—knew that their houses were not identical or monotonous, at least not for long. With space to expand and household goods available in welcome abundance, these first-time homeowners changed their "starters" into solid, middle-class houses. Typical postwar ads screamed: "Maytag's Making Washers Again!" and "Schick's Back—have you yours?" Encouraged by these come-ons, Americans went on a buying spree. With money saved during the war or credit recently acquired, they added furnishings, appliances, and entire rooms. Within record time, suburban homeowners could show off their country kitchens, garages, family rooms, and second (sometimes third) baths.[62]

During the 1950s, as family incomes increased along with family size, Americans began demanding more bathrooms in the average house. And once the Cape Cod and bungalow gave way to the spacious and informal ranch house, several bathrooms became commonplace. It was a way of ensuring privacy. Even inexpensive ranches usually included half-baths for guests, while expensive ones boasted luxurious bathroom suites (with both tub and shower) of "subtle colors and brass details" adjacent to master bedrooms. In *That Night* novelist Alice McDermott described a 1950s' master bedroom and bath: "Not a thing out of place, not a thing that didn't match. A gold swan spouting water in the bathroom sink, its wings Hot and Cold."[63]

As postwar kitchens became "all electric," they too, like bathrooms, became larger and more elaborate. In Levittown and elsewhere, the kitchen moved from the back of the house to the front; and in ranches, it usually found a place at the end of the house so that families could enter from the garage. Once inside, the most elaborate kitchens were "big, highly mechanized household factor[ies]," equipped with appliances "to make cooking and housework easy." During the 1950s the automatic washer (followed by the dryer and wash-and-wear fabrics in the 1960s) replaced the wringer washing machine. And the dishwasher, "the kitchen marvel that does dishes all by itself," became ubiquitous as did many other small, electric devices.[64]

It was this elaboration of rooms and "labor-saving" appliances that kept women as busy with housework as their mothers had been. This may seem obvious to us today, but the most routine habits have their beginnings and their history. And during the 1950s, despite the widespread availability of electric household tools, housewifery expanded to fill the time available. With washers and dryers at their command, more and more housewives began doing laundry every day; their husbands and children, as a result, learned to expect clean, pressed clothes every day, and often twice a day. Thus the new appliances, while reducing the drudgery, did not cut back the time women spent at the washtub and clothesline. Even with washers and dryers, women still had to load and unload the machines as well as sort, fold, iron, and put clothes away. Not to mention those compulsive super moms who began ironing sheets and underwear just to show how much they cared![65]

Growing sensitivity to smells also prompted homemakers to enlist themselves in "a clean fight" against "indoor odors"—household foes that seemed nearly as disturbing and pervasive as germs. Magazine advertisements and television commercials illustrated how unpleasant aromas presented "so many chances to offend." Cooking, bathroom, perspiration, smoking, and refrigerator odors were only a few of many that might embarrass or disgust family and friends. Thus "smart" housewives bought an excess of "freshening" products, tackled all those jobs nobody liked, and killed unwanted odors.[66]

At a time when women spent billions of dollars on toiletries, cosmetics, electric devices, and soaps, it is probably not surprising that the garbage disposer found its niche in the 1950s' kitchen. Presented as a "hunk of better living" that removed nauseous odors quickly and effortlessly, the disposer symbolized middle-class America's obsession with cleanliness and convenience. No other country became so captivated by this mundane household appliance, made it a public health benefit, and turned it into a required accoutrement of the Good Life. Not only did the disposer reduce the number of flies and rodents in and around houses, it also relieved housewives from the unsavory task of handling food wastes and freed their husbands and children from the distasteful chore of taking out the garbage.[67]

Although the disposer was never listed among the "glamour products" for the modern kitchen, it became a popular item, indeed a "must" for the "complete kitchen." In October 1958 the United Industry Committee for Housing and the National Association of Home Builders sponsored a Women's Conference on Housing in Washington, D.C. During the meeting, eighty-two women indicated how they would spend an imaginary $2500 on home improvements. From a list of nineteen items with their prices ($90 for a disposer), a majority selected the half-bath (41 votes) as their first need and a fireplace (25 votes) as second. The food-waste disposer took third place with 19 votes. Some of the items receiving 10 votes or less were dishwasher (10), dryer (6), central air conditioning (5), and a den or extra bedroom (2). There were no votes for the two-car garage. In 1959, in a "How's Your Home?" contest sponsored by the Home Improvement Council, the disposer again ranked third—after "more cabinets" and "clothes washer"—when 80,000 women listed their kitchen needs. That was the year when Vice President Nixon extolled the American way of life to Nikita Khrushchev—where else?—in a model kitchen.

Once it became apparent that the garbage disposer had "sales appeal," dealers staged colorful demonstrations to make their case to "Mrs. America." They cooperated with disposer manufacturers in putting together store window displays and exhibits at home shows, garnered free publicity in local newspapers, and developed long lists of leads. Direct mail campaigns told potential buyers how they could "refit" their kitchens at reasonable costs. Middle-class housewives responded well to these promotional efforts. In 1958 disposer sales topped $50 million for some half a million new units, and by 1959 figures showed that more than 4 million homes had garbage disposers. Two years later at least fourteen companies manufactured models ranging in price from $60 to $130 including installation.

When asked why they bought a disposer, women responded consistently that with it "there was no more garbage." And once they eliminated garbage they also did away with "insects and rodents," "trips to the back alley in rain and snow," "nauseous odors," "clutter in the sink," "nasty scrubbing and re-lining of garbage pails," and "arguments about 'whose turn it is to take out the garbage.'" Repeating again and again that the disposer was "indispensable" and that they "wouldn't trade it for anything," few women complained about the appliance's performance. Some disliked the grinding noise, but most said that it was only a minor annoyance. In short, the garbage disposer sold because it was "simple, safe, and sanitary."

For similar reasons, feminine hygiene products also sold in great quantities. Kotex was not only simple to use but promised a "special safety," while Tampax "never allow[ed] a hint of odor." Sanitary napkins were also disposable. Women who could afford them, when they first became available in the 1920s, no longer had to endure the unwelcome chore of laundering soiled cloths or rags. After World War II, most women could and did buy "sanitary protection." But freed from one burden, they discovered new and hidden dangers from 1950s' ads, which were far more threatening than the discreet ones of the 1930s. Vaginal odors and underarm wetness could not only spoil women's fun, but also undermine their confidence and make them unattractive and unlovable. To guard against such possibilities, a Veto deodorant ad urged women to "double check your charm everyday" since "you are the very air he breathes."[68]

The advertising industry did not exclude men and children from their reach. Dial soap, for example, promised it could help the whole family "stay fresh hour after hour," while Gleem sold itself as a "family" toothpaste for those "who can't brush after every meal." Yet marketers continued to assign women responsibility for cleanliness—it was their duty to see that "he wears the *cleanest* shirts in town." Clean clothes and clean bodies were now prerequisites for success and happiness.[69]

Considerations of health, which had been so important before World War II, ceased to be a primary reason for cleanliness after 1945. The contagious diseases that had plagued Americans for nearly all of their history had virtually disappeared. The Salk and Sabine polio vaccines and new antibiotics such as penicillin and streptomycin played major roles, as did better public works and housing. By the 1950s, three out of every four American families had indoor plumbing and water closets. Imaginative ways and reasons to use water (and waste it) proved boundless.[70]

Teenagers, who numbered eighteen million by 1960 and spent $10 billion a year on their culture, regarded access to the bathroom as essential to their appearance. There are no figures available to show that families with teenagers used more water and electricity than those without, but parents of the 1950s as well as those of today could testify that monthly water and electric bills were significantly higher when their teenage children lived at home. Girls, particularly readers of magazines like *Seventeen*, learned the intricacies of cleanliness as well as how to be women from advertising and high school "health" classes that placed increased emphasis on "good grooming." By the late 1950s, almost half of the nation's young women married after high school, when they were still teenagers—eighteen, in fact, was "the single most common age at which American girls married."[71]

"Often a bridesmaid . . . Never a bride," a popular Listerine ad slogan, unnerved scores of young women who feared rejection because of bad breath or some other infraction of cleanliness standards. The "right" appearance became everything, more important than personality or character in shaping one's fate. Advertisers knew it and played upon it. Thus, even though teenage girls averaged lower allowances and earned less money than boys, by 1957 they spent nearly three times as much on grooming and clothing. In 1958 alone they bought $25 million worth of deodorants and preferred an "antiseptic" soap like Dial because it "stops odor before its starts" and *"guarantees* . . . freshness round the clock."[72]

During the 1950s, American culture offered middle-class status to a large majority of its people. In a 1952 poll of high school teenagers, for example, 48 percent of all students with "low" incomes identified themselves as middle-class, as did 59 percent of those whose fathers had "mid-level jobs working with tools" and 52 percent of those whose mothers had only a grade-school education. Undoubtedly the increased prosperity and improved living conditions of the postwar years encouraged more American families to think of themselves as middle-class. And as they did so they "bought into" the culture of cleanliness. Afraid of backsliding and scared of offending, they became the main market for an endless supply of deodorants, mouthwashes, shavers, improved detergents, kitchen appliances, and bathroom fixtures.[73]

Although most rural whites and African-Americans were unable to share in this bounty for at least another decade or two, urban and suburban Americans had succeeded as dirt-chasers. In 1958 *Newsweek* reported that each year Americans not only spent about $200 million on products that made them smell better, but they also took more than 500 million baths each week. What the story didn't say, and probably saw no need to, was that Americans took their baths and used their deodorants in the privacy of their *own* homes. Nearly a century after their dirt chasing began in earnest, Americans were known worldwide for their cleanliness—sophisticated plumbing, luxurious bathrooms, daily habits of bathing or showering, soft toilet tissue, shiny teeth and hair, and spotless clothes. The "American Century" had arrived, with its luminous ideal—much less often the reality—that forgot the grimy, diseased nineteenth-century past and ignored the "other America" of the poor, which Michael Harrington revealed, as no one else had, in 1962.[74]

Yet, even as personal cleanliness was recognized as a quintessentially American value, public places became dirtier. According to Edna Ferber, the well-traveled novelist, New York City was "the most disgustingly filthy" city in the world in the mid-1950s, and litter and rubbish had already begun to turn "ribbons of green countryside along the highways into casual dumps." In the eyes of attentive observers, there were too many common spaces in urban areas and along public thoroughfares that were "a national disgrace."[75]

A Glimmer of Green

By the 1950s Americans had come to value cleanliness for personal reasons, but they failed to recognize the connection between how they behaved at home and what they did in public. They hardly ever heard the word "environment," and they considered "conservation" the responsibility of government officials and scientists rather than private citizens. With the disappearance of contagious diseases that had made earlier generations wary of the sanitary conditions of their streets and streams, Americans no longer worried that loved ones might die of cholera. Postwar prosperity brought more purchases of what had once been luxuries, more leisure time spent out-of-doors and on vacations, and more accumulations of trash and litter in public places. "Litterbags" had not yet sensitized Americans to the value of clean parks, beaches, or roadways, and most adults considered recycling a wartime conservation measure.[76]

The postwar rise in incomes and the acquisition of a family car made it possible for a great number of Americans to live outside industrial communities and to travel to locations they had only heard about or seen in photographs. In 1950, for the first time, eight million motor vehicles rolled off the assembly lines. Thus, even before the massive investment of federal funds into interstate highway construction that started in 1956, many Americans had become dependent on their cars. People who could not yet afford to buy one began to see it, along with the suburban tract house, as part and parcel of the American dream.

Automobile owners, like homeowners, took pride in the appearance of their purchases. Women especially wanted the family car to be safe, comfortable, and clean as well as stylish and well built. In fact, on car trips, they generally transferred their domestic routines to the road. Unlike their husbands and children, wives and mothers seldom escaped housekeeping chores; instead they found themselves buying groceries, doing laundry, and keeping the automobile and camping gear clean. But almost no one took responsibility for the highways, parks, and campsites they used while vacationing. In the 1950s few Americans understood how an unclean environment could harm them, and fewer still felt any sense of ownership over outdoor areas other than their backyards.[77]

Widespread ignorance was only part of the problem. The unprecedented growth in the packaging industry during the 1950s and 1960s was another. Between 1958 and 1976 packaging consumption rose 63 percent and contributed markedly to the "throwaway" ethic of postwar American society, one distinguished for its affluence as well as for its love of convenience and personal cleanliness. Paper cups, towels, and handkerchiefs had all been introduced after World War I; their disposable and sanitary features increasingly made them popular products in homes, schools, offices, and factories. But packaging—which included cans, bottles, and plastic as well as paper— became extremely important in the two decades after World War II. American consumers not only liked conveniently and securely wrapped goods, but they also sold more products as self-service supermarkets, department stores, and fast-food restaurants spread across the country.[78]

The proliferation of packaging aggravated the litter problem, both in cities and along rural roads and the thousands of miles of new interstate highways. Individuals who would never have thrown paper cups or beer cans in their own yard or their neighbor's garden unhesitatingly flung them from car windows; they also left large amounts of trash behind, especially in city streets. In 1954, one New York City observer remarked that "everything—but everything—finds its way to the streets"; however, instead of the "old-fashioned garbage," it was paper, cans, and bottles of every sort. And litter begot litter. It set up a "psychological chain reaction" that almost certainly made a dirty street dirtier.[79]

In an attempt to curb this nationwide problem before state legislatures took unwanted action against them, representatives of the packaging industry organized the "Keep Our Roadsides Clean Council" in October 1953 in New York City. Chaired by W. C. Stolk of the American Can Company, this group, which later chose the name "Keep America Beautiful," became the first national antilitter association. Although it had strong ties to the beverage container industry, KAB decided to focus attention on public education and emphasize individual and community responsibility. It did little to alter the packaging business itself; however, KAB did include individuals from outside the industry on an advisory council, stating that it wanted its programs against littering to "have the broadest support at the earliest possible date."[80]

In May 1954, at the advisory council's initial meeting, at least thirty people from government agencies and public interest groups joined the packaging executives and expressed a desire to clean up America and keep it beautiful. The "nonindustry" representatives came from such institutions as the U.S. Forest Service, the National Parks Association, the National Council of State Garden Clubs, the Girl and Boy Scouts of America, and the Nature Conservancy. Although only advisory, they made their presence felt from the beginning. Two women from the state garden clubs, for instance, tied their organization's future involvement to KAB's promise not to use billboards to remind motorists against littering.[81]

It is true that the nation's environmental consciousness was not adequately raised until the celebration of Earth Day on April 22, 1970. But it is untrue that the years immediately following World War II were entirely driven by "careless optimism and materialism" and were completely devoid of environmental concern. Despite KAB's connections to the packaging industry, its campaigns during the 1950s prompted many Americans to alter their ignorant outdoor habits—ones that KAB contended "offended our normal desire for neatness and cleanliness." "Litterbags" and "litterbugs," words that KAB made so popular and ultimately proved so effective in drawing attention to the need for public cleanliness, entered the language and began to change some people's behavior.[82]

During the 1960s KAB's "Crying Indian" proved even more influential. In a striking public-service television spot, Iron Eyes Cody paddled his canoe down an oil-drenched stream whose banks were laden with refuse and litter, and he shed a tear for the damage done to America ever since Columbus—and the Europeans who followed him—wrecked the pristine beauty of the landscape. The image was powerful, and millions took notice of the Indian's message: "People Start Pollution; People Can Stop It." KAB again stressed individual responsibility in achieving public cleanliness. And through a subsequent program, entitled the Clean Community System,

KAB showed local communities (265 had signed up by 1982) how to promote a sense of pride and ownership among their citizens. For, according to KAB-sponsored research, people littered when they believed someone else would clean up after them—usually the much maligned "garbageman"—or where trash had already accumulated. A litter-measuring technique developed by the American Public Works Association, one of the organizational members of KAB's Advisory Council, helped cities and counties identify major problem areas and develop practical ways of improving them.[83]

Antilittering campaigns, frequently overlooked or minimized in environmental histories, challenged ingrained habits and attitudes regarding outdoor cleanliness. They were not, however, the only force for change before the beginning of the environmental movement in the 1970s. The packaging industry, considered by some as a major source of pollution, may have been a surprising advocate of antilittering, but the long-haired hippies and unshaven students of the New Left were also unexpected champions of an endangered earth. These "revolutionaries," often sons and daughters of middle-class Americans, sought to overthrow the culture of cleanliness by their "countercultural" disregard of accepted standards of personal hygiene. In disavowing what they saw as the materialism, hypocrisy, and consumerism of their parents' generation, they hoped to create a "new order" in which life styles reflected a reverence for nature and consciousness-raising resulted in ecology centers.[84]

One of the best and most satisfying ways for young adults of the 1960s to thumb their noses at middle-class American values was to swear off soap and water. Personal cleanliness had become so embedded in national life that the hippies paid an unwitting, ironic tribute to its power when they ostentatiously junked it in favor of scraggly beards, stringy hair, and smelly bodies. In 1966, California Governor Ronald Reagan remarked that a hippie was somebody who " 'dresses like Tarzan, has hair like Jane, and smells like Cheetah.' " To mystified observers like Reagan, the behavior of the young signified bad manners and slovenliness; but to the "flower children" themselves, their appearance indicated "a turn from straight to curved, from uptight to loose, from cramped to free—above all, from contrived to natural."[85]

Drawn to the natural and unspoiled, the counterculture identified with the Native Americans. Their attractiveness emanated from their "primitiveness" as well as from the belief that they were oppressed, "nobly savage," and uniquely American. Many of the 1960s' fledgling ecologists also believed that the Native Americans, not unlike KAB's Iron Eyes Cody, cherished the earth and feared that its survival was at stake. In 1969, when an oil well exploded off the coast of Santa Barbara, California, these young people (among others) were predictably outraged. A year later, when 100,000 Americans came together for an environmental teach-in on Earth Day, college students—the majority of whom had been part of the counterculture or certainly influenced by it—formed the largest segment.[86]

Earth Day created a "tidal wave of public opinion in favor of cleaning up the environment." But the groundswell actually began in 1962 with publication of *Silent Spring*. This environmental classic alerted Americans to what its author, Rachel Carson, characterized as the "grim specter" that had "crept upon us almost unnoticed." She explained in powerful prose the dangers of pesticides to wildlife and made clear the worldwide disasters that would result from the indiscriminate use of toxic chemicals. Besides taking on the agricultural chemical industry, Carson introduced millions to the idea that the natural world was interconnected and that the destruction of nature included human life.[87]

Since the late nineteenth century, women sanitarians and conservationists had been instrumental in making the urban environment a cleaner and healthier place in which to live. None of them, however, received the measure of influence and recognition that Carson enjoyed before her death in 1964. Paradoxically, somewhat like the founders of Keep America Beautiful or the young radicals who formed rural communes to demonstrate their oneness with nature, Carson also seemed an unlikely defender of the earth and its living populations. Few of her contemporaries would have guessed that such a self-effacing, reclusive woman scientist and writer could have forced the world to take "a new direction." Yet, following the huge success of *The Sea Around Us* in 1951, one reader (who disregarded the name Rachel) believed so knowledgeable an author "must be a man." As in the past, women's efforts against outdoor pollution—especially those that fell into the broad, familiar categories of "municipal housekeeping" or "community beautification"—usually went unnoticed or were trivialized. Lady Bird Johnson, who shared with Carson an unusual concern for the natural environment, has only recently received the acknowledgment she deserves.[88]

Lady Bird's campaign to clean up and beautify America contributed substantively to a new consciousness about the environment. Despite the fact that outdoor advertising agencies continued to find ways to place billboards along the nation's roadsides, the 1965 Highway Beautification Act was a "significant legislative achievement." It focused an unusual amount of attention on the twin problems of billboards and junkyards. Lady Bird, who worked closely with Secretary of the Interior Stewart Udall, also committed herself to creating "a clean country" through conservation as well as beautification programs. She used her influence as First Lady to prepare the way for the conservation initiatives of the Johnson administration, which became a foundation of the environmental movement. Thus Lady Bird's causes served as a kind of bridge "from the older style of conservation to the ecological spirit of the 1970s."[89]

Earth Day ushered in "the heyday of environmentalism," and Congress responded to a vigorous public demand. In the early 1970s, it passed a surprising number of laws to clean up the nation—the National Environmental Policy Act, the Clean Air Act, the Water Pollution Control Act, the Safe Drinking Water Act, and the Resource Conservation and Recovery Act, to name the most important ones. Nearly all of the new statutes placed the burden of proof on polluters; they had to demonstrate that their actions did not damage or dirty their surroundings. Because Americans supported tough laws to protect the environment, politicians everywhere became "environmentalists," whatever their positions on particular policies. In the thirty years following World War II, the country underwent a revolution in favor of a cleaner, greener environment.[90]

Although the crusade to clean up and preserve the nation continues, the land, water, air, and wildlife are improved and, in many cases, better than they have been since the late nineteenth century. Americans still consume too great a proportion of the world's resources; they have rarely adopted recycling measures that would force both manufacturers and consumers to reuse half of what they produce or throw away; and they often leave litter in public places that are hard to keep clean or where they feel anonymous, most notably on the highways and in the streets of the largest cities. Nevertheless, in the 1950s and 1960s, Americans began to shift the balance from their obsession with personal cleanliness to a greater concern for the environment, which would define the 1970s.[91]

Cleanliness had come far and taken surprising turns since the advent of home economics and all-electric kitchens. During the 1950s, rural America embraced the culture of cleanliness as ardently as the cities and suburbs had done. Yet once cleanliness peaked nationwide, like so many other values of the Eisenhower era, it started to receive some knocks. Contagious diseases were no longer killers to be fought with detergents; "getting ahead" demanded a college degree more often than a gleaming smile; environmental littering proved more troublesome than rings-around-the-collar; and homemaking was seen as something less than every woman's total fulfillment. The old rationales for chasing dirt had lost some of their punch.

Are We as Clean as We Used to Be?

Probably not. At least, that's my quick and dirty answer to the one question I am most frequently asked. People who learn about my research—especially women in their forties and fifties—almost always tell me that they are not like their mothers; they are not as obsessed or as compulsive about cleanliness. They never arrange their spices in alphabetical order, iron their sheets and pillowcases, or scrub the kitchen floor on their hands and knees. Yet, most of them would agree that "a sparkling clean bathtub is truly a beautiful sight," and occasionally a few would admit to having found some satisfaction in the "scut work" of homemaking, especially if it were appreciated and they had the time to do it.[1]

In recent years, however, more women have had less time. By early 1986, 64 percent of all women under the age of sixty-five were part of the American labor force. Most of them did not have high-powered positions or enviable careers. A large majority had service, sales, or clerical jobs where the salaries were low, opportunities for advancement minimal, and the work generally routine. In 1990 about 20 million Americans, a large percentage of whom were women, held part-time jobs, and many needed full-time ones. Growing numbers of women supported themselves and their children without the help of a man.[2]

Nevertheless, when it came to cooking and cleaning, it seemed to matter very little whether there was a man around the house since so few husbands or fathers regularly cooked or cleaned—even those married to women at the top. Although they worked away from home, wives and mothers "usually remain[ed] the household's primary cook, dishwasher, and cleaner." As recent as 1990 the only chore that the sexes seemed to share equally was grocery shopping, and it was the woman's responsibility to make out the grocery list. When couples shared more than shopping for groceries, women did "two-thirds of the *daily* jobs . . . like cooking and cleaning up." In effect, they got the "second shift," which meant that they had to juggle housework and children as well as a job.[3]

A few women became "supermoms" and did it all, but the vast majority decided to put first things first—family and jobs over traditional standards of cooking and cleaning. They did not prepare elaborate meals, nor did they do the laundry every day. One woman, whose mother cleaned the house "from top to bottom before the maid came," said: "If I don't see dirt, it doesn't bother me. . . . So I just don't look." Some who chose to live among clutter and not see the dirt even learned to rid themselves of their cleanliness hang-ups. A wife and mother who has rejected the standards of the 1950s explained it this way: "There was this notion that your floor had to be so clean that you could eat off it. Well, that's ridiculous—we don't eat off floors." With less "antiseptic standards," husbands have sometimes been more willing to relieve their wives of the burden of cleanliness by doing the laundry, bathing the children, and cleaning up after dinner.[4]

Relief has also come from an age-old practice—*hiring* dirt chasers. Today's cleaners appear in a variety of forms that range from seasonal window washers to live-in maids. But, since dirt-chasing continues to bring little profit or pleasure, those who are employed as full-time housekeepers and nannies are almost always poor. Many are minority women who, if given a choice, would prefer working in their own homes. Many others are recent immigrants, whose presence in American households received unexpected attention in early 1993, when Zoe Baird had to withdraw her nomination for United States Attorney General because she had not paid the required Social Security taxes for her Peruvian servants. Unlike Baird, though, most working mothers cannot afford to hire live-in household help. Instead they are forced to rely more heavily on their husbands and older children, commercial dry cleaners, and housecleaning businesses.[5]

During the 1980s the housecleaning services industry boomed. By the end of the decade, 7200 franchised and non-franchised maid companies were doing business in the United States. Molly Maid, one of the fastest growing franchises, began in Canada in 1979; succeeding there, it spread to the United States during the mid-1980s. Because of the low start-up costs and five-day work weeks (with few evenings), Molly Maid franchises attracted as owners women and married couples who wanted "to be their own boss" and who knew how to clean. Their employees, who did the actual cleaning, were—as one would expect—all women. They worked in teams of two, wore blue-and-white uniforms modeled after those of English maids, and drove "Molly Maid" marked cars. Team leaders earned $8 to $10 an hour, and their assistants made between $6 and $8. Molly Maid owners, who were bonded and insured, charged clients between $45 and $95 a visit and paid their employees' Social Security taxes and workers' compensation.[6]

Whether housecleaning services become so successful and affordable that they actually free women (and some men) from time-consuming chores remains to be seen. We should not forget that commercial laundries were popular in the 1920s until the new electric washers and dryers put them out of business. And on and off for about fifty years before that, groups of feminists had experimented with ways to socialize domestic work by establishing neighborhood day-care centers and public kitchens as well as commercial laundries. But these alternatives failed to free middle-class women from the sole responsibility for housework for a variety of reasons. Above all, the reformers excused men from participating in their ventures and employed instead lower-income women to do the chores that nobody else would do. Second, middle-class families (men and women alike) refused to relinquish their privacy and autonomy for efficiency and leisure; they did not want to eat meals in community kitchens or wash clothes in public laundries. In the end, these experiments saved some women's labor, but they did so in a world where that labor cost very little.[7]

Twentieth-century women who worked at home—cleaning, cooking, caring for children—were, after all, *just* housewives. Since they were not compensated for their services, their work not only seemed less real than men's work but also less significant and increasingly less valued. Many women disliked "the triviality of housekeeping" and got tired of "looking at the eggy plates in the sink, at the dirt, the lost clothes balled up under the bed." It may have filled their days, but it kept them running on empty. As their families' need for income increased, especially during the 1970s and 1980s, more wives and mothers took jobs away from home. That, in short, explains the crack in the culture of cleanliness, which is definitely on the wane. But all is not completely lost. For most Americans can still rely on the much appreciated, ever available shower. "Oh, I don't clean the shower—I clean myself," said a man in Newton, Massachusetts. "At least, if my house is dirty, I'm clean."[8]

NOTES

INTRODUCTION

1. "Housing: What Can Be Done?," *Life*, Dec. 17, 1945, p. 36.

2. So did writers for women's magazines. See Carole Cleaver, "A Dirty Story," *Mademoiselle*, April 1958, p. 46. As late as 1985, a similar occurrence provoked "razor-sharp" judgments. One woman told "Dear Abby" that if "Rapunzel Legs" is "too lazy to shave, she should move to Europe"; another remarked that "in Europe it's considered sexy. But then Europeans . . . think sweat and other natural body odors are sexy. Pee—ooey!" Abigail Van Buren, "Non-Shaver Prompts Razor-Sharp Replies," *Raleigh Times*, July 17, 1985.

3. "Cleanliness: The Germ's Last Stand?," *Newsweek*, Nov. 24, 1958, p. 99.

CHAPTER 1. DREADFULLY DIRTY

1. Mark Twain, *Life on the Mississippi* [1883] (New York: Signet Classic, 1980), 29.

2. John Wesley, "Sermon XCIII.—On Dress," in *Sermons on Several Occasions* [1788] (2 vols.; New York, 1829), II: 259. Richard L. Bushman and Claudia L. Bushman, "The Early History of Cleanliness in America," *Journal of American History* 74 (March 1988): 1219, 1222.

3. As described by Faye E. Dudden, *Serving Women: Household Service in Nineteenth-Century America* (Middletown, Conn.: Wesleyan Univ. Press, 1983), 137–45.

4. Daniel T. Rodgers's phrase; see his *The Work Ethic in Industrial America, 1850–1920* (Chicago: Univ. of Chicago Press, 1978), 9–10 (quote).

5. Leonard W. Labaree, Ralph L. Ketcham, Helen C. Boatfield, and Helene H. Fineman, eds., *The Autobiography of Benjamin Franklin* (New Haven: Yale Univ. Press, 1964), 149–50, 202, 203, 207.

6. Norman S. Fiering, "Benjamin Franklin and the Way to Virtue," *American Quarterly* 30 (Summer 1978): 214, 216 (quote), 219 (quote); L. W. Labaree, Whitfield J. Bell, Jr., Helen C. Boatfield, and Helene H. Fineman, eds., *The Papers of Benjamin Franklin*, vol. I: *January 6, 1706 through December 31, 1734* (New Haven: Yale Univ. Press, 1959), 348 (quote). Rodgers, *The Work Ethic in Industrial America*, 9–10.

7. Michael C. Robinson, "Community Water Supply," in Ellis L. Armstrong, Michael C. Robinson, and Suellen M. Hoy, eds., *History of Public Works in the United States 1776–1976* (Chicago: American Public Works Association, 1976), 217–19.

8. Ibid., 219–22.

9. James Marston Fitch, *American Building*, vol. I: *The Historical Forces that Shaped It* (Boston: Houghton Mifflin, 1966), 22. Rose Lockwood, "Birth, Illness and Death in 18th-Century New England," *Journal of Social History* 12 (Fall 1978): 120.

10. Quoted in Harvey Green, *Fit for America: Health, Fitness, Sport and American Society* (New York: Pantheon, 1986), 10. See also Susan E. Cayleff, *Wash and Be Healed: The Water-Cure Movement and Women's Health* (Philadelphia: Temple Univ. Press, 1987); and Richard H. Shryock, "Sylvester Graham and the Popular Health Movement, 1830–1870," *Mississippi Valley Historical Review* 18 (Sept. 1931): 172–83.

11. Walter Nugent, *Structures of American Social History* (Bloomington: Indiana Univ. Press, 1981), 79–80; Tamara K. Hareven, "Family Time and Industrial Time: Family and Work in a Planned Corporation Town, 1900–1924," *Journal of Urban History* 1 (May 1975): 371.

12. Rodgers, *The Work Ethic in Industrial America*, 18; Nugent, *Structures of American Social History*, 81.

13. William Cobbett, *A Year's Residence in the United States of America* [1819] (Carbondale: Southern Illinois Univ. Press, 1964), 29; James Haines, "Social Life and Scenes in the Early Settlement of Central Illinois," *Transactions of the Illinois State Historical Society for the Year 1905* (Springfield: Illinois State Historical Society Library, 1906), 39; and R. Carlyle Buley, *The Old Northwest: Pioneer Period, 1815–1840* (Indianapolis: Indiana Historical Society, 1950), 210 (quote).

14. Jack Larkin, *The Reshaping of Everyday Life, 1790–1840* (New York: Harper & Row, 1988), 184–85; Cobbett, *A Year's Residence*, 32; Ruth Schwartz Cowan, *More Work for Mother: The Ironies of Household Technology from the Open Hearth to the Microwave* (New York: Basic Books, 1983), 26.

15. Quotations are from the following: W. Faux, *Memorable Days in America: Being a Journal of a Tour to the United States, Principally Undertaken to Ascertain, By Positive Evidence, The Condition and Probable Prospects of British Emigrants* [London, 1823], reprinted in Volume XI of Reuben Gold Thwaites, ed., *Early Western Travels, 1748–1846* (Cleveland: Arthur H. Clark, 1905), 198, 213, 214, 226, 230; James Stuart, *Three Years in North America* (2 vols.; Edinburgh: Oliver and Boyd, 1833), II: 273; and Harriet Martineau, *Society in America* (2 vols.; New York, 1837), II: 260.

16. Janet R. Walker and Richard W. Burkhardt, eds., *Eliza Julia Flower: Letters of an English Gentlewoman: Life on the Illinois-Indiana Frontier, 1817–1861* (Muncie, Ind.: Ball State University, 1991), 22, 23, 41 (quote), 44 (quote), 153 (quote).

17. Explicit descriptions of everyday life in the early nineteenth century include Buley, *Old Northwest*, 210–34; Christiana Holmes Tillson, *A Woman's Story of Pioneer Illinois* (Chicago: R. R. Donnelley & Sons, 1919), xiv, 104; Larkin, *Reshaping of Everyday Life 1790–1840*, 127–32; and Cobbett, *A Year's Residence*, 178.

18. Louis B. Wright and Marion Tinling, eds., *Quebec to Carolina in 1785–1786: Being the Travel Diary and Observations of Robert Hunter, Jr., a Young Merchant of London* (San Marino: Huntington Library, 1943), 7, 236, 281, 282, 288–89.

19. Frederick Law Olmsted first sent a series of dispatches to the *New York Times*, then brought them out in three volumes between 1856 and 1860; he finally published *The Cotton Kingdom*, a two-volume version in 1861. Quotations are from

Frederick Law Olmsted, *The Cotton Kingdom: A Traveller's Observations on Cotton and Slavery in the American Slave States. Based on Three Former Volumes of Journeys and Investigations by the Same Author* (2 vols.; New York: Mason Brothers, 1861), I: 168, 181, 202, 206, 368; II: 9–10, 56, 148–49.

20. "Summer Conveniences," *Harper's Bazaar* 2 (Aug. 21, 1869): 531.

21. Helen Stuart MacKay-Smith Marlatt, ed., *Stuart Letters of Robert and Elizabeth Sullivan Stuart and Their Children, 1819–1864* (Privately printed, 1961), 558; and William Oliver, *Eight Months in Illinois: With Information to Immigrants* [1843] (Chicago: Walter M. Hill, 1924), 76–77.

22. Quotations are from Harriet Connor Brown, *Grandmother Brown's Hundred Years, 1827–1927* (Boston: Little, Brown, 1930), 57–58; Buley, *Old Northwest*, 233; Fredrika Bremer, *The Homes of the New World: Impressions of America* (2 vols.; New York: Harper & Brothers, 1853), I: 281.

23. Joseph C. Robert, *The Story of Tobacco in America* [1949] (Chapel Hill: Univ. of North Carolina Press, 1967), 101–5; Buley, *Old Northwest*, 364; Paul M. Angle, "The Hardy Pioneer: How He Lived in the Early Middle West," in Davis Lecture Committee, ed., *Essays in the History of Medicine: In Honor of David J. Davis* (Chicago: Univ. of Illinois Press, 1965), 141; Martineau, *Society in America*, I: 310; II: 200; Isabella Lucy Bird, *The Englishwoman in America* [1856] (Madison: Univ. of Wisconsin Press, 1966), 147–48; Charles Dickens, *American Notes for General Circulation* (New York, 1842), 44 (quote); Frances Trollope, *Domestic Manners of the Americans* [1832] (New York: Dodd, Mead, 1949), 58 (quote).

24. Larkin, *Reshaping of Everyday Life*, 157–58.

25. "Washing Made Easy," *Godey's Magazine and Lady's Book*, 48 (April 1854): 379 (quote). See also Susan Strasser, *Never Done: A History of American Housework* (New York: Pantheon, 1982), especially "Blue Monday," 104–24; Francis H. Underwood, *Quabbin: The Story of a Small Town with Outlooks upon Puritan Life* (Boston: Lee and Shepard), 162; and Eliza Leslie, *The House Book: Or, A Manual of Domestic Economy for Town and Country* (Philadelphia: Cary & Hart, 1845), 8 (quote).

26. Walker and Burkhardt, eds., *Eliza Julia Flower*, 90.

27. Quotations are from Linda J. Borish, "Farm Females, Fitness, and the Ideology of Physical Health in Antebellum New England," *Agricultural History* 64 (Fall 1990): 24 and 23 respectively.

28. Buley, *Old Northwest*, 234–35.

29. Ibid., 236; Larkin, *Reshaping of Everyday Life*, 131–32; Frances Anne Kemble, *Journal of a Residence on a Georgian Plantation in 1838–1839* [1863] (New York: Alfred A. Knopf, 1961), 100 (quote).

30. Joel A. Tarr, "Urban Pollution—Many Long Years Ago," *American Heritage* 22 (Oct. 1971): 65–66; and Trollope, *Domestic Manners*, 39.

31. Angle, "The Hardy Pioneer," 143; Buley, *Old Northwest*, 236; Edgar W. Martin, *The Standard of Living in 1860: American Consumption Levels on the Eve of the Civil War* (Chicago: Univ. of Chicago Press, 1942), 89.

32. Buley, *Old Northwest*, 233; Larkin, *Reshaping of Everyday Life*, 163.

33. Susan Warner, *The Wide, Wide World* [1850] (New York: Feminist Press, 1987), 103–5, 174–75, 584; and Jane Tompkins, *Sensational Designs: The Cultural Work of American Fiction, 1790–1860* (New York: Oxford Univ. Press, 1985), 148.

34. Lucy Larcom, *A New England Girlhood* [1889] (Gloucester, Mass.: Peter Smith, 1973), 168.

35. Catherine Cebra Webb, "Diary, 1815–1816," in Emily Noyes Vanderpoel and Elizabeth C. Barney Buel, eds., *Chronicles of a Pioneer School: From 1792 to 1833, Being the History of Miss Sarah Pierce and Her Litchfield School* (Cambridge, Mass.: Univ. Press, 1903), 150; and Underwood, *Quabbin*, 80.

36. E. Douglas Branch, *The Sentimental Years, 1836–1860* (New York: D. Appleton-Century, 1934), 59; Harold Donald Eberlein, "When Society First Took a Bath," *Pennsylvania Magazine of History and Biography* 67 (Jan. 1943): 45–46; and Jacqueline S. Wilkie, "Submerged Sensuality: Technology and Perceptions of Bathing," *Journal of Social History* 19 (Summer 1986): 650.

37. By 1860 the nation's sixteen largest cities had waterworks, with a total of 136 systems; 57 were public, 79 private. The majority of nineteenth-century cities, however, had no underground drains. Street gutters of wood or stone removed stormwater and sometimes human wastes. Armstrong, Robinson, and Hoy, eds., *History of Public Works in the United States, 1776–1976*, 217–22, 399–402. Nelson Manfred Blake, *Water for the Cities: A History of the Urban Water Supply Problem in the United States* (Syracuse: Syracuse Univ. Press, 1956), 265–71; Stanley Lebergott, *The American Economy: Income, Wealth, and Want* (Princeton: Princeton Univ. Press, 1976), 163–64.

38. May N. Stone, "The Plumbing Paradox: American Attitudes toward Late Nineteenth-Century Domestic Sanitary Arrangements," *Winterthur Portfolio* 14 (Autumn 1979): 285 (quote). See also Martin, *Standard of Living in 1860*, 89–90; and Joel A Tarr, James McCurley, and Terry F. Yosie, "The Development and Impact of Urban Wastewater Technology: Changing Concepts of Water Quality Control, 1850–1930," in Martin V. Melosi, ed., *Pollution & Reform in American Cities, 1870–1930* (Austin: Univ. of Texas Press, 1980), 59–63.

39. Lebergott, *The American Economy*, 263.

40. Jean H. Baker, *Mary Todd Lincoln: A Biography* (New York: W. W. Norton, 1987), 114–15.

41. Eliza W. Farnham, *Life in Prairie Land* (New York: Harper & Brothers, 1846), 116–17, 126–28, 149–50.

42. See chap. 3 on "Domesticity" in Witold Rybczynski, *Home: A Short History of an Idea* (New York: Viking, 1986), especially 62, 64–66, 70–75 (quote on p. 74).

43. Christine Stansell, *City of Women: Sex and Class in New York, 1789–1860* (Urbana: Univ. of Illinois Press, 1987), 46–50 (quote on p. 48); and Earl F. Niehaus, *The Irish in New Orleans* (Baton Rouge: Louisiana State Univ. Press, 1965), 93.

44. Hasia R. Diner, *Erin's Daughters in America: Irish Immigrant Women in the Nineteenth Century* (Baltimore: Johns Hopkins Univ. Press, 1983), 30–42, 74. See also Mary Doyle Curran, *The Parish and the Hill* [1948] (New York: Feminist Press, 1986), a fictional account of three generations of Irish immigrants.

45. "The New York Labor Market: Female House Servants," *Harper's Weekly* 1 (July 4, 1857): 418–19; Jennie June, *Jennie Juneiana: Talks on Women's Topics* (Boston: Lee and Shepard, 1864), 45.

46. MacKay-Smith Marlatt, ed., *Stuart Letters*, ix, xi, 312–13.

47. "Domestic Management," *Godey's Lady's Book and Magazine* 52 (April 1861): 313.

48. Stansell, *City of Women*, 159 (quote), 160–63; and Clifford E. Clark, Jr., "Domestic Architecture as an Index to Social History: The Romantic Revival and the Cult of Domesticity in America, 1840–1870," *Journal of Interdisciplinary History* 7 (Summer 1976): 49–53.

49. Cowan, *More Work for Mother*, 26.

50. Laurel Thatcher Ulrich, *Good Wives: Image and Reality in the Lives of Women in Northern New England, 1650–1750* (New York: Oxford Univ. Press, 1983), 9.

51. Cowan, *More Work for Mother*, 28–29; see also Dudden, *Serving Women*, 143.

52. Cowan, *More Work for Mother*, 42, 63–68.

53. A. B., "Doing Her Own Washing," *Godey's Lady's Book and Magazine* 62 (June 1861): 516–19; and Barbara Welter, "The Cult of True Womanhood: 1820–1860," *American Quarterly* 18 (Summer 1966): 161–74.

54. Rybczynski, *Home*, 158–60; and Kathryn Kish Sklar, *Catharine Beecher: A Study in American Domesticity* (New York: W. W. Norton, 1976), 161 (quote).

55. Allen Johnson, ed., *Dictionary of American Biography* (11 vols.; New York: Scribner, 1946–58), I: 133 (quote). This volume contains sketches of Catharine, 125–26; Charles, 126–27; Henry Ward, 129–35; Lyman, 135–36; and Thomas, 136–37.

56. James Marston Fitch, *Architecture and the Esthetics of Plenty* (New York: Columbia Univ. Press, 1961), 70–71 (quote), 74–75; and Sklar, *Catharine Beecher*, 151 (quote).

57. Catharine E. Beecher, *A Treatise on Domestic Economy for the Use of Young Ladies at Home and at School* (Boston: Marsh, Capen, Lyon, & Webb, 1841), 2; and Sklar, *Catharine Beecher*, 155–59 (quote p. 158).

58. Beecher, *Treatise*, 15, 16 (quotes).

59. Catharine E. Beecher, *Letters to Persons Who Are Engaged in Domestic Service* (New York: Leavitt & Trow, 1842), 211. In her *Treatise* (149–50), she says essentially the same thing less succinctly.

60. Beecher, *Treatise*, 367 (on kitchen sink), 308 (on clean clothes), 270 (on cock and pump), and 269 (on additional rooms).

61. Ibid., 272 (quote); and 100–105. See also Wilkie, "Submerged Sensuality," 652.

62. Harriet Beecher Stowe, "Our Houses—What Is Required to Make Them Healthful," *Herald of Health* 6 (Oct. 1865): 109–11; it is quoted in Cayleff, *Wash and Be Healed*, 144. On Catharine's visits to spas, see Cayleff, 148–51; and Sklar, 205–9. Catharine Beecher and Harriet Beecher Stowe, *The American Woman's Home: Or, Principles of Domestic Science; Being a Guide to the Formation and Maintenance of Economical, Healthful, and Christian Homes* (New York, 1869), 156 (quote).

63. Shryock, "Sylvester Graham and the Popular Health Movement," 174; and Buley, *Old Northwest*, 361 (quote).

64. Beecher, *Treatise*, 103.

65. Jonas Frykman and Orvar Lofgren, *Culture Builders: A Historical Anthropology of Middle-Class Life* (New Brunswick: Rutgers Univ. Press, 1987), 181–82.

66. Green, *Fit for America*, 46–49.

67. Charles E. Rosenberg, *The Cholera Years: The United States in 1832, 1849, and 1866* (Chicago: Univ. of Chicago Press, 1962), 5.

68. Wm. A. Alcott, ed., *The Moral Reformer and Teacher on the Human Constitution* (Boston: Light & Stearns, 1836), 340–42; Louis B. Salomon, "The Least-Remembered Alcott," *New England Quarterly* 34 (March 1961): 87–93; and Johnson, ed., *Dictionary of American Biography*, I: 142–43.

69. Wm. A. Alcott, *The Young Woman's Book of Health* (Boston: Tappan, Whittemore and Mason, 1850), 57, 59–60.

70. Wm. A. Alcott, *Health Tracts: For the Diffusion of Knowledge on the Preservation of Health, and the Laws of the Human Constitution* (Boston: George W. Light, 1841), 26, 28.

71. Quotations are from Wm. A. Alcott, *The Young Mother: Or Management of Children in Regard to Health* (Boston: Light & Stearns, 1836), 89; and Wm. A. Alcott, *The Laws of Health: Or Sequel to "The House I Live In"* (Boston: John P. Jewett, 1860), 245.

72. Alcott, *Young Mother*, 92–93.

73. Wm. A. Alcott, *The Young House-Keeper: Or Thoughts on Food and Cookery* (Boston: George W. Light, 1838), 19, 53 (quote); and Wm. A. Alcott, *The Young Husband: Or Duties of the Man in the Marriage Relation* (Boston: George W. Light, 1841), 362–63.

74. Alcott, *Young Mother*, 93–94.

75. James H. Cassedy, "The Roots of American Sanitary Reform 1843–47: Seven Letters from John H. Griscom to Lemuel Shattuck," *Journal of the History of Medicine* 30 (April 1975): 137–38; and Dorothy G. Becker, "The Visitor to the New York City Poor, 1843–1920," *Social Service Review* 35 (Dec. 1961): 386.

76. John H. Griscom, *The Sanitary Condition of the Laboring Population of New York: With Suggestions for Its Improvement* (New York, 1845), 3, 6.

77. On Lemuel Shattuck's career, see Barbara Gutmann Rosenkrantz, *Public Health and the State: Changing Views in Massachusetts, 1842–1936* (Cambridge: Harvard Univ. Press, 1972), 14–36.

78. [Lemuel Shattuck], *Report of a General Plan for the Promotion of Public and Personal Health, Devised, Prepared and Recommended by the Commissioners Appointed under a Resolve of the Legislature of Massachusetts, Relating to a Sanitary Survey of the State* (Boston: Dutton & Wentworth, 1850), 275 (first quote), 161–62 (second quote).

79. Griscom, *Sanitary Condition*, 46.

80. [Shattuck], *Report of a General Plan*, 162.

81. Howard D. Kramer, "The Beginnings of the Public Health Movement in the United States," *Bulletin of the History of Medicine* 21 (May–June 1947): 362–63, 369–70.

82. Harold M. Cavins, "The National Quarantine and Sanitary Conventions of 1857 to 1860 and the Beginnings of the American Public Health Association," *Bulletin of the History of Medicine* 13 (April 1943): 404–26.

CHAPTER 2. A WIDER WAR

1. Frederick Law Olmsted to the United States Sanitary Commission, Sept. 5, 1861, in Jane Turner Censer, ed., *The Papers of Frederick Law Olmsted*, vol. 4: *Defending the Union: The Civil War and the U.S. Sanitary Commission, 1861–1863* (Baltimore: Johns Hopkins Univ. Press, 1986), 179.

2. "War and Hygiene," *American Medical Times*, Aug. 22, 1863, pp. 89–90.

3. "Military Hospitals and Nursing," ibid., May 11, 1861, p. 306.

4. Frederick Edge, *A Woman's Example: And a Nation's Work.—A Tribute to Florence Nightingale* (London: William Ridgway, 1864), 41. Henry Wadsworth Longfellow immortalized Florence Nightingale as the "lady with a lamp" in the sixth and tenth stanzas of his poem, "Santa Filomena," which first appeared in the *At-*

lantic Monthly 1 (Nov. 1857): 22–23. See Virginia M. Dunbar, "Foreword," to Florence Nightingale, *Notes on Nursing: What It Is, and What It Is Not* [1860] (New York: Dover, 1969), xviii, for the publication figures.

5. (London) *Times*, Oct. 9 and 12, 1854.

6. Quotations are from Florence Nightingale, *Notes on Hospitals: Being Two Papers Read Before the National Association for the Promotion of Social Science at Liverpool, in October, 1858. With Evidence Given to the Royal Commissioners on the State of the Army in 1857* (London: John W. Parker and Son, 1859), 38; and Florence Nightingale to Sidney Herbert, Dec. 25 and 28, 1854, in Sue M. Goldie, ed., *"I have done my duty": Florence Nightingale in the Crimean War* (Iowa City: Univ. of Iowa Press, 1987), 60.

7. Ibid., 69. See also Nightingale to Herbert, Jan. 8 and 28, 1855, in ibid., 73 (quote)-75, 79 (quote). Anne Summers, *Angels and Citizens: British Women as Military Nurses, 1854–1914* (London: Routledge & Kegan Paul, 1988), 47–52, explains the close relationship between "good housekeeping and medical science" in the mid-1850s.

8. Florence Nightingale to her mother, Feb. l, 1855, in Goldie, ed., *"I have done my duty,"* 81. Here she again described herself as "Purveyor, Scavenger, everything to these colossal calamities, as the Hospitals of Scutari will come to be called in History."

9. Quotation from Lytton Strachey, *Eminent Victorians* (Garden City, N.Y.: Garden City Publishing, 1918), 154. See Nancy Boyd, *Three Victorian Women Who Changed Their World: Josephine Butler, Octavia Hull, Florence Nightingale* (New York: Oxford Univ. Press, 1982), 210, on Nightingale's sanitary reforms. For biographical information on Nightingale, see Edward Cook's standard work: *The Life of Florence Nightingale* (2 vols.; London: Macmillan, 1913); also important is Cecil Woodham-Smith's *Florence Nightingale, 1820–1910* (London: Constable, 1950). Indispensable to any study of Nightingale is W. J. Bishop and Sue Goldie, comps., *A Bio-Bibliography of Florence Nightingale* (London: Dawsons of Pall Mall, 1962).

10. Charles E. Rosenberg, "Florence Nightingale on Contagion: The Hospital as Moral Universe," in Charles E. Rosenberg, ed., *Healing and History: Essays for George Rosen* (New York: Science History Publications, 1979), 116–36. See also Charles E. Rosenberg, *The Care of Strangers: The Rise of America's Hospital System* (New York: Basic Books, 1987), 128–35; and Martha Vicinus, *Independent Women: Work and Community for Single Women, 1850–1920* (Chicago: Univ. of Chicago Press, 1985), 85–101.

11. Nightingale, *Notes on Hospitals*, 26, 29, 35. In a letter to Herbert, Nightingale reported that the Sanitary Commission had arrived and was "really doing something"; it had "set to work burying dead dogs & white washing infected walls, two prolific causes of fever." Nightingale to Herbert, March 18, 1855, in Goldie, ed., *"I have done my duty,"* 108.

12. Catharine E. Beecher, *A Treatise on Domestic Economy for the Use of Young Ladies at Home and at School* (Boston: Marsh, Capen, Lyon, & Webb, 1841), 144; and Catharine E. Beecher, *Miss Beecher's Domestic Recipt-Book Designed as a Supplement to Her Treatise on Domestic Economy* [1846] (New York: Harper & Brothers, 1871), 212.

13. For this description of Nightingale's war work, see Mary Cowden Clarke, "Biographical Sketch," *New York Times*, Dec. 18, 1857; and Agatha Young, *The Women and the Crisis: Women of the North in the Civil War* (New York: McDowell, Obolensky, 1959), 18.

14. "Florence Nightingale before the Army Medical Reform Commission," *New York Times*, March 11, 1858. See also Nightingale's "Answers to Written Questions Addressed to Miss Nightingale by the Commissioners Appointed to Inquire into the Regulations Affecting the Sanitary Condition of the Army," in *Notes on Hospitals*, 54.

15. *Godey's Lady's Book and Magazine* 61 (Sept. 1860): 269. It regarded *Notes on Nursing* as truly singular: "Few medical books, produced by the most eminent men, equal it in usefulness and in the good it must initiate and produce for the sick and suffering." See also *New York Times Supplement*, March 10, 1860.

16. Quotations are from Jane E. Schultz, "The Inhospitable Hospital: Gender and Professionalism in Civil War Medicine," *Signs: Journal of Women in Culture and Society* 17 (Winter 1992): 364; and Young, *The Women and the Crisis*, 18. See also James H. Cassedy, "Numbering the North's Medical Events: Humanitarianism and Science in Civil War Statistics," *Bulletin of the History of Medicine* 66 (Summer 1992): 213–17.

17. Susan M. Reverby, *Ordered to Care: The Dilemma of American Nursing, 1850–1945* (Cambridge: Cambridge Univ. Press, 1987), 44. On Southern women inspired by Nightingale's example, see J. Fraise Richard, comp., *The Florence Nightingale of the Southern Army: Experiences of Mrs. Ella K. Newsom, Confederate Nurse in the Great War of 1861–65* (New York: Broadway Publishing, 1914). Ella Newsom described a visit from a group of women from Mobile, Alabama—the "Florence Nightingale Brigade"—who wanted "to revolutionize the bad management" (p. 44).

18. Robert H. Bremner, "The Impact of the Civil War on Philanthropy and Social Welfare," *Civil War History* 12 (Dec. 1966): 293–94. Women like Chicago's Mary Livermore and Jane Hoge, who would organize one of the Sanitary Commission's most successful fairs in 1864, were "veterans of community service." See Nina Bennett Smith, "The Women Who Went to the War: The Union Army Nurse in the Civil War" (Ph.D. dissertation, Northwestern Univ., 1981), 24–25; and Beverly Gordon, "'A Furor of Benevolence,'" *Chicago History* 15 (Winter 1986–87): 48–64.

19. C. Vann Woodward, ed., *Mary Chesnut's Civil War* (New Haven: Yale Univ. Press, 1981), 85.

20. *American Medical Times*, April 27, 1861, p. 276.

21. Marjorie Barstow Greenbie, *Lincoln's Daughter of Mercy* (New York: Putnam's, 1944), 49. There was also strong public pressure in the North and the South against women working in hospitals for fear that they would lose their virtue by caring for strange men. Kate Cumming, a nurse with the Confederate Army of Tennessee, lamented in May 1862: "As soon as Miss Nightingale went to the Crimean war, the whole world resounded with her praises; and here I have been nearly two months, and have scarcely heard Miss N.'s name mentioned." Kate Cumming, *A Journal of Hospital Life in the Confederate Army of Tennessee from the Battle of Shiloh to the End of the War: With Sketches of Life and Character, and Brief Notices of Current Events during That Period* (Louisville: John P. Morthon, 1866), 29. See also Francis Butler Simkins and James Welch Patton, *The Women of the Confederacy* (Richmond: Garrett and Massie, 1936), 89.

22. George C. Rable, *Civil Wars: Women and the Crisis of Southern Nationalism* (Urbana: Univ. of Illinois Press, 1991), 47, 138–40 (quote on pp. 138–39).

23. Cassedy, "Numbering the North's Medical Events," 211; and Rable, *Civil Wars*, 76–77.

24. Quotations are from Mrs. Sarah Edwards Henshaw, *Our Branch and Its Tributaries: Being a History of Work of the Northwestern Sanitary Commission* (Chicago: A. L. Sewell, 1868), 21; and Young, *The Women and the Crisis*, 65. Frederick Law Olmsted, general secretary of the Sanitary Commission, would write Louisa Lee Schuyler, chairman of the Committee of Correspondence of the Woman's Central Association of Relief, in July that an acquaintance who had spent time in Europe and India had never seen "the things called havelocks . . . and never heard the term used until he met with it here." Frederick Law Olmsted to Louisa Lee Schuyler, July 12, 1861, United States Sanitary Commission (USSC) Papers, Box 654 (New York Public Library). See also Elisha Harris to Louisa Lee Schuyler, July 15, 1861, USSC Papers, ibid. (quote).

25. The first two quotations are from Mary Bache Walker to Alexander Dallas Bache, May 12, 1861, William Jones Rhees Papers (Henry E. Huntington Library, San Marino, Calif.). Alexander Dallas Bache, superintendent of the United States Coast Survey, later became vice president of the Sanitary Commission. The last quotation is from Katharine P. Wormeley, *The United States Sanitary Commission: A Sketch of Its Purposes and Its Work* (Boston: Little, Brown, 1863), 2.

26. "An Appeal," *New York Times*, April 28, 1861; also Document 1 in Charles J. Stillé, *History of the United States Sanitary Commission, Being the General Report of Its Work during the War of the Rebellion* (Philadelphia: J. B. Lippincott, 1866), 523.

27. Stillé, *History of the United States Sanitary Commission*, 42, 524.

28. The quotation is from Elizabeth Blackwell, *Pioneer Work in Opening the Medical Profession to Women: Autobiographical Sketches* [1895] (New York: Schocken Books, 1977), 176. On the subject of immunity from smallpox, for instance, Elizabeth Blackwell believed: "Pure air, cleanliness, and decent house-room secured to all our people, form the true prophylaxis of small-pox." Elizabeth Blackwell, "Why Hygienic Congresses Fail," in *Essays in Medical Sociology* [1902] (2 vols.; New York: Arno Press, 1972), II: 73.

29. Dorothea Dix's letter to Mrs. William Rathbone, April 10, 1856, is given in its entirety in Francis Tiffany, *Life of Dorothea Lynde Dix* (Boston: Houghton, Mifflin, 1891), 299. See Victor Robinson, *White Caps: The Story of Nursing* (Philadelphia: J. B. Lippincott, 1946), 127, who writes that "William Rathbone of Liverpool used to say: 'In any matter of nursing, Miss Nightingale is my Pope, and I believe in her infallibility.' "

30. Quotations are from Margaret Leech, *Reveille in Washington: 1860–1865* (New York: Harper & Brothers, 1941), 76–77. See also Mary C. Gillett, *The Army Medical Department 1818–1865* (Washington: Center of Military History, 1987), 158.

31. Henshaw, *Our Branch and Its Tributaries*, 41 (quote); "Military Hygiene," *American Medical Times*, May 25, 1861; Theodore Winthrop, "Washington as a Camp," *Atlantic Monthly* 8 (July 1861): 105–18; and Leech, *Reveille in Washington*, 77 (quote).

32. Stillé, *History of the United States Sanitary Commission*, 33 (quote); and William Quentin Maxwell, *Lincoln's Fifth Wheel: The Political History of the United States Sanitary Commission* (New York: Longmans, Green, 1956), 32–33. Bellows also recalled that, because of the uncooperativeness of the army's Medical Department, he and his colleagues were convinced that "the objects which had brought" the group to Washington were "even more important" than they had initially

thought. See Henry W. Bellows to Charles J. Stillé, Nov. 15, 1865, Henry W. Bellows Papers (Massachusetts Historical Society, Boston).

33. The quotations are from: Bellows et al., "Address to the Citizens of the United States," July 21, 1861, United States Sanitary Commission, *Documents of the U.S. Sanitary Commission* (2 vols.; New York: n.p., 1866), I: Document 4, p. 1; Bellows to Stillé, Nov. 15, 1865, Bellows Papers; and Stillé, *History of the United States Sanitary Commission*, 51, 52.

34. On the month's struggle, see Elisha Harris, "The Sanitary Commission," Part I, *North American Review* 98 (Jan. 1864): 167. From the beginning, the government considered the plan "troublesome, impracticable, and dangerous." See also Censer, ed., *Papers of Frederick Law Olmsted*, IV: 4–5, as well as several other accounts of the organization of the United States Sanitary Commission: William Y. Thompson, "The U.S. Sanitary Commission," *Civil War History* 2 (June 1956): 41–63; Maxwell, *Lincoln's Fifth Wheel*, 4–9; George Fredrickson, *The Inner Civil War: Northern Intellectuals and the Crisis of Union* (New York: Harper & Row, 1965), especially 98–112; and Robert H. Bremner, *The Public Good: Philanthropy and Welfare in the Civil War Era* (New York: Alfred A. Knopf, 1980), 35–46. Also Stillé's *History of the United States Sanitary Commission*, cited above; and Henry W. Bellows, *The United States Sanitary Commission* (New York, [ca. 1870s]), which was reprinted from *Johnson's Universal Encyclopedia*.

35. Some historians have imputed to Bellows, Olmsted, and others a desire for "social control"—to fasten reforms upon potentially unruly immigrants and poor people, thus making the mass of Americans conform to their own upper-middle-class values to preserve law and order and, of course, their own privileged postion. See, for example, George Fredrickson, *The Inner Civil War*, 102–3. Other historians have taken these bourgeois reformers more at face value; they may have acted to "contain disorder" but they also hoped to benefit society through literacy programs, aid to dependent widows, etc. See, for example, Carroll Smith-Rosenberg, *Disorderly Conduct: Visions of Gender in Victorian America* (New York: Oxford Univ. Press, 1986), 86–87. Since the 1960s and 1970s, "social control" explanations of reformers have been used increasingly less.

Elizabeth Blackwell, who emigrated from England with her parents at age eleven, fought her way from less than prosperous English immigrant origins to become the first female graduate of an American medical college in 1849, opened a dispensary and then a hospital in New York City, became accredited as a physician in England, and by 1859 had discussed nurses' training, hygiene, and the role of women in public health with Nightingale herself. In 1869 she returned to England for the rest of her life. She established a successful practice in London and founded the National Health Society; its motto was "Prevention is better than cure." See Elizabeth H. Thomson, "Elizabeth Blackwell," in Edward T. James, Janet Wilson James, and Paul S. Boyer, eds., *Notable American Women* (4 vols.; Cambridge: Belknap Press, 1971), I: 161–63.

36. Censer, ed., *The Papers of Frederick Law Olmsted*, IV: 5. Censer also provides a useful "Biographical Directory," which includes essays on some of the major figures (pp. 78–114). See too Bremner, *The Public Good*, 40.

37. Bellows et al., "An Address to the Secretary of War," in Stillé, *History of the United States Sanitary Commission*, Appendix 2, p. 528. Nightingale indirectly assisted the Sanitary Commission in this purpose through her friend, statistician William Farr. He sent copies of reports, folios containing calculations and diagrams,

and an old edition of her *Notes on Hospitals* to E. B. Elliott, a Boston statistician hired by the Sanitary Commission as its actuary. William Farr to Florence Nightingale, Sept. 21, 1864; Nightingale to Farr, Sept. 28, 1864; and Farr to Nightingale, Sept. 30, 1864, Florence Nightingale Papers (British Library, London). Earlier, in 1861, Nightingale had given copies of the Royal Commission's Sanitary Report of 1858, Army Medical Regulations of 1859, and Army Purveyor's Regulations of 1861 to her friend, Harriet Martineau, who forwarded them to Secretary of War Simon Cameron. Martineau also wrote several articles ("Health in the Camp" and "Health in the Hospital"), based on material supplied by Nightingale, that appeared in the *Atlantic Monthly* in November and December 1861 respectively. As a result, according to Martineau, many Americans were "learning from us." Harriet Martineau to Florence Nightingale, Sept. 20, 1861; and Nightingale to Martineau, Sept. 24, 1861, Nightingale Papers.

38. Elisha Harris, "The Sanitary Commission," Part II, *North American Review* 98 (April 1864): 371, 381. Here too Harris describes the considerations and spirit that guided the commission in its work: first, *prevention* from disease; second, *relief* from suffering.

39. Bellows, *The United States Sanitary Commission*, 3–5.

40. Quotations are from ibid., 7; and Dorothea Dix to Elisha Harris, May 13, 1861, USSC Papers, Box 661. In a letter to Elizabeth Blackwell's Registration Committee (of the Woman's Central Association of Relief in New York City), Commissioner Elisha Harris reported that he had talked to Dix and explained to her the goal of the Registration Committee—"of admitting to the Army Hospitals none but carefully selected & qualified nurses"—and that she seemed "ready to join heartily" in their "good works." Harris then suggested that the committee "open a correspondence with her." Elisha Harris to the Ladies of the Registration Comee. of Association of Relief, May 15, 1861, USSC Papers, Box 661.

41. Bellows to Stillé, Nov. 15, 1865, Bellows Papers.

42. Dix to Harris, May 13, 1861, USSC Papers, Box 661.

43. Bellows to Stillé, Nov. 15, 1865, Bellows Papers (quote); and Censer, ed., *Papers of Frederick Law Olmsted*, IV: 2 (quote), 5–6. He believed especially in the importance of "thorough-drainage" to sound health. "Thorough-drainage" refers to the practice of draining swampy lands with underground tile pipes.

44. Fred Albert Shannon, *The Organization and Administration of the Union Army, 1861–1865* (2 vols.; Cleveland: Arthur H. Clark, 1928), I: 195 (quote); and Bremner, *The Public Good*, 42 (quote).

45. Leech, *Reveille in Washington*, 111 (quote); Frederick Law Olmsted to Mary Perkins Olmsted, July 2, 1861, in Censer, ed., *Papers of Frederick Law Olmsted*, IV: 125 (quote); T. W. Higginson, "Regular and Volunteer Officers," *Atlantic Monthly* 14 (Sept. 1864): 350 (quote). Higginson observed that for the volunteer war was "an episode in life, not a profession"; thus few recently elected officers wished to risk offending their neighbors. See also Henry W. Bellows to Executive Committee of the Central Financial Committee in New York, July 9, 1861, United States Sanitary Commission, *Documents*, I: Document 15, p. 3 (quotes).

46. Gillett, *Army Medical Department*, 27, 35, 82, 99–125 (quotation from 124), 140–41, 153.

47. Quotations are from Stillé, *History of the United States Sanitary Commission*, 85–86; Elbert L. Porter to George T. Strong, July 18, 1862, USSC Papers, Box 655; and Frank Hamilton, "Report of a Preliminary Survey of the Camps of a Por-

tion of the Volunteer Forces Near Washington," July 9, 1861, United States Sanitary Commission, *Documents*, I: Document 17, p. 5.

48. Quotations are from S. G. Howe, *A Letter on the Sanitary Condition of the Troops in the Neighborhood of Boston, Addressed to His Excellency the Governor of Massachusetts* (Washington: Government Printing Office, 1861), 4, 11–12; and Laura E. Richards, *Letters and Journals of Samuel Gridley Howe* (2 vols.; Boston: Dana Estes, 1909), II: 481.

49. "The Necessity of War," *Harper's Weekly* 5 (Aug. 17, 1861): 514; and Frederick Law Olmsted to John Olmsted, August 3, 1861, in Censer, ed., *Papers of Frederick Law Olmsted*, IV: 138, 139. He also told his father that he had dined earlier that day with William Howard Russell, the London *Times* correspondent whose articles on the unsanitary conditions of British soldiers in the Crimea led to Nightingale's tour of duty there. See also Frederick Law Olmsted to Mary Perkins Olmsted, July 29, 1861, in Censer, ibid., 130.

50. Frederick Law Olmsted, "Report on the Demoralization of the Volunteers," Sept. 5, 1861, in ibid., 153–94. Quotations appear on 153, 162, 164–65.

51. Ibid., 170–71, 173, 174–75, 179–80, and 184–85. Although Olmsted complained about the army's maladministration, he was encouraged by the accession of George B. McClellan to the command of the Army of the Potomac.

52. Executive Committee of the United States Sanitary Commission to the President of the United States, July 21, 1862, United States Sanitary Commission, *Documents*, I: Document 43, p. 4. See also Frederick Law Olmsted, "A Report to the Secretary of War of the Operations of the Sanitary Commission, and upon the Sanitary Condition of the Volunteer Army, Its Medical Staff, Hospital, and Hospital Supplies," Dec. 1861, ibid., I: Document 40, pp. 27 and 28.

53. Cassedy, "Numbering the North's Medical Events," 224–25. The quotes are from Frederick Law Olmsted to Lewis Henry Steiner, Aug. 12, 1861, in Censer, ed., *Papers of Frederick Law Olmsted*, IV: 143; and Frederick Law Olmsted, "Revised General Instructions for Camp Inspections," United States Sanitary Commission, *Documents*, I: Document 51, p. 2. Lewis Henry Steiner served the commission as an inspector of camps and hospitals for three years.

54. James Mann, *Medical Sketches of the Campaigns of 1812, 13, 14: To Which Are Added, Surgical Cases; Observations on Military Hospitals; and Flying Hospitals Attached to a Moving Army . . .* (Dedham, Mass.: H. Mann, 1816), 36.

55 Gerald F. Linderman, *Embattled Courage: The Experience of Combat in the American Civil War* (New York: Free Press, 1987), 36. Gerald Linderman argues persuasively that the "extraordinary lack of formal discipline within the Civil War armies sprang from the strength, vitality, and persistence of soldiers' local sources of identity and support." Ibid. See also Harriet Martineau, "Health in the Camp," *Atlantic Monthly* 8 (Nov. 1861): 578, 580.

56. Edward Jarvis, "Sanitary Condition of the Army," *Atlantic Monthly* 10 (Oct. 1862): 486 (quote). See also James M. McPherson, *Ordeal by Fire: The Civil War and Reconstruction* (New York: Alfred A. Knopf, 1982), 383; and Bell Irvin Wiley, *The Life of Billy Yank: The Common Soldier of the Union* (Indianapolis: Bobbs-Merrill, 1951), 120.

57. Stuart Brooks, *Civil War Medicine* (Springfield, Ill.: Charles C. Thomas, 1966), 108. Quotes are from Robert Ware to J. S. Jenkins, Jan. 21, 1862, USSC Papers, Box 737; and Charles Beneulyn Johnson, *Muskets and Medicine: Or Army Life in the Sixties* (Philadelphia: F. A. Davis, 1917), 159.

58. "Camp Inspection Return," United States Sanitary Commission, *Documents*, I: Document 19a, pp. 1–4.

59. Ibid., 5–8, 15.

60. Stillé, *History of the United States Sanitary Commission*, 98–99; and Frederick Law Olmsted, *Books and Printed Papers Relating to Concerns of the United States Sanitary Commission in the War of the Rebellion* (n.p., 1890), x (quote).

61. Olmsted, "A Report to the Secretary of War of the Operations of the Sanitary Commission . . . ," *Documents*, I: Document 40, pp. 12–13, 23–28, 39.

62. Ibid., 12–13, 23–28, 39. See also Hale, "The United States Sanitary Commission," 426; Stillé, *History of the United States Sanitary Commission*, 111–25; and George Worthington Adams, *Doctors in Blue: The Medical History of the Union Army in the Civil War* (New York: Henry Schuman, 1952), 199.

63. "Ignorant and Uneducated Contract Surgeons," *Medical and Surgical Reporter* 11 (June 11, 1864): 377–78; and Stillé, *History of the United States Sanitary Commission*, 110–11. For a complete listing of these publications, see Olmsted, *Books and Printed Papers*, xxiv.

64. "Hospital Construction," *American Medical Times*, Oct. 26, 1861; Rosenberg, *The Care of Strangers*, 136–37; Bremner, *The Public Good*, 43.

65. Edward Everett Hale, "The United States Sanitary Commission," *Atlantic Monthly* 19 (April 1867): 422.

66. Jenkin Lloyd Jones, *An Artilleryman's Diary* (Madison: Wisconsin History Commission, 1914), 166–68; Stephen E. Ambrose, ed., *A Wisconsin Boy in Dixie: The Selected Letters of James K. Newton* (Madison: Univ. of Wisconsin Press, 1961), 25; and Joseph Burt Holt to Julia Rollins Holt, June 9, 1863, Holt-Messer Family Papers (Schlesinger Library, Radcliffe College, Cambridge, Mass.).

67. Quotes are from Chauncey H. Cooke, "Letters of a Badger Boy in Blue: The Atlantic Campaign," *Wisconsin Magazine of History* 5 (Sept. 1921): 82–83, 90; William Prock Landon, "Prock's Letters from the Eastern Front (July 1862 to May 1863)," *Indiana Magazine of History* 33 (Sept. 1937): 325, 330; and Margaret Brobst Roth, ed., *Well Mary: Civil War Letters of a Wisconsin Volunteer* (Madison: Univ. of Wisconsin Press, 1960), 54.

68. Quotes can be found in Henry G. Clark, "Department of Special Inspection of the General Hospitals of the Army: First Report to the Commission," United States Sanitary Commission, *Documents*, I: Document 56, p. 1; and Henry G. Clark, "Plan of the Inspection of General Hospitals," Sept. 24, 1862, USSC Papers, Box 38.

69. Bellows, "The United States Sanitary Commission," 40; Henry G. Clark, "Department of Special Inspection of the General Hospitals of the Army: Second Report to the Commission," United States Sanitary Commission, *Documents*, II: Document 65, p. 5 (quote), 6; and William A. Hammond, "Reports on the Condition of Military Hospitals in Virginia and Maryland," ibid., I: Document 41, p. 3 (quote).

70. The ratings can be found in "Special Inspection of General Army Hospitals," USSC Papers, Box 37. See also Gillett, *Army Medical Department*, 166, 231–32 (quote).

71. Stephen Smith, "Inspection of the Warehouse Hospital, Georgetown," Sept. 27, 1862, USSC Papers, Box 37; and Elisha Harris, "2nd Report on the General Hospital at Fort Schuyler," Feb. 3, 1863, ibid., Box 38.

72. In a letter to an unidentified woman, Superintendent Dix admitted that "the cause has suffered seriously by some indiscretions on the part of many good persons" who were unable to control their feelings. She wanted instead "your best in-

structed reliable nurses" to "fill places of important trust." Dorothea L. Dix to "My dear Madam," June 4, 1861, USSC Papers, Box 661. See also Helen E. Marshall, *Dorothea Dix: Forgotten Samaritan* (Chapel Hill: Univ. of North Carolina Press, 1937), 206, 208.

73. The estimate of 2000 nurses is from Isabel M. Stewart and Anne L. Austin, *A History of Nursing from Ancient to Modern Times: A World View* (5th ed., New York, 1962), 132; the number 3200 is given in Mary Elizabeth Massey, *Bonnet Brigades* (New York: Alfred A. Knopf, 1966), xiv. Jane E. Schultz, "The Inhospitable Hospital," 363–64 (note 2), estimates over 20,000 women served in military hospitals, but since these are from Union records only, and "reliable statistics for Confederate hospital workers are unavailable, the total number of female hospital workers in both [armies] is likely to be much greater." On matrons and other women workers, see Schultz, 369–70.

74. Rable, *Civil Wars*, 118–28 (quotes on pp. 119, 122, and 127).

75. Madeleine B. Stern, "Louisa M. Alcott: Civil War Nurse," *Americana* 37 (April 1943): 298–99.

76. H. Bowditch and C. Ellis, "Inspection of Union Hospital," Oct. 10, 1862, USSC Papers, Box 37; Ednah D. Cheney, ed., *Louisa May Alcott: Her Life, Letters and Journals* (Boston: Little, Brown, 1928), 117; and Joseph Janvier Woodward, *The Hospital Steward's Manual: For the Instruction of Hospital Stewards, Ward-Masters, and Attendants, in Their Several Duties* (Philadelphia: J. B. Lippincott, 1862), 39.

77. Stern, "Louisa M. Alcott," 303; and John R. Brumgardt, ed., *Civil War Nurse: The Diary and Letters of Hannah Ropes* (Knoxville: Univ. of Tennessee Press, 1980), 55.

78. L. M. Alcott, *Hospital Sketches* (Boston: James Redpath, 1863), 33–36. When Louisa May Alcott returned to Concord, she wrote a children's story about Nurse Nelly who began a "hospital" in a backyard summerhouse by scrubbing, cleaning, and ventilating the place; it later becomes a branch of the Sanitary Commission. See Louisa May Alcott, *Nelly's Hospital* (Boston: Ticknor and Fields, 1866), 2, 3.

79. Sheila M. Rothman, *Woman's Proper Place: A History of Changing Ideals and Practices, 1870 to the Present* (New York: Basic Books, 1978), 70. Rothman correctly observes in her footnotes (pp. 296–97) that Fredrickson's *Inner Civil War* neglects the important role of women in the Sanitary Commission's operations. For this reason and others, Fredrickson incorrectly portrays the commission and its auxiliaries as cold-hearted and inhumane—saving "the soldier in the hospital so that he could die a useful death on the battlefield." Fredrickson, *The Inner Civil War*, 102–3.

80. Alcott, *Hospital Sketches*, 38–39.

81. Sophronia E. Bucklin, *In Hospital and Camp: A Woman's Record of Thrilling Incidents among the Wounded in the Late War* (Philadelphia: J. E. Potter, 1869), 67–70 (quotes on pp. 68 and 70). See also Smith, "The Women Who Went to the War," 29, 60; and Ann Douglas Wood, "The War Within a War: Women Nurses in the Union Army," *Civil War History* 18 (Sept. 1972): 197–212. The only American women who had gained nursing experience by caring for strangers prior to 1861 were Roman Catholic nuns, many of whom served with dedication and distinction during the Civil War. See Sister Mary Denis Maher, *To Bind Up the Wounds: Catholic Sister Nurses in the U.S. Civil War* (New York: Greenwood Press, 1989).

82. Quotations are from Bucklin, *In Hospital and Camp*, 70; and Georgeanna Woolsey Bacon and Eliza Woolsey Howland, eds., *Letters of a Family during the War for the Union, 1861–1865* (2 vols.; New Haven, Conn.: Privately printed, 1899), I: 143.

83. Ibid., 143–44. For biographical data on Georgeanna Woolsey and the second quotation, see Censer, ed., *Papers of Frederick Law Olmsted*, IV: 324.

84. Bacon and Howland, eds., *Letters of a Family*, I: 202; see also 143–44.

85. Ibid., 310–12, 313; and Frederick Law Olmsted, *Hospital Transports: A Memoir of the Embarkation of the Sick and Wounded from the Peninsula of Virginia in the Summer of 1862* (Boston: Ticknor and Fields, 1863), xiii-xiv, 25, 36–37.

86. Olmsted, *Hospital Transports*, esp. 35, 40–41, 81, and 84. Besides the four women nurses, Olmsted's staff included 6 medical students, 20 male nurses (volunteers), 4 surgeons, 12 "contrabands," 3 carpenters, 8 military officers, 90 soldiers (convalescents), some quartermaster's mechanics, a short ship's crew and officers, and 5 members of the Sanitary Commission and central staff (including Olmsted). Bacon and Howland explained how Olmsted organized his people: "We were all assigned to duty by Mr. Olmsted wherever he thought we fitted in best, and his large printed placards put up on the steamers gave orders for the 'watches' and hours for 'relief,' meals, etc., etc., so that the work went on as in a city hospital." Bacon and Howland, eds., *Letters of a Family*, I: 347.

87. Quotations can be found in Katharine Prescott Wormeley, *The Other Side of War: With the Army of the Potomac* (Boston: Ticknor, 1889), 57, 102; and Bacon and Howland, eds., *Letters of a Family*, I: 348. On the commission "leading the way," see Wormeley, *The United States Sanitary Commission*, 92. Of more recent treatments, Bremner's evaluation of the Sanitary Commission and its leadership in *The Public Good* is the most helpful. He shows its benevolent side as well as how useful programs and services—camp inspections, hospital transports, railway ambulance cars, pavilion hospitals—were inaugurated by the commission and then adopted by the military (p. 53). The means employed by the commission to carry out a mission intended to be efficient as well as humane demonstrated a larger commitment to a "'professional ethic'" as described by Jane Turner Censer in her introduction to the *Frederick Law Olmsted Papers*, IV: 1–69 (see especially p. 5).

88. I first came across this quotation at the Huntington Library in *Spirit of the Fair*, a bound volume of newspapers published daily from April 5 to 23, 1864, in New York City during the Metropolitan Sanitary Fair. See a column entitled "How I Came To Be a Nurse—No. V," in *Spirit of the Fair*, April 18, 1864, p. 137; a similar version also appears in Bacon and Howland, eds., *Letters of a Family*, II: 402. This idea can also be found in a description of the effect of a woman's visit to a hospital in Cairo, Illinois. See Mary A. Livermore, *My Story of the War: A Woman's Narrative of Four Years Personal Experience as Nurse in the Union Army, and in Relief Work at Home, in Hospitals, Camps, and at the Front, during the War of the Rebellion* (Hartford, Conn.: A. D. Worthington, 1888), 202–3.

89. Wormeley, *The Other Side of War*, 17, 62, 101. Another description of the "housekeeping" work of women nurses appears in Jane Stuart Woolsey, *Hospital Days* (New York: Van Nostrand, 1870), 47. During the American Revolution, according to Linda K. Kerber, women who followed the troops and eventually secured employment as "nurses" almost always found themselves washing clothes or patients. Only in the absence of male surgeon's mates did women administer medi-

cines. Linda K. Kerber, *Women of the Republic: Intellect and Ideology in Revolutionary America* (Chapel Hill: Univ. of North Carolina Press, 1980), 55–60.

90. For the *Herald* quote, see Massey, *Bonnet Brigades*, 43; and for the number of auxiliary groups, see Wormeley, *The United States Sanitary Commission*, 2, and Stillé, *History of the United States Sanitary Commission*, 172–73. There was a "Florence Nightingale Association" in Paterson, New Jersey, and a "Wisconsin Florence Nightingale Union" in Berlin, Wisconsin. See USSC Papers, Boxes 658–59, 661. On how supplies were collected and distributed, consult Bremner, *The Public Good*, 55; and Stillé, *History of the United States Sanitary Commission*, 178–79. And, finally, on the kind of disciplined giving that the commission encouraged is Bellows' plea: "Let the homes of the land abandon the preparation of comforts and packages for *individual* soldiers. . . . If they contain eatables, they commonly spoil; if they do not spoil, they enervate the soldier; if made up of extra clothing, they crush him on the march. All this kindness kills. . . . " See Woman's Central Association of Relief, *Second Semi-Annual Report* (New York, 1862), 10.

91. Quotations are from George Augustus Sala, *My Diary in America in the Midst of War* (2 vols.; London: Tinsley Brothers, 1865), II: 358; and Henry W. Bellows, "Introduction," in L. P. Brockett and Mary C. Vaughan, *Woman's Work in the Civil War: A Record of Heroism, Patriotism, and Patience* (Philadelphia: Zeigler, McCurdy, 1867), 41. See also Stillé, *History of the United States Sanitary Commission*, 172–73; and O. B. Frothingham, "Civil War and Social Beneficence," *Harper's New Monthly Magazine* 34 (Feb. 1867): 360. On "the woman in America" during the Civil War, he says: "The country is her country; the war was her war; the Sanitary Commission was as much her protege as it was her patron."

92. New England Women's Auxiliary Association, *Fourth Report of the Executive Committee*, April 7, 1862, Papers of the New England Women's Auxiliary Association, Box 2 (Massachusetts Historical Society); and *Thirtieth Report of the Executive Committee*, Oct. 17, 1864, ibid. (These reports were signed by Abby W. May, Chairman.) See also issues of the *Sanitary Bulletin* beginning Dec. 5, 1863 (Vol. I, No. 4) intermittently to Aug. 1, 1864 (Vol. I, No. 19). Louisa L. Schuyler served as chairman of the Woman's Central Association of Relief's Committee of Correspondence. Having persuaded Bellows to begin the publication, she became responsible for it. Robert D. Cross, "The Philanthropic Contribution of Louisa Lee Schuyler," *Social Service Review* 35 (Sept. 1961): 292–93.

93. Quotations are from Maxwell, *Lincoln's Fifth Wheel*, 299; and Hale, "The United States Sanitary Commission," 422.

94. Bremner, *The Public Good*, 47.

95. Benjamin F. Butler, "Some Experiences with Yellow Fever and Its Prevention," *North American Review* 147 (Nov. 1888): 533 (quote), 536–37; and Carrigan, "Yankees Versus Yellow Jack," 257–60. For more discussion of government's involvement in public health matters during the Civil War, see Harold M. Hyman, *A More Perfect Union: The Impact of the Civil War and Reconstruction on the Constitution* (New York: Alfred A. Knopf, 1973), 314–25.

96. Sandra E. Small, "The Yankee Schoolmarm in Freedmen's Schools: An Analysis of Attitudes," *Journal of Southern History* 45 (Aug. 1979): 381–402 (quote on p. 391). For another good discussion of the "Yankee Schoolmarm," see Robert C. Morris, *Reading, 'Riting, and Reconstruction: The Education of the Freedmen in the South, 1861–1870* (Chicago: Univ. of Chicago Press, 1981), esp. pp. 56–59. Sojourner Truth, black abolitionist and reformer, also preached cleanliness to freed-

men. See *Narrative of Sojourner Truth* [1850] (New York: Arno Press, 1968), 182–83; and Hertha Pauli, *Her Name Was Sojourner Truth* (New York: Appleton-Century-Crofts, 1962), 208–10.

97. Cornelia Hancock to William Hancock, Jan. 1864, in Henrietta Jacquette, ed., *South after Gettysburg: Letters of Cornelia Hancock from the Army of the Potomac, 1863–1865* (Philadelphia: n.p., 1937), 41, 43.

98. Rupert Sargent Holland, ed., *Letters and Diary of Laura M. Towne: Written from the Sea Islands of South Carolina, 1862–1884* (New York: Negro Universities Press, 1969), 5, 6, 8.

99. Quotations are from Jacqueline Jones, *Labor of Love, Labor of Sorrow: Black Women, Work, and the Family from Slavery to the Present* (New York: Vintage Books, 1986), 86; Anne Raver, "In Georgia's Swept Yards, a Dying Tradition," *New York Times*, Aug. 8, 1993; and Bishop William Henry Elder to the Reverend Thomas Bennett, Oct. 17, 1865, All Hallows Collection of Letters from Bishops and Priests, 1843–77 (All Hallows College Archives, Dublin, Ireland).

100. Quotations are from Henry L. Swint, ed., *Dear Ones at Home: Letters from Contraband Camps* (Nashville: Vanderbilt Univ. Press, 1966), 134; Henry N. Sherwood, ed., "Journal of Miss Susan Walker March 3d to June 6th, 1862," *Quarterly Publication of the Historical and Philosophical Society of Ohio* 7 (Jan.-March 1912): 20; and E. P. Breck to M. A. Cochran and Education Committee of the New England Freedmen's Aid Society, Dec. 23, 1864, Papers of New England Freedmen's Aid Society—Reconstruction, Sophia Smith Collection, Box 35 (Smith College Archives).

101. Quotations can be found in *Freedmen's Record* 3 (May 1867): 80 (quote); an untitled speech given in 1894 by Mary Ellen Peirce on her work in the Sea Islands, South Carolina, John Bachelder Peirce Family Papers, Box 1 (Massachusetts Historical Society); Elizabeth Hyde Botume, *First Days Amongst the Contrabands* [1893] (New York: Arno Press, 1968), 236; and *Freedmen's Record* 5 (April 1872): 120. See also Mary Ames, *From a New England Woman's Diary in Dixie in 1865* (Springfield, Mass.: n.p., 1906), 25; and Holland, ed., *Letters and Diary of Laura M. Towne*, 227. Laura Towne gave bookmarks "as rewards for clean books."

102. Morris, *Reading, 'Riting, and Reconstruction*, 182. For quotations, see L. Maria Child, *The Freedmen's Book* [1865] (New York: Arno Press, 1968), introduction, 247, 270–72.

103. I. W. Brinckerhoff, *Advice to Freedmen* [1864] (New York: American Tract Society, 1865), 12, 29; and J. B. Waterbury, *Friendly Counsels for Freedmen* (New York: American Tract Society, 1864), 7–8, 26. An example of an American Tract Society reader that gives the same kind of advice is Mrs. H. E. Brown, *John Freeman and His Family* (Boston: American Tract Society, 1864), 28–30. For a fuller discussion of these texts, see Ronald E. Butchart, *Northern Schools, Southern Blacks, and Reconstruction: Freedmen's Education, 1862–1875* (Westport, Conn.: Greenwood Press, 1980), 141–54.

104. This quotation is from W. E. B. Du Bois, who believed these New England teachers were the unsung heroines of the Civil War. See McPherson, *Ordeal by Fire*, 399.

105. On servant Rose, see Elizabeth Ware Pearson, *Letters from Port Royal: Written at the Time of the Civil War* (Boston: W. B. Clarke, 1906), 213. For these comments (and others) on students' improvements, see Ames, *From a New England*

Woman's Diary in Dixie in 1865, 36; Swint, ed., *Dear Ones at Home*, 120; Holland, ed., *Letters and Diary of Laura M. Towne*, 32; and Botume, *First Days Amongst the Contraband*, 92.

106. Quotations are from Dixon Wecter, *When Johnny Comes Marching Home* (Boston: Houghton Mifflin, 1944), 153; Ambrose, ed., *A Wisconsin Boy in Dixie*, 142; and David Lane, *A Soldier's Diary: The Story of a Volunteer* (printed by author, 1905), 210.

107. Wecter states that the Union army's soap ration of four pounds daily per hundred men seemed "prodigal" to Europeans. Wecter, *When Johnny Comes Marching Home*, 153; and John D. Billings, *Hardtack and Coffee: Or, the Unwritten Story of Army Life* (Boston: G. M. Smith, 1887), 82, 343–44. See also "A Soldier's Retrospect," in *The Soldiers' and Sailors' Half-Dime Tales, of the Late Rebellion* (2 vols.; New York: n.p., 1868), II: 234.

108. Smith, "War and Hygiene," 90 (quote). John Shaw Billings responded on Jan. 4, 1876, to a questionnaire sent to him by Henry I. Bowditch, a Boston physician who served as an inspector in the Civil War and then as a member of the Massachusetts State Board of Health for a decade. Henry I. Bowditch, *Public Hygiene in America: Being the Centennial Discourse Delivered before the International Medical Congress, Philadelphia, September 1876* [1877] (New York: Arno Press, 1972), 36 and 147 (quotes).

109. Cassedy, "Numbering the North's Medical Events," 225–27 (quote).

110. Gillett, *Army Medical Department*, 124, for information on the the the Mexican war. Of all Union deaths, 61.4 percent resulted from disease, 38.5 percent from battle; in World War II, with the germ theory, sulfa drugs, and other improvements in place, the ratio was 28.1 percent from disease, 71.9 percent from battle. U.S. Bureau of the Census, *Historical Statistics of the United States, from Colonial Times to 1970* (Washington: Government Printing Office, 1975), II: 1140. See also Gillett, *Army Medical Department*, 203–5, 277; and Maris Vinovskis, "Have Social Historians Lost the Civil War? Some Preliminary Demographic Considerations," *Journal of American History* 76 (June 1989): 41 n. 14.

111. Howard D. Kramer, "Effect of the Civil War on the Public Health Movement," *Mississippi Valley Historical Review* 35 (Dec. 1948): 451, 456 (quote); Bowditch, *Public Hygiene in America*, 38; and Rebecca Harding Davis, *Bits of Gossip* (Boston: Houghton Mifflin, 1904), 34 (quote).

CHAPTER 3. CITY CLEANSING

1. Helen Campbell, *Household Economics: A Course of Lectures in the School of Economics of the University of Wisconsin* (New York: G. P. Putnam's Sons, 1897), 206.

2. Henry I. Bowditch, physician and longtime member of the Massachusetts Board of Health, referred to the "immense strides" made in matters of hygiene in his book, *Public Hygiene in America: Being the Centennial Discourse Delivered before the International Medical Congress, Philadelphia, September 1876* [1877] (New York: Arno Press, 1972), 36. However, it was Elisha Harris, co-founder of the United States Sanitary Commission and the American Public Health Association, that encouraged Americans to continue their warfare. See his pamphlet entitled

"How to Cleanse and Disinfect," which was reprinted in the *Southern Workman* 8 (Nov. 1879): 115 (quote).

3. Stephen Smith, *The City That Was* (New York: Frank Allaben, 1911), 127.

4. Howard D. Kramer, "Effect of the Civil War on the Public Health Movement," *Mississippi Valley Historical Review* 35 (Dec. 1948): 458–59.

5. *Harper's Weekly*, Sept. 28, 1878, p. 755. Families that could not flee were often "reduced to absolute want," and large relief efforts were organized to supply them with medicine, food, and clothing. See also George C. Whipple, *Typhoid Fever: Its Causation, Transmission, and Prevention* (New York: John Wiley & Sons, 1908), 214 (quote).

6. Jon A. Peterson, "The Impact of Sanitary Reform upon American Planning, 1840–1890," *Journal of Social History* 13 (Fall 1979): 83. Quotations are from Harris, "How to Cleanse and Disinfect," 116; and Stephen Smith, *Doctor in Medicine: And Other Papers on Professional Subjects* [1872] (New York: Arno Press, 1972), 275.

7. C.-E.A. Winslow, "Of What Use Are Our Voluntary Health Agencies" (undated copy), Charles-Edward Amory Winslow Papers (Yale University Archives).

8. Robert H. Bremner, *The Public Good: Philanthropy and Welfare in the Civil War Era* (New York: Alfred A. Knopf, 1980), 89. For quotation, see Gert H. Brieger, "Sanitary Reform in New York City: Stephen Smith and the Passage of the Metropolitan Health Bill," *Bulletin of the History of Medicine* 40 (Sept.-Oct. 1966): 421.

9. Quotations are from Smith, *The City That Was*, 137; and Elisha Harris, comp., *Report of the Council of Hygiene and Public Health of the Citizens' Association of New York, upon the Sanitary Condition of the City* [1866] (New York: Arno Press, 1970), x, xi, and xii. Chap. 4, "New York, the Unclean," in *The City That Was* contains Smith's testimony given to a committee of the New York state legislature on Feb. 13, 1865. For Harris and Smith's opinion on the 1863 draft riots, see Harris, *Report of the Council*, xv-xvi; and Smith, *The City That Was*, 99–100.

10. The details leading up to passage of the Metropolitan Health Bill are best told by Brieger, "Sanitary Reform in New York City," 407–29; and Howard D. Kramer, "Early Municipal and State Boards of Health. Part I: The New York Metropolitan Health Bill of 1866," *Bulletin of the History of Medicine* 24 (Nov.-Dec. 1950): 503–29.

11. The classic study of cholera in the United States is Charles E. Rosenberg, *The Cholera Years: The United States in 1832, 1849, and 1866* (Chicago: Univ. of Chicago Press, 1962). It explains how Americans' views regarding the causes of cholera changed in important ways during several decades.

12. In addition to Rosenberg's *Cholera Years*, see Richard J. Evans, *Death in Hamburg: Society and Politics in the Cholera Years, 1830–1910* (Oxford: Clarendon Press, 1987). See especially pages 226–30 on "The Challenge of Cholera."

13. Quotations are from G. B. Thornton, "Memphis Sanitation and Quarantine, 1879 and 1880," *Public Health: Papers and Reports Presented at the Meetings of the American Public Health Association in the Year 1880* (Boston: 1881), 193; and George E. Waring, Jr., comp., *Report on the Social Statistics of Cities. Part II: The Southern and the Western States* [1887] (New York: Arno Press, 1970), 286. See also Gerald M. Capers, Jr., "Yellow Fever in Memphis in the 1870s," *Mississippi Valley Historical Review* 24 (1937–38): 484; Henry H. Moore, *Public Health in the United*

States: An Outline with Statistical Data (New York: Harper & Brothers, 1923), 79; and Bernard A. Weisberger, "Epidemic," *American Heritage* 35 (Oct.-Nov. 1984): 57–64.

14. "Is New-York Safe?," *New York Times*, Sept. 4, 1878, p. 4 (quote). See also Gerald M. Capers, Jr., *The Biography of a River Town: Memphis, Its Heroic Age* (Chapel Hill: Univ. of North Carolina Press, 1939), 164, 195–97. The quotation describing the homes freed slaves built for themselves is found in Leon F. Litwack, *Been in the Storm So Long: The Aftermath of Slavery* (New York: Vintage Books, 1980), 314.

15. Stephen Smith, "The History of Public Health, 1871–1921," in Mazyck P. Ravenel, ed., *A Half Century of Public Health: Jubilee Historical Volume of the American Public Health Association in Commemoration of the Fiftieth Anniversary Celebration of Its Foundation, New York City, November 14–18, 1921* (New York: American Public Health Association, 1921), 9–10; and Stephen Smith, "Historical Sketch of the American Public Health Association," in *Public Health: Papers and Reports Presented at the Meetings of the American Public Health Association in the Year 1879* (Boston, 1880), x.

16. John Duffy gives an almost day-by-day account of the actions of the Metropolitan Health Board in *A History of Public Health in New York City, 1866–1966* (New York: Russell Sage Foundation, 1974), 6–19.

17. Ibid., 12–13, 18–19.

18. Lewis H. Steiner, "A Sanitary View of the Question,—'Am I My Brother's Keeper?,'" *Public Health: Papers and Reports Presented at the Meetings of the American Public Health Association in the Year 1874–75* (New York, 1876), 525.

19. Max Von Pettenkofer (the famous German sanitarian), "Value of Health to a City," *Sanitarian* 4 (Jan. 1876): 21.

20. Sam B. Warner, Jr., "Public Health Reform and the Depression of 1873–1878," *Bulletin of the History of Medicine* 29 (Nov.-Dec. 1955): 505–6.

21. Martin V. Melosi, *Garbage in the Cities: Refuse, Reform, and the Environment, 1880–1980* (College Station: Texas A&M University Press, 1981), 43. After the dirt and debris were swept up, they were sometimes collected by local farmers, private contractors, or scavengers employed by municipalities. For the quotation, see William Dean Howells, *A Hazard of New Fortunes* [1890] (New York: New American Library, 1965), 260.

22. William P. Gerhard, *On Bathing and Different Forms of Baths* (New York: William Comstock, 1895), 23; and Henry F. Lyster, "Baths and Bathing," *Fifth Annual Report of the Secretary of the State Board of Health of the State of Michigan, for the Fiscal Year Ending September 30, 1877* (Lansing, 1878). I am grateful to Ronald L. Numbers at the University of Wisconsin for sending me a copy of the Michigan report.

23. The best reference to 200 years of public works development in the United States is Ellis L. Armstrong, Michael C. Robinson, and Suellen M. Hoy, eds., *History of Public Works in the United States, 1776–1976* (Chicago: American Public Works Association, 1976). The best monographic studies on sewer and wastewater technology are the many articles and essays by Joel A. Tarr. See, for example, "The Separate vs. Combined Sewer Problem: A Case Study in Urban Technology Design Choice," *Journal of Urban History* 5 (May 1979): 308–39. An important complement to these is Stanley K. Schultz, *Constructing Urban Culture: American Cities and City Planning, 1800–1920* (Philadelphia: Temple Univ. Press, 1989).

24. Howard D. Kramer, "Agitation for Public Health Reform in the 1870's: The National Board of Health of 1879," *Journal of the History of Medicine & Allied Sciences* 4 (Winter 1949): 75–89.

25. For a contemporary, laudatory, and brief biography of George Waring, see Albert Shaw, *Life of Col. Geo. E. Waring, Jr.: The Greatest Apostle of Cleanliness* (New York: Patriotic League, 1899). Two solid articles on Waring's career are those by James H. Cassedy, "The Flamboyant Colonel Waring: An Anti-Contagionist Holds the American Stage in the Age of Pasteur and Koch," *Bulletin of the History of Medicine* 36 (March–April 1962): 163–72; and Martin V. Melosi, "Pragmatic Environmentalist: Sanitary Engineer George E. Waring, Jr.," *Essays in Public Works History* 4 (April 1977): 1–18. The quotation can be found in Cassedy, "The Flamboyant Colonel Waring," 166.

26. See Tarr, "The Separate vs. Combined Sewer Problem," 308–9, 316. See also Melosi, "Pragmatic Environmentalist," 9; and George E. Waring, Jr., "The National Board of Health," *Atlantic Monthly* 44 (Dec. 1879): 732–33 (quotes).

27. On the friendship between Waring and Olmsted, see Laura Wood Roper, *FLO: A Biography of Frederick Law Olmsted* (Baltimore: Johns Hopkins Univ. Press, 1973), 148, 162, 164, 299, 320, and 462. On Waring's military career, see "The Military Element in Colonel Waring's Career," *Century* 59 (Feb. 1900): 544–55.

28. Cassedy, "The Flamboyant Colonel Waring," 164.

29. Thornton, "Memphis Sanitation and Quarantine," 193 (quote); Lynette B. Wrenn, "The Memphis Sewer Experiment," *Tennessee Historical Quarterly* 44 (Fall 1985): 341–42, 349; John Duffy, *The Sanitarians: A History of American Public Health* (Urbana: Univ. of Illinois Press, 1990), 146; and Tarr, "The Separate vs. Combined Sewer Problem," 317–18.

30. Tarr, "The Separate vs. Combined Sewer Problem," 318–22; and Armstrong, Robinson, and Hoy, eds., *History of Public Works*, 402. Waring's sewers were smaller because two sets of pipes—rather than one large one—separated sewage from storm water.

31. Cassedy, "The Flamboyant Colonel Waring," 170. For a concise history of the National Board of Health, see Duffy, *Sanitarians*, 162–72.

32. Quotations are from *Sanitarian* 4 (Aug. 15, 1884); and George E. Waring, Jr., "The Sewering and Draining of Cities," *Public Health: Papers and Reports Presented at the Meetings of the American Public Health Association in the Year 1879* (Boston, 1880), 40.

33. See U.S. Bureau of the Census, *Historical Statistics of the United States, Colonial Times to 1970* [Bicentennial Edition] (2 vols.; Washington, D.C.: Government Printing Office, 1975), I: 58 (Series B149-B166).

34. J. S. Billings, "The President's Address," in *Public Health: Papers and Reports Presented at the Eighth Annual Meeting of the American Public Health Association in the Year 1880* (Boston, 1881), 4.

35. See the first two chapters in Robert H. Wiebe, *The Search for Order, 1877–1920* (New York: Hill and Wang, 1967); the quotation is on p. 45.

36. Phyllis Allen Richmond, "American Attitudes Toward the Germ Theory of Disease (1860–1880)," in Gert H. Brieger, ed., *Theory and Practice in American Medicine: Historical Studies from the Journal of the History of Medicine & Allied Sciences* (New York: Science History Publications, 1976), 60.

37. *Chicago Inter Ocean*, Sept. 23, 1892.

38. "Modern Sanitation," *Sanitary News* 6 (June 27, 1885): 74.

39. Quotations are from Frank Hastings Hamilton, "Sewer-Gas," *Popular Science Monthly* 22 (Nov. 1882): 15–17: and Charles F. Chandler to C.-E.A. Winslow, Dec. 20, 1909, Winslow Papers.

40. Quotations are from George E. Waring, Jr., *The Sanitary Drainage of Houses and Towns* (New York: Hurd and Houghton, 1876), 94; and Hamilton (on Waring), "Sewer-Gas," 17. For a discussion of Waring's advocacy of the filth theory of disease and his belief in sanitary reform, see Melosi, *Garbage in the Cities*, 60–62.

41. Quotations can be found in George F. Waring, Jr., "The Causation of Typhoid Fever," *Boston Medical and Surgical Journal* 99 (July 25, 1878): 107: *Sanitary News* 5 (April 11, 1885): 138; and Charles F. Wingate, "The Unsanitary Homes of the Rich," *North American Review* 132 (1883): 177.

42. Duffy, *Sanitarians*, 129, 187; David P. Handlin, *The American Home: Architecture and Society, 1815–1915* (Boston: Little, Brown, 1979), 471. Handlin writes that "it often took city authorities many decades to update their codes. . . . In this respect George Waring was right, if only for the wrong reasons." *Sanitary News* is a rich source of information on the plumbers' movement. See, for example, volumes 1 (Nov. 15, 1882), 15; 2 (June 15, 1883), 73; 4 (July 15, 1884), 78; 5 (Feb. 15 and March 14, 1885), 88 and 105; and 6 (July 18, 1885), 95.

43. See "Mrs. Harriette M. Plunkett," in Frances E. Willard and Mary A. Livermore, eds., *A Woman of the Century: Fourteen Hundred-Seventy Biographical Sketches Accompanied by Portraits of Leading American Women in All Walks of Life* (Chicago: Charles Wells Moulton, 1893), 576–77. Quotations are on pages 10, 165, and 227 of Mrs. H. M. Plunkett, *Women, Plumbers, and Doctors; Or, Household Sanitation* (New York: D. Appleton, 1885). Whole chapters of this book are devoted to such topics as "Sewerage and Plumbing," "Sewer-Gas and Germs," "Our Neighbor's Premises," and "Public Sanitation." The inscription on the title page reads: "Showing that, if women and plumbers do their whole sanitary duty, there will be comparatively little occasion for the services of the doctors."

44. Mrs. John Hays Hammond, "Woman's Place in Civic Life," *American Club Woman* 2 (Nov. 1911): 406 (quote); and Mary Caroline Robbins, "Village Improvement Societies," *Atlantic Monthly* 79 (Feb. 1897): 212 (quote).

45. George F. Waring, Jr., "Village Improvement Associations," *Scribner's Monthly* 14 (May 1877): 98.

46. Ruth Bordin, *Women and Temperance: The Quest for Power and Liberty, 1873–1900* [1981] (New Brunswick: Rutgers Univ. Press, 1990), 58. By 1890, the WCTU was "the goliath of women's organizations" with its 150,000 dues-paying members and a national budget of about $30,000. But Ruth Bordin points out that this was only a small part of the total budget; local unions had reported raising $317,345 in 1890. There were also auxiliary groups for young women and children.

47. Frances E. Willard, "How to Win: A Book for Girls [1888]," in Aileen S. Kraditor, ed., *Up from the Pedestal: Selected Writings in the History of American Feminism* (Chicago: Quadrangle Books, 1968), 318 (quote); and Bordin, *Woman and Temperance*, 160. Portions of this story have been told in Suellen M. Hoy, "'Municipal Housekeeping': The Role of Women in Improving Urban Sanitation Practices, 1880–1917," in Martin V. Melosi, ed., *Pollution & Reform in American Cities, 1870–1920* (Austin: Univ. of Texas Press, 1980), 173–98. See also Maureen A. Flanagan, "Gender and Urban Political Reform: The City Club and the Woman's City Club of Chicago in the Progressive Era," *American Historical Review* 95 (Oct.

1990): esp. 1036–39 and 1046–50; and Nancy Tomes, "The Private Side of Public Health: Sanitary Science, Domestic Hygiene, and the Germ Theory, 1870–1900," *Bulletin of the History of Medicine* 64 (Winter 1990): esp. 536.

48. All quotations, except one, are from Robbins, "Village Improvement Societies," 213, 214, and 217. For the quotation on Mary Hopkins's motivation, see William H. Wilson, *The City Beautiful Movement* (Baltimore: Johns Hopkins Univ. Press, 1989), 42. For a fuller description of the Stockbridge changes by a "hometown boy," see B. G. Northrop, "The Work of Village-Improvement Societies," *Forum* 19 (March 1895): 95–96.

49. William H. Wilson makes the important distinction between preventing decline and controlling growth. See Wilson, *The City Beautiful Movement*, 42. And Robbins, for example, notes that Olmsted's early reports showed "that much of the unhealthiness of New York's suburbs arose from the neglect of proper precautions about drainage." Robbins, "Village Improvement Societies," 214.

50. *New York Times*, Jan. 23 and April 21, 1881. Many such accounts appeared prior to the creation of a street-cleaning department in the spring of 1881. New York City's Citizens' Committee of Twenty-one had promoted this change as a matter "better calculated to advance political interests than to secure cleanliness and health." Melosi, *Garbage in the Cities*, 35.

51. The pile of manure weighed 20,000 tons and was 30 feet high and 200 feet long! Mary E. Trautmann, "Women's Health Protective Association," *Municipal Affairs* 2 (Sept. 1898): 439–40; and (for all quotations) Ladies' Health Protective Association, *Memorial of the New York Ladies' Health Protective Association, to the Hon. Abram S. Hewitt, Mayor of New York, on the Subject of Street-Cleaning* (New York: n.p., 1887), 3–4, 5.

52. Ladies' Health Protective Association, *Memorial*, 5–11 (quotation on last page).

53. Duffy, *Public Health in New York City, 1866–1966*, 130–32; Melosi, *Garbage in the Cities*, 35–36; and Ladies' Health Protective Association, *Memorial*, 4–5 (quote).

54. Duffy, *Public Health in New York City, 1866–1966*, 124; "Clean for Once" (on the Street Cleaning Aid Association, an organization of women assisted by an advisory board of men), *Woman's Journal* 22 (Sept. 19, 1891): 299; and William Howe Tolman, *Municipal Reform Movements in the United States* (New York: Fleming H. Revell, 1895), 172–73, 174–76.

55. See the following articles from the Chicago *Tribune*: "City Officials and the Fair," Feb. 26, 1890; "A Hint to the Women of Chicago," May 2, 1890 (quote); "Clean the City Alleys," June 22, 1890; and "Filth and Inefficiency," July 5, 1890. See too Melosi, *Garbage in the Cities*, 28–29.

56. *Daily Inter Ocean*, March 21 and 28, 1892. The *Inter Ocean* even suggested that Sweet be made the new street-cleaning superintendent. See "Clean Up" and "Why Not Ada C. Sweet," *Daily Inter Ocean*, July 20, 1892 (quotes). Members of the Hull-House Women's Club were among those who inspected streets and alleys "through the Municipal Order League." See Residents of Hull-House, *Hull-House Maps and Papers* (New York: Thomas Y. Crowell, 1895), 220. The health department previously had responsibility for street cleaning; then in March 1893 this new street-cleaning department was named the Bureau of Street and Alley Cleaning and placed in the Department of Public Works. See *Daily Inter Ocean*, March 15, 1893, and Bessie Louise Pierce, *A History of Chicago: The Rise of a Modern City, 1871–1893* (New York: Alfred A. Knopf, 1957), 321.

57. "Women versus Garbage," *Woman's Journal* 23 (July 23, 1892): 236 (quote); Melosi, *Garbage in the Cities*, 47; and "Clean Up," *Daily Inter Ocean*, July 20, 1892 (quote).

58. "Women and Street Cleaning" (Sweet's letter published by Stanton), *Woman's Journal* 24 (Aug. 19, 1893): 257 (quote); and Willard and Livermore, eds., *A Woman of the Century*, 702–3. For petitions, see "Ada C. Sweet" folders, Illinois Pension Agency, Chicago, U.S. Department of Interior, RG 48 (National Archives, Washington, D.C.).

59. For motto, see stationery heading in letter of Ada C. Sweet to B. F. Mc-Clure, Jan. 26, 1889, Illinois Pension Agency, Chicago, U.S. Department of Interior RG 48 (National Archives). In Sweet's published letter to Elizabeth Cady Stanton, Sweet stressed the importance of understanding current waste disposal practices and "the local state of public feeling" before making recommendations to correct certain conditions. *Woman's Journal*, Aug. 19, 1893. See also *Daily Inter Ocean*, Oct. 10, 1892.

In early 1893 Stanton published a pamphlet entitled "Important Work to Get Ready for the World's Fair" in which she encouraged people of influence—city officials, teachers, railroad authorities, ministers, and women (particularly those on the Fair's Board of Lady Managers)—to "see that the city has such a thorough cleaning as it has never had before." While she wanted to impress foreign visitors, she too was especially worried about an outbreak of disease in the summer months. See *Woman's Tribune*, March 18, 1893. The editors of the Papers of Elizabeth Cady Stanton and Susan B. Anthony believe that this text is identical to the pamphlet that appeared as an issue of the *National Bulletin* (probably Vol. 2, No. 4) in April 1893. It is not certain how this pamphlet was distributed, but the editors of the Stanton-Anthony Papers have an advertisement that shows that "Work for Women before the World's Fair" was available as a separate pamphlet.

60. Bessie Louise Pierce, *A History of Chicago . . . 1871–1893*, 321; and *Daily Inter Ocean*, Aug. 25 and 26, 1892 (on "plague spots" and the contract system). "Plague spots" were extremely serious; the Chicago Department of Health reported nearly 2000 deaths from typhoid fever in the year ending Feb. 29, 1892. Daniel H. Burnham, *The Final Official Report of the Director of Works of the World's Columbian Exposition* (2 parts; New York: Garland, 1989), I: 71. For the final quotes, see "Minutes," Dec. 28, 1892, Box 2, Chicago Woman's Club Ms. Collection (Chicago Historical Society). And for a significant study that demonstrates how the purposes of women reformers frequently differed from that of their male counterparts, see Flanagan, "Gender and Urban Political Reform," 1032–50.

In Sweet's letter to Stanton noted above (*Woman's Journal*, Aug. 19, 1893), Sweet fell short of demanding the municipal ballot for women. Stanton, however, used her letter to demonstrate the need. She argued that if the women who had established municipal sanitary leagues "could express their opinions in votes, and select officers who would carry out their wishes, their influence would be increased four-fold." Before long most municipal housekeepers would agree.

61. Wilson, *The City Beautiful Movement*, 57; David F. Burg, *Chicago's White City of 1893* (Lexington: Univ. Press of Kentucky, 1976), 87, 337–38; and Wm. S. MacHarg, Water Supply, Sewerage, and Fire Protection Engineer, to Daniel H. Burnham, Director of Works, *Final Offical Report*, I: 84. MacHarg also proudly reported that "there has been no dissemination of disease, like typhoid fever through-

out the country, such as resulted from the use of impure water at the Centennial [in Philadelphia in 1876]." Ibid., 72.

62. *New York Times*, Dec. 30, 1894 (quote). On Eleanora Kinnicutt's overall influence, see the obituary of "Mrs. F. P. Kinnicutt" (her husband was Dr. Francis P. Kinnicutt), ibid., Oct. 27, 1919. See also Richard Welling, *As the Twig Is Bent* (New York: G. P. Putnam's Sons, 1942), 69 (quote); and Richard Skolnik, "George F. Waring, Jr.: A Model for Reformers," *New-York Historical Society Quarterly* 52 (Jan. 1968): 357. For Kinnicutt's role in the 1892 reorganization, she was compared to Governor DeWitt Clinton, who gave canals to the state; "Mrs. Kinnicutt," for her part, was "giving clean streets to its metropolis." See "Clean Streets for New York," *Woman's Journal* 23 (May 7, 1892): 148.

Kinnicutt was not acquainted with William L. Strong until after the election, although she had supported his candidacy. She then asked Seth Low for a letter of introduction: "A word from you would perhaps take away from Mr. Strong's very natural fear of petticoat meddling & would certainly give me courage to undertake a disagreeable & difficult task, which should not be shirked." Eleanora Kinnicutt to Seth Low, Nov. 10, 1894, Seth Low Papers (Columbia University Rare Book and Manuscript Library, New York City). I am grateful to Daniel E. Burnstein for sending me a copy of this letter.

63. The most recent account of Waring's career as commissioner by a historian is Martin Melosi's " 'The Apostle of Cleanliness' and the Origins of Refuse Management," in Melosi, *Garbage in the Cities*, 51–78. Two other fine articles by historians are Cassedy's, "The Flamboyant Colonel Waring," 163–76; and Skolnik's, "George Edwin Waring, Jr.," 354–78 (full citations are given above). For accounts written by contemporaries, see Charles A. Meade, "City Cleansing in New York: Some Advances and Retreats," *Municipal Affairs* 4 (Dec. 1900): 723–33; and Shaw, *Life of Col. Geo. Waring, Jr.* (citation above). See also George E. Waring, Jr., to Frederick Law Olmsted, Jan. 6, 1895, General Correspondence Series, Frederick Law Olmsted Papers (Manuscript Division, Library of Congress). This letter is touching; Waring recalls their days together in Central Park and thanks Olmsted for the training and example he provided.

64. Ibid.; and George E. Waring, Jr., "The Cleaning of a Great City," *McClure's Magazine* 9 (Sept. 1897): 924 (quote). On Waring's style, see "Colonel Waring's 'White Angels': A Sketch of the Street-Cleaning Department of New York," *Outlook* 53 (June 27, 1896): 1191–93; "Clean Streets at Last: Fruitless Search for Derelict Wagons and Stray Bits of Paper—A Drive with Colonel Waring," *New York Times*, July 28, 1895, p. 28; and Skolnick, "George Edwin Waring, Jr.," 359–69.

65. Reuben S. Simons, "The Juvenile Street Cleaning Leagues of New York," *American City* 3 (Oct. 1910): 163–66; Waring, "The Cleaning of a Great City," 922; Melosi, *Garbage in the Cities*, 74–76; and David Willard, "The Juvenile Street-Cleaning Leagues," in George E. Waring, Jr., *Street-Cleaning and the Disposal of a City's Wastes: Methods and Results and the Effect upon Public Health, Public Morals, and Municipal Prosperity* (New York: Doubleday & McClure, 1899), 177–86.

66. I am especially indebted to Martin V. Melosi for his analysis of Waring as an environmentalist and as a model for turn-of-the-century reformers. See chap. 2 in Melosi, *Garbage in the Cities*, particularly pp. 60–62 and 77–78. See also Charles V. Chapin, "The End of the Filth Theory of Disease," *Popular Science Monthly* 60 (1902): 235 (quote).

67. *New York Times*, July 7, 1896.

68. Timothy J. Gilfoyle, *City of Eros: New York City, Prostitution, and the Commercialization of Sex, 1790–1920* (New York: W. W. Norton, 1992), 181, 197, 223; and David J. Pivar, "A Walk on the Dark Side," *Reviews in American History* 21 (Sept. 1993): 432–33.

69. Besides Gilfoyle's *City of Eros*, see David J. Pivar, *Purity Crusade: Sexual Morality, and Social Control, 1868–1900* (Westport, Conn.: Greenwood Press, 1973); James F. Gardner, "Microbes and Morality: The Social Hygiene Crusade in New York City, 1892–1917" (Ph.D. dissertation, Indiana University, 1974); David J. Pivar, "Cleansing the Nation: The War on Prostitution," *Prologue* 12 (Spring 1980): 29–40; and Mary P. Ryan, *Women in Public: Between Banners and Ballots, 1825–1880* (Baltimore: Johns Hopkins Univ. Press, 1990), 95–129.

70. See Gilfoyle's *City of Eros*, 306–15, for a thorough discussion of "The End of the Century of Prostitution." Besides what I have already mentioned, he shows that premarital sex increased (making prostitution less necessary or attractive), and within marriage, Americans saw sex more as a basic expression of mutual love and less a technique of reproduction. Better working conditions and wages for women also made prostitution less appealing and served to cleanse cities of it. The quotations from government pamphlets are in Gardner, "Microbes and Morality," 372.

71. Mary Ritter Beard, *Woman's Work in Municipalities* (New York: D. Appleton, 1916), 84 (quotes). For a history of women's clubs, see Karen J. Blair, *The Clubwoman as Feminist: True Womanhood Redefined, 1868–1914* (New York: Holmes & Meier, 1980); and for the municipal housekeeping contributions of various women's groups and especially the work of Mary McDowell in Chicago, Kate Gordon in New Orleans, Sarah Platt Decker in Denver, and Sarah A. Evans in Portland, see Hoy, " 'Municipal Housekeeping,' " 173–98. On African-American women's groups, see Cynthia Neverdon-Morton, "Self-Help Programs as Educative Activities of Black Women in the South, 1895–1925: Focus on Four Key Areas," *Journal of Negro Education* 51 (Summer 1982): 217–18 as well as her monograph, *Afro-American Women of the South and the Advancement of the Race, 1895–1925* (Knoxville: Univ. of Tennessee Press, 1989), esp. pp. 145–48; and Gerda Lerner, "Early Community Work of Black Club Women," *Journal of Negro Education* 59 (April 1974): 158–67.

72. Charles R. Starring, "Caroline Julia Bartlett Crane," in Edward T. James, Janet Wilson James, and Paul S. Boyer, eds, *Notable American Women, 1607–1950* (3 vols.; Cambridge: Harvard Univ. Press, 1971), I: 402 (quote); and Hoy, " 'Municipal Housekeeping,' " 181–88 (used here with permission).

73. Caroline Bartlett Crane, "The Story and the Results," typescript autobiography, ca. 1925, Caroline Bartlett Crane Papers (Western Michigan University Archives and Regional History Collections, Kalamazoo), 1–15. For a discussion of Crane as a Progressive, see Alan S. Brown, "Caroline Bartlett Crane and Urban Reform," *Michigan History Magazine* 56 (Winter 1972): 287–301.

74. Caroline Bartlett Crane, "Interest in Meat Inspection," typescript, 1909, Crane Papers, 1–13; and *Kalamazoo Gazette*, March 28, 1902. The bill was Senate Bill No. 306, which became effective on Sept. 17, 1903.

75. Quotations appear in Caroline Bartlett Crane, "The Work for Clean Streets," *Women's Forum* (Sept. 1905): 2; and Crane, "The Making of an Ideal City," Crane Papers.

76. Crane, "Work for Clean Streets," 3. See also clippings from the Kalamazoo newspapers in the Crane Papers.

77. Caroline Bartlett Crane to Mrs. C. G. Higbee, Sept. 21, 1910, Crane Papers.

78. Caroline Bartlett Crane, "Questions about Your City," Crane Papers.

79. Caroline Bartlett Crane to Mrs. [?] Atwood, Aug. 13, 1910, Crane Papers.

80. See, for example, Crane to Atwood, Aug. 13 and 27, and Sept. 10, 1910, Crane Papers; "Cleaning Up American Cities," *Survey* 25 (Oct. 8, 1910): 83–84; and Crane, "The Making of an Ideal City."

81. Helen Christine Bennett, *American Women in Civic Work* (New York: Dodd, Mead, 1915), 41–42; Caroline Bartlett Crane, typescript on Kentucky surveys and clippings from Kentucky newspapers, 1909, Crane Papers; and *Journal of the American Medical Association* 53 (Sept. 11, 1909): 887–88. Katherine C. Halley of Nashville, Tennessee, wrote to Crane following her visit: "Plans are already on foot to clean up and paint the market house and the mayor wishes the city council to appropriate money for a three-storied market house. . . . There are also recommendations for flushing the streets two or three times a week." Halley to Crane, May 6, 1910, Crane Papers, which are filled with such letters.

82. Crane was hardly alone among women reformers of the Progressive era in her desire for "clean" government. See "The Feminine Version of Civil Service Reform" in Theda Skocpol, *Protecting Soldiers and Mothers: The Political Origins of Social Policy in the United States* (Cambridge: Belknap Press, 1992), 355–61, as well as Caroline Bartlett Crane, *Clean Streets for Chicago* [pamphlet] (Chicago, 1907), 3; and Crane, *General Sanitary Survey of Erie, Pennsylvania* (Erie, 1910), 21–22. Quotations are from William O'Neill, *Everyone Was Brave: A History of Feminism in America* (New York: Quadrangle, 1976), 143; Martha E. D. White, "The Work of the Women's Club," *Atlantic Monthly* 93 (May 1904): 615; and Edith Parker Thomson, "What Women Have Done for the Public Health," *Forum* 24 (Sept. 1897): 54–55.

83. See, for example, the 1907 garbage workers' strike in New York City. Before the strike the Women's Municipal League had cooperated with the New York Academy of Medicine and the City Club to improve the Street Cleaning Department's operations as directed by a new commissioner. Once the strike occurred, New Yorkers grew more offended each day by the growing mounds of garbage. Not only did they fear epidemic disease (most were still influenced by a miasma theory of disease that also incorporated aspects of the newer germ theory), but they also complained that the garbage threatened their orderly way of life. For cleanliness had become "popularly associated with wholesomeness, good character, and social order." Daniel Eli Burnstein, "Progressivism and Urban Crisis: The New York City Garbage Workers' Strike of 1907," *Journal of Urban History* 16 (Aug. 1990): 386–423 (quotation on pages 400–401).

CHAPTER 4. THE AMERICAN WAY

1. Anzia Yezierska, *Bread Givers* [1925] (New York: Persea Books, 1975), 6.

2. Quotations are from "Disease in Filth—Health in the Bath," *Sanitarian* 6 (Oct. 10, 1885): 196; and *The Immigrant's Guide to Cleveland, Ohio* (Cleveland: City Hall, n.d.), 10. A copy can be found on microfilm in the "Y.M.C.A. Papers Dealing with Immigration," Folder 35, Immigration History Research Center (University of Minnesota, St. Paul).

3. Mary Antin, *The Promised Land* (Boston: Houghton Mifflin, 1912), 271. A group of Boston immigrants said they studied English for "the personal benefits de-

rived from it" and because they did not want to be considered "inferior" or "animals." These same motives encouraged habits of cleanliness. See "Report of the Armenian Secretary for the Year 1925," Papers of the International Institute of Boston, Immigration History Research Center.

4. For quotations, see "The Greatest Virtue," *Ladies' Home Journal* 27 (May 1910): 5; William T. Sedgwick, "The Philosophy of Cleanness," *Current Literature* 33 (Sept. 1902): 345; and Theodore Hough and William T. Sedgwick, *The Human Mechanism: Its Physiology and Hygiene and the Sanitation of Its Surroundings* (Boston: Ginn, 1906), 413. Sedgwick, a prominent sanitary engineer and pioneering bacteriologist, understood clearly the cause of disease. As an advocate of the "new public health," he was one of the first to emphasize the importance of personal cleanliness over public cleanliness. See also Alan M. Kraut, *The Huddled Masses: The Immigrant in American Society, 1880–1921* (Arlington Heights, Ill.: Harlan Davidson, 1982), 2.

5. John F. McClymer, "The Americanization Movement and the Education of the Foreign-Born Adult, 1914–25," in Bernard J. Weiss, ed., *American Education and the European Immigrant, 1840–1940* (Urbana: Univ. of Illinois Press, 1982), 109 (quote). On a list of "Characteristics of the Uneducated Foreign-Born," numbers one and two are "Little appreciation of sanitation and its benefits" and "Have habits of disorder in their homes and the work of the home." See Edith May Garretson, *Home and Health in a New Land: English Lessons for Women First and Second Years* (New York: Charles Scribner's Sons, 1927), xix. For other examples of English language books that offered instruction in hygiene, see Rose M. O'Toole, *Practical English for New Americans* (Boston: D.C. Heath, 1920) and John A. Long, *Reader for New Americans: Book One* (New York: American Book Company, 1923).

"Americanization" did not necessarily mean repressive Anglo conformity. Otis Graham and Elizabeth Koed distinguish between the "100 percent Americanism" of the sometimes hysterical World War I years and the earlier "liberal Americanization," which sought through "social activism . . . to hasten individual and group advancement and social assimilation, and promote national unity." Otis L. Graham, Jr., and Elizabeth Koed, "Americanizing the Immigrant, Past and Future: History and Implications of a Social Movement," *Public Historian* 15 (Fall 1993): 41.

6. Booker T. Washington, *Up from Slavery: An Autobiography* (New York: Doubleday, Page, 1901), 58.

7. "To the Students of Hampton: For Young Men," *Southern Workman* 4 (May 1875): 36.

8. Edith Armstrong Talbot, *Samuel Chapman Armstrong: A Biographical Study* [1904] (New York: Negro Universities Press, 1969), 47, 104–5, 106, 114, 115. For a concise biographical sketch of Armstrong, see Louis Harlan et al., eds., *The Papers of Booker T. Washington*, vol. 2: *1860–89* (Urbana: Univ. of Illinois Press, 1972), 40–41.

9. Quotations are from Louis R. Harlan, *Booker T. Washington: The Making of a Black Leader, 1856–1901* (New York: Oxford Univ. Press, 1972), 60–61; and Talbot, *Samuel Chapman Armstrong*, 156, 202.

10. Harlan, *Booker T. Washington*, 58, 62–64.

11. For quotations, see Raymond W. Smock, ed., *Booker T. Washington in Perspective: Essays of Louis R. Harlan* (Jackson: Univ. Press of Mississippi, 1988), 11; and Washington, *Up from Slavery*, 44.

12. Washington, *Up from Slavery*, 52–53.

13. See ibid., 58; letter from "W," *Southern Workman* 7 (July 1878): 52; and "To the Students of Hampton: For Young Men," 36. Hampton's young men were also taught about their underclothes. Heavy in winter and light in summer, they were to be changed "at least, once a week." And young women were told to prefer "cleanliness" over "finery"—to buy a "proper change of underclothing" rather than "ribbons." See "To the Students of Hampton: For Young Women," *Southern Workman* 4 (March 1875): 20.

14. Washington, *Up from Slavery*, 126 and 174 (quote); and Booker T. Washington, *Working with the Hands: Being a Sequel to "Up from Slavery" Covering the Author's Experiences in Industrial Training at Tuskegee* (New York: Doubleday, Page, 1904), 183 (quote). For an extended discussion of the purpose and methods of the Armstrong-Washington schools and their place in the history of southern black education, see James D. Anderson, "The Hampton Model of Normal School Industrial Education, 1868–1915," in *The Education of Blacks in the South, 1860–1935* (Chapel Hill: Univ. of North Carolina Press, 1988), 33–78.

15. On Booker T. Washington and his social philosophy, see C. Vann Woodward, *Origins of the New South, 1877–1913* (Baton Rouge: Louisiana State Univ. Press, 1951), 356–68. The three quotations are from *Origins* and may be found respectively on pages 357, 359, and 365. For a description of the poor living and working conditions in Georgia's Black Belt in the 1890s, see W. E. Burghardt Du Bois, "Of the Quest of the Golden Fleece," in *The Souls of Black Folk: Essays and Sketches* (Chicago: A. C. McClurg, 1903), 135–62.

16. Woodward, *Origins*, 325. For an example of Anglo-Saxonist nativism at this time, see William Allen White's *Emporia Gazette* editorial for Feb. 23, 1898: " . . . as between Cuba and Spain there is little choice. Both crowds are yellow-legged, garlic-eating, dagger-sticking, treacherous crowds—a mixture of Guinea, Indian, and Dago. One crowd is as bad as the other. It is folly to spill good Saxon blood for that kind of vermin." Quoted in Walter T. K. Nugent, *The Tolerant Populists: Kansas Populism and Nativism* (Chicago: Univ. of Chicago Press, 1963), 214.

17. Edward Bok, "The Morals of the Bathtub," *Ladies' Home Journal* 13 (Nov. 1896): 14.

18. Winthrop D. Jordan, *White over Black: American Attitudes toward the Negro, 1550–1812* (Chapel Hill: Univ. of North Carolina Press, 1968), esp. 252–59. Francis A. Walker, "Immigration," *Yale Review* 1 (Aug. 1892): 125–45 (quotations are on pp. 126, 132, 133, and 137). In the same vein, see Madison Grant and Chas. Stewart Davison, eds., *The Alien in Our Midst: Or "Selling Our Birthright for a Mess of Pottage"* (New York: Galton, 1930). "Mudsill" was a term commonly used by better-off Southerners to describe poor whites and blacks.

19. Quotation is from Antin, *The Promised Land*, 187. See also Walter Nugent, *Crossings: The Great Transatlantic Migrations, 1870–1914* (Bloomington: Indiana Univ. Press, 1992), chap. 15. Nativists especially resented the "birds of passage."

20. Emily Greene Balch, *Our Slavic Fellow Citizens* (New York: Charities Publication Committee, 1910), 107. See too John Bodnar, *The Transplanted: A History of Immigrants in Urban America* (Bloomington: Indiana Univ. Press, 1985), 13; and Ewa Morawska's discussion of the "American option" in *For Bread with Butter: The Life-Worlds of East Central Europeans in Johnstown, Pennsylvania, 1890–1940* (Cambridge: Cambridge Univ. Press, 1985), 63–78.

21. 61 Cong., 3rd Sess., S. Doc. 747, *Reports of the Immigration Commission:*

Abstracts of Reports of the Immigration Commission (2 vols.; Washington: Government Printing Office, 1911), II: 300–301. The number of toilets varied from ship to ship. Some early vessels had only 21 toilets per thousand immigrants; later ones had one toilet for every 47 passengers. Kraut, *Huddled Masses*, 49. See also Philip A. M. Taylor, *The Distant Magnet: European Migration to the U.S.A.* (New York: Harper & Row, 1971), 138 (quote). Prior to 1892, migrants to New York disembarked at Castle Garden.

22. Michael La Sorte, *La Merica: Images of Italian Greenhorn Experience* (Philadelphia: Temple Univ. Press, 1985), 26; Salvatore J. LaGumina, *The Immigrants Speak: Italian Americans Tell Their Story* (New York: Center for Migration Studies, 1979), 116; and Transcript of Oral Interview with Angela Mischke (undated), Polish American Collection, Immigration History Research Center.

23. "Where the World Was New: Immigrants Recall Ellis Island," *New York Times*, Sept. 9, 1990.

24. LaGumina, *The Immigrants Speak*, 116. Kraut, *Huddled Masses*, 43–63, provides a detailed and readable account of the "gruelling inspection procedure" that immigrants confronted at Ellis Island; he also explains the treatment given to those persons detained or not admitted. See also Alan M. Kraut, "Healers and Strangers: Immigrant Attitudes Toward the Physician in America—A Relationship in Historical Perspective," *Journal of the American Medical Association* 263 (April 4, 1990): 1808.

25. Anzia Yezierska, "How I Found America," in *Hungry Hearts* (Boston: Houghton Mifflin, 1920), 263. I am grateful to Alice Kessler-Harris for introducing me to Anzia Yezierska.

26. Antin, *The Promised Land*, 183 (quote). Antin also recalled the trauma of a steam shower when she left Gdansk for America at age 12, quoted in Sydney Stahl Weinberg, *The World of Our Mothers: The Lives of Jewish Immigrant Women* (New York: Schocken Books, 1990), 79. Weinberg is rich with references and quotations from young eastern-European Jewish women struggling to preserve their own standards of cleanliness while learning to become "good Americans." See also Transcript of Oral Interview with Sophie Kosciolowski (undated), Polish American Collection, Immigration History Research Center; and Viola Paradise, "The Jewish Immigrant Girl in Chicago," *Survey* 30 (Sept. 6, 1913): 701–2. And, finally, Yezierska, "How I Found America," 263 (quote). On the absence of urban amenities, see Esther G. Barrows, *Neighbors All: A Settlement Notebook* (Boston: Houghton Mifflin, 1929), 107; A Polish Trade Unionist, "Impressions of America," *Life and Labor* 6 (Nov. 1916): 172–73; and Jane Addams, *Twenty Years at Hull-House: With Autobiographical Notes* (Urbana: Univ. of Illinois Press, 1990), 66.

27. Quotations are quoted in Valentine Rossilli Winsey, "The Italian Immigrant Women Who Arrived in the United States Before World War I," in Francesco Cordasco, ed., *Studies in Italian American Social History: Essays in Honor of Leonard Covello* (Totowa, N.J.: Rowman and Littlefield, 1975), 201; and in Dorothy Schwieder, *Black Diamonds: Life and Work in Iowa's Coal Mining Communities, 1895–1925* (Ames: Iowa State Univ. Press, 1983), 89.

28. Walter Nugent, *Structures of American Social History* (Bloomington: Indiana Univ. Press, 1979), 103–5; and Leonard Dinnerstein, Roger L. Nichols, and David M. Reimers, *Natives and Strangers: Blacks, Indians, and Immigrants in America* (2nd ed., New York: Oxford Univ. Press, 1990), 132 (quote). By the 1920s,

according to these authors, Chicago's diverse population included the largest colonies of Scandinavians, Persians, Poles, Czechs, Serbo-Croatians, and Lithuanians in the nation; and it had the second highest number of Germans, Greeks, Slovaks, Jews, and African-Americans.

29. See "The Laborers' Lot" in Dinnerstein, Nichols, and Reimers, *Natives and Strangers*, 149–60 (esp. 150–51 and 157). Except for scattered enclaves, European immigrants generally shunned the South, which already had its cheap labor supply in African-Americans. Ibid., 134; and Woodward, *Origins*, 199.

30. On "Packingtown's" flies, smoke, and odor, see Upton Sinclair, *The Jungle* [1906] (New York: Bantam Books, 1981), 23–25, 28–29. On the succession and number of immigrants, see Sophonisba P. Breckinridge and Edith Abbott, "Housing Conditions in Chicago, III: Back of the Yards," *American Journal of Sociology* 16 (Jan. 1911): 437; and Robert A. Slayton, *Back of the Yards: The Making of a Local Democracy* (Chicago: Univ. of Chicago Press, 1986), 12.

31. The general description is quoted in Breckinridge and Abbott, "Housing Conditions in Chicago," 434. See also pp. 438, 446–48. Breckinridge and Abbott found private water closets within apartments clean, while those located outdoors were "in the majority of cases dirty and out of order" (p. 448). On the high incidence of tuberculosis, see Dominic A. Pacyga, "Crisis and Community: The Back of the Yards 1921," *Chicago History* 6 (Fall 1977): 170. See also Thomas J. Jablonsky, *Pride in the Jungle: Community and Everyday Life in Back of the Yards Chicago* (Baltimore: Johns Hopkins Univ. Press, 1993), for descriptions of washing clothes in kitchens (69, 71), garbage and vermin in alleys (81–82), and bathrooms (113).

32. Breckinridge and Abbott, "Housing Conditions in Chicago," 465–66; and Slayton, *Back of the Yards*, 27–28.

33. The quotation is from Mary Gulevaty, "An Immigrant Autobiography" (Feb. 16, 1914). A copy can be found on microfilm in the "Y.M.C.A. Papers Dealing with Immigration," Folder 33, Immigration History Research Center. See also Katharine Anthony, *Mothers Who Must Earn* (New York: Survey Associates, 1914), 70–80.

34. Anthony, *Mothers Who Must Earn*, 1, 67. A tenement mother in New York City, who was employed as a scrubwoman in a hospital, said that "every woman in the twenty-family house where she lived worked away from home more or less regularly" (p. 1). See also Albion Fellows Bacon, "American Housing and the Immigrant," *Immigrants in Review* 2 (July 1916): 43–44; and Frances Kellor, "Standard of Living," ibid. 1 (March 1915): 48.

35. 61 Cong., 2nd Sess., S. Doc. 338, *Reports of the Immigration Commission: Immigrants in Cities* (2 vols.; Washington: Government Printing Office, 1911), I: 98, 100, and 559.

36. Ibid., 160, 250. Several Chicago Poles interviewed in 1977 remembered these toilets "under the sidewalks." See transcripts of oral interviews with Victor Harackiewicz and Bessie Leniek, Oral History Archives of Chicago Polonia, Chicago Historical Society. Quotations can be found in Robert Hunter, *Tenement Conditions in Chicago: Report by the Investigating Committee of the City Homes Association* (Chicago: City Homes Association, 1901), 88; and Helen L. Wilson and Eunice W. Smith, "Chicago Housing Conditions, VIII: Among the Slovaks in the Twentieth Ward," *American Journal of Sociology* 20 (Sept. 1914): 155.

37. See especially Anzia Yezierska, "Soap and Water and the Immigrant," *New Republic* 18 (Feb. 22, 1919): 117–19. See also *Reports of the Immigration Commis-*

sion: Abstracts, I: 37 and 729; and Miriam Cohen, *Workshop to Office: Two Generations of Italian Women in New York City, 1900–1950* (Ithaca: Cornell Univ. Press, 1992), 102–3.

38. Balch, *Our Slavic Fellow Citizens*, 89; and Donna R. Gabaccia, *From Sicily to Elizabeth Street: Housing and Social Change among Italian Immigrants, 1880–1930* (Albany: State Univ. of New York Press, 1984), 38, 39, and 44.

39. Gabaccia, *From Sicily to Elizabeth Street*, 74. See also Sophonisba P. Breckinridge, *New Homes for Old* [1921] (Montclair, N.J.: Patterson Smith, 1971), 15, 55–56 (quote); and Transcript of Oral Interview with Rose Tellerino (quote), Italians in Chicago Project, Chicago Historical Society.

40. Slayton, *Back of the Yards*, 69–72.

41. Phyllis H. Williams, *South Italian Folkways in Europe and America: A Handbook for Social Workers, Visiting Nurses, School Teachers, and Physicians* (New Haven: Yale Univ. Press, 1938), 5. Jews, of course, were the exception, as I will note later. See too Yezierska, *Bread Givers*, 5 and 212 (quote); and Transcript of Oral Interview with Anonymous Female (ANON-111/quote), Oral History Archives of Chicago Polonia; and Transcript of Oral Interview with Mario Avignone, Italians in Chicago Project, Chicago Historical Society.

42. On contagion, see: E. B. Borland, "The Danger of Contagion in Street Cars," *Sanitarian* 24 (1896): 508–11; "Books, Paper Money and Disease Germs," *Architects' and Builders' Magazine* 1 (Dec. 1899): 95–96; Gardner Maynard Jones, "Contagious Diseases and Public Libraries," *Library Journal* 16 (1891): 35–38; and "Killing Germs in Books," *Scientific American* 77 (Aug. 28, 1897): 138. See also Blanche Wiesen Cook, *Eleanor Roosevelt: 1884–1933* (New York: Viking Press, 1992), 136 (quote); Mrs. H. M. Plunkett, *Women, Plumbers, and Doctors; or, Household Sanitation* (New York: D. Appleton, 1885), 203 (quote); and Cyrus Edson, M.D., "The Microbe as a Social Leveller," *North American Review* 161 (Oct. 1895): 425.

43. Josiah Quincy, "Public Baths and Gymnasia," *New York Times*, Jan. 24, 1899.

44. Neil M. Cowan and Ruth Schwartz Cowan, *Our Parents' Lives: The Americanization of Eastern European Jews* (New York: Basic Books, 1989), 57–58, 62 (quote); and Susan A. Glenn, *Daughters of the Shtetl: Life and Labor in the Immigrant Generation* (Ithaca: Cornell Univ. Press, 1990), 16, 18, and 58–59.

45. James Hurt, "Introduction," in Addams, *Twenty Years at Hull-House*, ix (quote). See also Dinnerstein, Nichols, and Reimers, *Natives and Strangers*, 161. This explains why Hull-House opened Chicago's first free public bath in 1894 (with help from the Municipal Order League and Chicago City Council). The bath contained 17 showers, a swimming tank, and tub. See Residents of Hull-House, *Hull-House Maps and Papers: A Presentation of Nationalities and Wages in a Congested District of Chicago Together with Comments and Essays on Problems Growing Out of the Social Conditions* (New York: Thomas Y. Crowell, 1895), 219.

46. For quotations, see Barrows, *Neighbors All*, 36; and Lillian D. Wald, *The House on Henry Street* (New York: Henry Holt, 1915), 9 (quote), 10–12. A little boy from the basement apartment, who ate a "simple" dinner with Wald and Brewster one evening, told his mother that " 'them ladies live like the Queen of England and eat off of solid gold plates.' " See also Mina Carson, *Settlement Folk: Social Thought and the American Settlement Movement, 1885–1930* (Chicago: Univ. of Chicago Press, 1990), 58.

Carson's book is one of three recent monographs on the settlement-house movement; the other two are Rivka Shpak Lissak, *Pluralism & Progressives: Hull House and the New Immigrants, 1890–1919* (Chicago: Univ. of Chicago Press, 1989), and Ruth Hutchinson Crocker, *Social Work and Social Order: The Settlement Movement in Two Industrial Cities, 1889–1930* (Urbana: Univ. of Illinois Press, 1992). Lissak's continues in the "social control" interpretation of settlement workers which, as I noted earlier, was more prevalent in the 1970s than today. Carson and Crocker, however, "return to social control as an interpretative device, but with a new complexity that dismisses the nearly conspiratorial version. . . . " (From Eileen Boris, "The Settlement Movement Revisited: Social Control with a Conscience," in *Reviews in American History* 20 (June 1992): 217.) For Crocker, settlement workers were social democrats as well as social controllers, both Americanizers and admirers of immigrants, not true cultural pluralists but "missionaries of the American way" (p. 213). Crocker also contributes fresh information on seven settlements in Indianapolis and Gary. For her linkage of cleanliness with Americanization, see especially pages 135, 138, 141, 147–48, and 154–55.

47. On settlement workers as interpreters of America, see John Daniels, *America via the Neighborhood* (New York: Harper & Brothers, 1920), 168–69. See also Mary Ann Johnson, ed., *The Many Faces of Hull-House: The Photographs of Wallace Kirkland* (Urbana: Univ. of Illinois Press, 1989), 50–51; Addams, *Twenty Years at Hull-House*, 166–68, 170; "Sanitary Work in the Ward," *Chicago Commons* 1 (April 1896): 2; and "The Drinking Trough," ibid. (July 1896): 9. *Chicago Commons* was published monthly by the Chicago Commons Settlement House, founded by Graham Taylor in 1894 in Chicago's Seventeenth Ward. All ten volumes of the publication are located in the Newberry Library (Chicago, Illinois).

48. Charity Organization Society [of the City of New York], comp., *Hand-Book for Friendly Visitors among the Poor* (New York: G. P. Putnam's Sons, 1883), 1–2. See also Robert H. Bremner, *The Public Good: Philanthropy and Welfare in the Civil War Era* (New York: Alfred A. Knopf, 1980), 156–58, 202, 206–7; and Sheila M. Rothman, *Woman's Proper Place: A History of Changing Ideals and Practices, 1870 to the Present* (New York: Basic Books, 1978), 70–73.

49. Quotations can be found in Josephine Shaw Lowell, *The True Aim of Charity Organization Societies* (New York: Forum, 1895), 1–2; Paul Boyer, *Urban Masses and Moral Order in America, 1820–1920* (Cambridge: Harvard Univ. Press, 1978), 146; and Josephine Shaw Lowell, "Duties of Friendly Visitors" (May 1883), in William Rhinelander Stewart, ed., *The Philanthropic Work of Josephine Shaw Lowell: Containing a Biographical Sketch of Her Life Together with a Selection of Her Public Papers and Private Letters* (New York, 1911), 145.

50. Addams, *Twenty Years at Hull-House*, 121 (quote). On page 103, there is another description of a local woman scrubbing the corridor of an office building at eleven o'clock at night. See also Boyer, *Urban Masses and Moral Order*, 158.

51. "Relieving the Unemployed," *Review of Reviews* 9 (Jan. 1894): 5; and Carson, *Settlement Folk*, 75. Carson also quotes residents of the Rivington Street Settlement in New York City as admitting that "only the most positive determination to keep our minds away from any suffering that we could not relieve made it possible for us to do our work." See too Addams, *Twenty Years at Hull-House*, 95–96 (quotes). The English journalist William T. Stead spent six months in Chicago during 1893, and in 1894 he published *If Christ Came to Chicago*, an indictment of the city's social conditions. During his stay he visited Hull-House frequently.

52. Neva R. Deardorff, "Women in Municipal Activities," in *Women in Public Life: The Annals of the American Academy of Political and Social Science* 4 (Nov. 1914): 75 (quote). On "public motherhood," see Paula Baker, "The Domestication of Politics: Women and American Political Society, 1780–1920," *American Historical Review* 89 (June 1894): 640–41; and on "growth from remedy to prevention" and "justice rather than charity," see Mary Ritter Beard, *Woman's Work in Municipalities* (New York: D. Appleton, 1915), 221. For a discussion of Addams's view of government, see Daniel Levine, *Varieties of Reform Thought* (Madison: State Historical Society of Wisconsin, 1964), 27–32; and for a discussion of how municipal housekeepers linked themselves ever more closely to City Hall, see Maureen A. Flanagan, "Gender and Urban Political Reform: The City Club and the Woman's City Club of Chicago in the Progressive Era," *American Historical Review* 95 (Oct. 1990): 1048–50.

53. American settlement workers were supposedly more concerned with garbage than drains, the preoccupation of English settlements. Paul Kellogg, "Semi-Centennial of the Settlements," *Survey Graphic* (Jan. 1935): 31, in Mary Lynn Mc-Cree Bryan, ed., *The Jane Addams Papers* (Chicago and Ann Arbor: Univ. of Illinois and University Microfilms International, 1984), Reel 34. See also Alice Hamilton, "The Social Settlement and Public Health," *Charities and the Commons* 17 (March 9, 1907): 1037–39; Florence Kelley, "Hull House," *New England Magazine* 18 (July 1898): 550–51; and Carson, *Settlement Folk*, 72.

54. Charles-Edward A. Winslow, "Florence Nightingale and Public Health Nursing," *Public Health Nursing* 38 (1946): 332.

55. Martha Vicinus and Bea Nergaard, *Ever Yours, Florence Nightingale: Selected Letters* (Cambridge: Harvard Univ. Press, 1990), 424–25. The quotation appears on page 424 in a letter from Nightingale to George H. De'ath, May 20, 1892. See also Florence Nightingale, *Rural Hygiene: Health Teaching in Towns and Villages* (London: Spotteswood, 1894), 21 (quote).

56. Addams, *Twenty Years at Hull-House*, 166–67 (quote).

57. Ibid.

58. *Chicago Times-Herald*, July 5 and 29, 1895; and *Omaha Bee*, June 2, 1895. Because of Addams's success, the Chicago Commons Settlement in the Seventeenth Ward also secured the garbage inspector position for one of its residents along with five tenement house inspectorships. See "Sanitary Work in the Ward," *Chicago Commons* 1 (April 1896): 2.

59. Addams, *Twenty Years at Hull-House*, 168.

60. Alice Hamilton to Agnes Hamilton, July 16, 1893, in Barbara Sicherman, *Alice Hamilton: A Life in Letters* (Cambridge: Harvard Univ. Press, 1984), 59. For a concise biographical sketch of Hamilton by Sicherman, see Barbara Sicherman and Caroline Hurd Green, eds., *Notable American Women: The Modern Period* (Cambridge: Harvard Univ. Press, 1980), 303–6.

61. Hamilton stayed at the Woman's Medical School until it closed in 1902; she then accepted a position as bacteriologist at the new Memorial Institute for Infectious Disease. Alice Hamilton, *Exploring the Dangerous Trades: The Autobiography of Alice Hamilton, M.D.* (Boston: Little, Brown, 1943), 115 (quote).

62. Sicherman, *Alice Hamilton*, 118–19; and Hamilton, *Exploring the Dangerous Trades*, 69 (quote).

63. Hamilton, *Exploring the Dangerous Trades*, 98 (quote). Hamilton describes the entire episode on pages 98–100. See also Sicherman, *Alice Hamilton*, 145–46; *Hull-House Bulletin* 5 (Semi-Annual 1902): 14–15; and Hull-House Residents, "An

Inquiry into the Causes of the Recent Epidemic of Typhoid Fever in Chicago," *The Commons* 8 (May 1903): 3–7.

64. Hamilton, *Exploring the Dangerous Trades*, 99.

65. Sicherman, *Alice Hamilton*, 146.

66. Hamilton, *Exploring the Dangerous Trades*, 99 (quote)–100. For the number of people who died, see Hull-House Residents, "An Inquiry into the Causes of the Recent Epidemic," 3. Hamilton recalled in her autobiography that because Chicago's water supply was not chlorinated (and would not be until 1916), housewives were often instructed by the city's health department to boil water as a precaution against pollution. Hamilton, *Exploring the Dangerous Trades*, 98.

67. See "Ours Is the Age of Plumbing," in Henry Hartshorne, *Our Homes* (Philadelphia: Presley Blakiston, 1880), 101. Good housekeeping practices in middle-class and immigrant homes could make a difference. On domestic hygiene in middle-class homes, see Nancy Tomes, "The Private Side of Public Health: Sanitary Science, Domestic Hygiene, and the Germ Theory, 1870–1900," *Bulletin of the History of Medicine* 64 (Winter 1990): 509–39. On immigrant practices, see Michael P. McCarthy, "Urban Optimism and Reform Thought in the Progressive Era," *Historian* 52 (Feb. 1989): 239–62. McCarthy explains that city dwellers became typhoid victims by drinking infected water or eating contaminated food (p. 249). He then shows that in the densely populated Tenth Ward of New York's Lower East Side there was a very low death rate because "nearly all the residents were Russian and Polish Jews, who observed strict kosher laws of cleanliness in their eating and drinking" (p. 255).

68. The Visiting Nurses of Chicago, for example, began in 1889 with private funding; its purpose was "to furnish visiting nurses to those otherwise unable to secure skilled attendance in time of illness, to teach cleanliness and proper care of the sick." See the 1889 pamphlet, *The Visiting Nurse Association of Chicago,* in the Visiting Nurse Association of Chicago Papers, Box 1 (Chicago Historical Society). Charles V. Chapin, "Dirt, Disease, and the Health Officer: Address to the American Public Health Association, New Orleans, Louisiana, December 1902," in Frederic P. Gorham and Clarence L. Scamman, eds., *Papers of Charles V. Chapin, M.D.: A Review of Public Health Realities* (New York: Commonwealth Fund, 1934), 20 (quote). The quote from Sedgwick can be found in Elizabeth Fee, *Disease and Discovery: A History of the Johns Hopkins School of Hygiene and Public Health, 1916–1939* (Baltimore: Johns Hopkins Univ. Press, 1987), 19.

69. For quotations, see Charles-Edward Amory Winslow, *The Conquest of Epidemic Disease: A Chapter in the History of Ideas* (Princeton: Princeton Univ. Press, 1943), 364; Charles V. Chapin, "The End of the Filth Theory of Disease," *Popular Science Monthly* 60 (Jan. 1902): 236; and ibid., "Dirt, Disease, and the Health Officer," 22. Chapin believed most cleanup measures could be justified on the grounds of public comfort, not public health. See James H. Cassedy, *Charles V. Chapin and the Public Health Movement* (Cambridge: Harvard Univ. Press, 1962), 96. Chapin's efforts (and others) to link the new bacteriology to public health practice is described skillfully by Judith Walzer Leavitt, " 'Typhoid Mary' Strikes Back: Bacteriological Theory and Practice in Early Twentieth-Century Public Health," *Isis* 83 (Dec. 1992): 608–29.

70. For quotations, see Chapin, "The End of the Filth Theory of Disease," 237; and Charles V. Chapin, *How to Avoid Infection* (Cambridge: Harvard Univ. Press, 1917), 61–62.

71. See, for example, Grace Abbott, *The Education Needs of Immigrants in Illinois* (Springfield: State of Illinois, Department of Registration and Education, 1920), 17–18, on "The Special Problem of the Immigrant Mother." Abbott argued that "no public health program can be carried out without her cooperation" (p. 17). On the convergence of sanitary science and domestic hygiene practices, see Tomes, "The Private Side of Public Health," 535–37.

72. On the Italian woman in Chicago, see Addams, *Twenty Years at Hull-House*, 148. See too Charles V. Chapin, "How Shall We Spend the Health Appropriation? Address to the Massachusetts Association of Boards of Health, Boston, January 1913," in Gorham and Scamman, eds., *Papers of Charles V. Chapin*, 33; and "Pasteurization for Chicago," *New York Times*, Jan. 2, 1909. For an excellent overview of what American cities did to improve their milk supply, see Richard A. Meckel, *Save the Babies: American Public Health Reform and the Prevention of Infant Mortality, 1850–1929* (Baltimore: Johns Hopkins Univ. Press, 1990), 62–91.

73. V. W. Greene, *Cleanliness and the Health Revolution* (New York: Soap and Detergent Association, 1984), 7. The purification of urban water supplies in the early twentieth century was the chief factor in reducing death rates from diseases such as typhoid and diarrhea. See Metropolitan Life Insurance Company, "Typhoid Fever in Relation to Filtration and Chlorination of Municipal Water Supplies in American Cities, 1900 to 1924," *Statistical Bulletin* 8 (March 1927): 5–12. See too Michael P. McCarthy, *Typhoid and the Politics of Public Health in Nineteenth-Century Philadelphia* (Philadelphia: American Philosophical Society, 1987). McCarthy points out that Philadelphia spent $28 million in its quest for pure water—a good deal less than Chicago and New York, which spent about $100 million and $188 million respectively (p. 96). The medical examination of school children is discussed in the next chapter.

74. The first quotation is from "Medical Lectures for Polish Mothers," *Narod Polski*, July 25, 1915 (more a middle-class than a peasant-class source in the Polish context), in Box 34, Chicago Foreign Language Press Survey (University of Chicago Special Collections, Joseph Regenstein Library, Chicago, Illinois). See also Breckinridge, *New Homes for Old*, 54–58, 60–64. The second quotation is quoted in Doris Groshen Daniels, *Always a Sister: The Feminism of Lillian Wald* (New York: Feminist Press, 1989), 28. Lillian Wald remarked that "it is very rare to find a woman who cannot learn the lesson when made to understand its importance to her children." Wald, *The House on Henry Street*, 56.

75. Balch, *Our Slavic Fellow Citizens*, 59; and for the 1910 statistics and Children's Bureau report, see Molly Ladd-Taylor, *Raising a Baby the Government Way: Mothers' Letters to the Children's Bureau, 1915–1932* (New Brunswick: Rutgers Univ. Press, 1986), 6 and 19. See also Greene, *Cleanliness and the Health Revolution*, 46; and Richard A. Meckel, *Save the Babies*.

76. Robert Coit Chapin, *The Standard of Living among Workingmen's Families in New York City* (New York: Charities Publication Committee, 1909), 79.

77. C.-E.A. Winslow, "The Parent, The Strategic Point of the Present," *Bulletin of the American Academy of Medicine* 11 (Dec. 1910): 610 (quote; copy in the Winslow Papers, Yale University Archives). Settlement workers and public health nurses who taught immigrant women how to care for their babies were not middle-class meddlers, "insinuating bourgeois ideals into the authentic culture of the work-

ing-class." See Paul Starr, *The Social Transformation of American Medicine* (New York: Basic Books, 1982), 192. Starr argues forcefully that these women were not agents of social control nor was their work "secondary or irrelevant." Catholic nuns also instructed immigrant women in child care and homemaking. For example, the Sisters of Notre Dame de Namur in Boston, working among Irish women, taught "the untaught and overworked creatures how to make everything clean, tidy, and bright about them." Quoted in Hasia Diner, *Erin's Daughters in America* (Baltimore: Johns Hopkins Univ. Press, 1983), 131.

78. Although the United States death rate for infants (babies less than one year old) dropped between 1880 and 1910 from about 200 to 120 per thousand, New York City experienced a sharp increase. In 1903, 1,222 infant deaths occurred in New York City; the number leapt to 1,712 deaths a year later. This increase persisted until 1908, when the Division of Child Hygiene was established in the city's health department. S. Josephine Baker, "The Reduction of Infant Mortality in New York City," *American Journal of Diseases of Children* 5 (1913): 151. In her autobiography, Baker remembered that immigrant women in New York City believed that "babies always died in summer and there was no point in trying to do anything about it." S. Josephine Baker, *Fighting for Life* (New York: Macmillan, 1939), 58.

79. Patricia Mooney-Melvin, "Milk to Motherhood: The New York Milk Committee and the Beginning of Well-Child Programs," *Mid-America* 65 (Oct. 1983): 121–23; and New York Milk Committee, *Milk: Its Value to the Home* (New York: New York Milk Committee, n.d.) A copy can be found in the Winslow Papers, Box 33, Yale University Archives.

80. Mooney-Melvin, "Milk to Motherhood," 124–27. She points out that the New York Milk Committee's work also demonstrated the value of pasteurized milk. In 1912 New York City adopted a compulsory pasteurization ordinance.

81. On the infant welfare station, see Wald, *The House on Henry Street*, 55–56. For a good explanation of the relationship between the Henry Street nurses and Metropolitan Life, see Diane Hamilton, "The Cost of Caring: The Metropolitan Life Insurance Company's Visiting Nurse Service, 1909–1953," *Bulletin of the History of Medicine* 63 (Fall 1989): 414–34.

82. Quotations can be found in C.-E.A. Winslow, *Man and Epidemics* (Princeton: Princeton Univ. Press, 1952), 26; and Hamilton, "The Cost of Caring," 419. See also p. 415 for her description of the nurse as messenger. The chief financial backer of Wald's Henry Street work was Jacob Schiff, a German-Jewish immigrant who became a successful banker. See Ellen Condliffe Lagemann, "Lillian D. Wald, 1867–1940," in *A Generation of Women: Education in the Lives of Progressive Reformers* (Cambridge: Harvard Univ. Press, 1979), 77–78.

83. Lee K. Frankel, "Insurance Companies and Public Health Activities," *American Journal of Public Health* 4 (Jan. 1914): 1–10.

84. A very good discussion of Metropolitan as a "social institution" appears in Olivier Zunz, *Making America Corporate, 1870–1920* (Chicago: Univ. of Chicago Press, 1990), 93–100. On the connections of Frankel and Dublin to progressive reformers, see pages 93–94. The quotation is taken from a one-page printed blurb that explains how doctors in China are engaged by the year so they will keep their patients in good health and not simply give treatment in illness. See *Chinese Doctors* (New York: Metropolitan Life Insurance Company, 1915). A copy can be found in

the Metropolitan Life Insurance Company Archives, New York City. I am grateful to Alan M. Kraut for encouraging me to visit this archives and to Daniel B. May for assisting me while there.

85. Hamilton, "The Cost of Caring," 241. In his autobiography, Louis Dublin explains that when the welfare program was begun in 1909 Metropolitan was "a relatively small organization" and "far behind the giants of those days—the New York Life, the Equitable, and the Mutual." Within a decade, however, Metropolitan had taken the lead in "amounts of new business written each year, total insurance coverage, and total assets." Louis I. Dublin, *After Eighty Years: The Impact of Life Insurance on the Public Health* (Gainesville: Univ. of Florida Press, 1966), 49.

86. *The War Upon Consumption: The Nature of the Disease, Its Extent, Growth and Spread* (New York: Metropolitan Life Insurance Company, 1909), esp. 3; Louis I. Dublin, *A Family of Thirty Million: The Story of the Metropolitan Life Insurance Company* (New York: Metropolitan Life Insurance Company, 1943), 429; and Zunz, *Making America Corporate*, 95. The Metropolitan Archives retains one of the 1915 fly swatters plus numerous company handouts explaining the dangers of the fly.

87. *Educating for Longer Life: Service Record of the Welfare Division, Metropolitan Life Insurance Company, 1909–1928* (New York: Metropolitan Life Insurance Company, c. 1929), 9 (quote); Dublin, *A Family of Thirty Million*, 429; and Andrew R. Heinze, *Adapting to Abundance: Jewish Immigrants, Mass Consumption, and the Search for American Identity* (New York: Columbia Univ. Press, 1990), 171. Heinze reports that "the public response to Metropolitan's bold departure in the marketing of insurance was expressed by a flood of approving letters. . . . " On the Borden Company, see Susan L. Braunstein and Jenna Weissman Joselit, *Getting Comfortable in New York: The American Jewish Home, 1880–1950* (New York: Jewish Museum, 1990), 39. Almost all of Borden's foreign-language ads had coupons at the bottom. The company replied to a returned coupon with booklets in the appropriate languages on the feeding and care of infants. According to company lore, Gail Borden, a stickler for cleanliness at the dairies where he purchased milk, first thought about the possibility of condensed milk on board a slow-sailing emigrant ship from England to the United States in 1851. The ship carried cows for fresh milk; on this particular voyage, the cows became sick as did the babies who depended on them for their milk. Then and there, Borden supposedly resolved to find a way to preserve pure milk. See Frank Crane, "The Borden Company," *Current Opinion* 77 (1924): 235–36; and Joe B. Frantz, *Gail Borden: Dairyman to a Nation* (Norman: Univ. of Oklahoma Press, 1951), 243–45; 251.

88. *Educating for Longer Life*, 10; Dublin, *A Family of Thirty Million*, 440; and Zunz, *Making America Corporate*, 98.

89. Zunz, *Making America Corporate*, 99; Lisabeth Cohen, *Making a New Deal: Industrial Workers in Chicago, 1919–1939* (Cambridge: Cambridge Univ. Press, 1990), 65–67, 110. See too Elsa G. Herzfeld, *Family Monographs: The History of Twenty-four Families Living in the Middle West Side of New York City* (New York: James Kempster, 1905), 101, 114. The quotation appears in Frankel, "Insurance Companies and Public Health," 8.

90. New York–New Jersey Committee of the North American Civic League for Immigrants, "Domestic Education" [three-page press release] (New York: n.p., c. 1911). A copy can be found on microfilm in the "Y.M.C.A. Papers Dealing with Immigration," Folder 32, Immigration History Research Center. See also S. P. Breck-

inridge, "Education for the Americanization of the Foreign Family," *Journal of Home Economics* 11 (May 1919): 191; Grace Abbott, "The Education of the Immigrant," in Winthrop Talbot, ed., *Americanization: Principles of Americanism, Essentials of Americanization, Technic of Race-Assimilation, and Annotated Bibliography* (New York: H. W. Wilson, 1917), 15 (quote); and Annie L. Hansen, "Two Years as a Domestic Educator in Buffalo, New York," *Journal of Home Economics* 5 (Dec. 1913): 434.

91. Hansen, "Two Years as a Domestic Educator," 434–35; and Olivia Howard Dunbar, "Teaching the Immigrant Woman," *Harper's Bazaar* 47 (June 1913): 277–78.

92. H. H. Wheaton, "Education of Immigrants," in Talbot, ed., *Americanization*, 209. The California Commission of Immigration and Housing sponsored the "Home Teacher Act." By 1917 home teachers worked in San Francisco, Los Angeles, Sacramento, Ontario, and South Pasadena; in 1918 home teaching began in Oakland, Tulare County, and Santa Barbara. See State Commission of Immigration and Housing, *A Manual for Home Teachers* (Sacramento: California State Printing Office, 1918), 8, 10–12, 19, 29–30. Certified teachers selected for this work had some ability to speak the language of the immigrant groups they would be instructing. The main purpose of their work was "to broaden, elevate and *Americanize* the viewpoint and life of the homes" they entered. See also James Barrett, "Americanization from the Bottom Up," *Journal of American History* 79 (Dec. 1992): 1012–13 (quote); and John McClymer, "Gender and the 'American Way of Life': Women in the Americanization Movement," *Journal of American Ethnic History* 10 (Spring 1991): 3–20, esp. 9, 14–16.

93. Mabel H. Kittredge, "The Training of the Domestic Educator," in *Education of the Immigrant* (Washington, D.C.: Bulletin No. 51, United States Bureau of Education, 1913), 12 (quote); and Barrows, *Neighbors All*, 115–17. Americanizers also taught Indian and Mexican women how to keep model houses and maintain standards of cleanliness and good nutrition. See Robert A. Trennert, "Educating Indian Girls at Nonreservation Boarding Schools, 1878–1920," in Ellen Carol DuBois and Vicki L. Ruiz, *Unequal Sisters: A Multicultural Reader in U.S. Women's History* (New York and London: Routledge, 1990), 230–31; and George J. Sanchez, " 'Go after the Women': Americanization and the Mexican Immigrant Woman, 1915–1929," in ibid., 257–58.

94. Mabel Hyde Kittredge, *Housekeeping Notes: How to Furnish and Keep House* (Boston: Mabel Hyde Kittredge, 1911), 1 and 14 (quotes); and Kittredge, "Housekeeping Centers in Settlements and Public Schools," *Survey* 30 (May 3, 1913): 192. Kittredge was so convinced of the need for model American apartment-homes that she wanted to build one at Ellis Island. On Kittredge and Wald's relationship, see Blanche Wiesen Cook, "Female Support Networks and Political Activism," in Nancy Cott and Elizabeth Pleck, eds., *A Heritage of Her Own* (New York: Simon and Schuster, 1979), 424–27.

95. Kittredge, *Housekeeping Notes*, 1–13 (on furnishings), and 18–62 (housekeeping lessons I through XII).

96. Heinze, *Adapting to Abundance*, 137–38. See also Morawska, *For Bread with Butter*, 137. Morawska quotes one immigrant who wrote to his family in Galicia and said: "Don't worry about me, 'cause I live here like a *pan* [gentleman]."

97. Kittredge, "Housekeeping Centers in Settlements and Public Schools," 190;

Braunstein and Joselit, *Getting Comfortable in New York*, 33 (quote); Antin, *The Promised Land*, 274 (quote); and Lisabeth A. Cohen, "Embellishing a Life of Labor: An Interpretation of the Material Culture of American Working-Class Homes, 1885–1915," in Thomas J. Schlereth, *Material Culture Studies in America* (3rd ed., Nashville: American Association for State and Local History, 1986), 301–4.

98. Colleen McDannell, *The Christian Home in Victorian America, 1840–1900* (Bloomington: Indiana Univ. Press, 1986), 66–70. Much of this ornamentation characterized Irish immigrant homes as well as those of Poles, Slavs, and Italians. See also Braunstein and Joselit, *Getting Comfortable in New York*, 31.

99. Yezierska, *Bread Givers*, 8 (quote). On New York City's 1901 Tenement House Law, see Roy Lubove, *The Progressives and the Slums: Tenement House Reform in New York City, 1890–1917* (Pittsburgh: Univ. of Pittsburgh Press, 1962), 134. See also Marilyn Thornton Williams, *Washing "The Great Unwashed": Public Baths in Urban America, 1840–1920* (Columbus: Ohio State Univ. Press, 1991), 137; and Cowan and Cowan, *Our Parents' Lives*, 62. They say that "by 1905, virtually all American cities had banned outdoor privies and required landlords to install indoor toilets, connected to sewer lines."

100. Chicago's "New Tenement" ordinance, which required every apartment to have a kitchen sink and private toilet, passed in December 1902. But old tenements built before this date were largely exempt; and, as housing reformers found out, it was "one thing to legislate reform and quite another thing to enforce it." Thomas Lee Philpott, *The Slum and the Ghetto: Immigrants, Blacks, and Reformers in Chicago, 1880–1930* (paper ed., Belmont, Calif.: Wadsworth Publishing, 1991), 102–4 (quote). See also Thomas Neville Bonner, *Medicine in Chicago, 1850–1950: A Chapter in the Social and Scientific Development of a City* (Madison, Wisc.: American History Research Center, 1957), 23–24; and Jacob A. Riis, *The Battle with the Slums* (New York: Macmillan, 1902), 90. On public baths, see Williams, *Washing "The Great Unwashed*," 203–20. She states that the poor "did not reject the gospel of cleanliness, although they did not use the public baths to the extent that the bath reformers expected. What they wanted and what they eventually got was what the middle-class reformers already had—baths in their own homes" (p. 137).

101. For "deadening dirt," see Yezierska, *Bread Givers*, 163. See also "Tiled Bathroom of My Own," in Anzia Yezierska, *Red Ribbon on a White Horse* (New York: Charles Scribner's Sons, 1950), 36–40 (esp. 37).

102. Herzfeld, *Family Monographs*, 48; Cowan and Cowan, *Our Parents' Lives*, 62; Bodnar, *The Transplanted*, 180–82; and Morawska, *For Bread with Butter*, 136, 188.

103. Stanley Lieberson, *A Piece of the Pie: Blacks and White Immigrants since 1880* (Berkeley: Univ. of California Press, 1980), 381–83; and Philpott, *The Slum and the Ghetto*, xiv. "A city within a city" is the description given the Black Belt by the 1919 Chicago Commission on Race Relations. See its final report, *The Negro in Chicago: A Study of Race Relations and a Race Riot* (Chicago: Univ. of Chicago Press, 1922), 612.

104. Philpott, *Slum and the Ghetto*, 121, 135. See especially pages 139–40 for a discussion of how the Jewish and African-American ghettos differed.

105. See Steven J. Diner, "Chicago Social Workers and Blacks in the Progressive Era," *Social Service Review* 44 (Dec. 1970): 393–410. For a longer and more satisfying explanation, see "Settlement Workers and Blacks: A 'Valid Difference'" and

"The Color Line in Neighborhood Work," in Philpott, *Slum and the Ghetto*, 295–345.

106. James R. Grossman, *Land of Hope: Chicago, Black Southerners, and the Great Migration* (Chicago: Univ. of Chicago Press, 1989), 4 (quote), 74, 81.

107. Roi Ottley, *The Lonely Warrior: The Life and Times of Robert S. Abbott* (Chicago: Henry Regnery, 1955), 125–30. The actual paid circulation of the *Defender* was over 230,000 by 1920. Two-thirds of this number was sent outside Chicago, and copies were passed on and circulated among those who could not afford to subscribe (pp. 138–39). See also "Personal: Robert Sengstacke Abbott," *Journal of Negro History* 25 (April 1940): 261–62; and Mary E. Stovall, "The Chicago *Defender* in the Progressive Era," *Illinois Historical Journal* 83 (Autumn 1990): 159–72.

108. See, for example, Dr. A. Wilberforce Williams, "Keep Healthy," *Defender*, Aug. 30, 1913; Sept. 12, April 4, 1914; March 20, 1915; April 1, 1916; March 30, 1918; and June 22, 1918. By 1914 the column bore the title "Dr. A. Wilberforce Williams Talks on Preventative Measures, First Aid Remedies, Hygienics, and Sanitation." For biographical information on Williams, see "Personal: A. Wilberforce Williams," *Journal of Negro History* 25 (April 1940): 262–63.

109. Abbott, *Tenements of Chicago*, esp. 121–25; and Alzada P. Comstock, "Chicago Housing Conditions, VI: The Problem of the Negro," *American Journal of Sociology* 18 (Sept. 1912): 245–48, 250–52.

110. Richard R. Wright, Jr., "The Economic Condition of Negroes in the North v. Recent Improvement in Housing among Negroes in the North," *Southern Workman* 37 (Nov. 1908): 601 (quote); Barbara Bates, *Bargaining for Life: A Social History of Tuberculosis, 1876–1938* (Philadelphia: Univ. of Pennsylvania Press, 1992), 288–96, 329–34; and H. L. Harris, Jr., "Negro Mortality Rates in Chicago," *Social Service Review* 1 (March 1927): 58–77. From 1900 to 1950 African-American mortality rates were a good deal higher nationwide than the rates for foreign-born whites and native whites. Lieberson, *A Piece of the Pie*, 41; David McBride, "Medicine and the Health Crisis of the Urban Black American Family, 1910–1945," in Jean E. Hunter and Paul T. Mason, eds., *The American Family: Historical Perspectives* (Pittsburgh: Duquesne Univ. Press, 1988), 113, 118. See also *Defender*, Dec. 5, 1914, and Feb. 12, 1916; Arvarh E. Strickland, *History of the Chicago Urban League* (Urbana: Univ. of Illinois Press, 1966), 44–45; and Philpott, *Slum and the Ghetto*, 349–50.

111. Quotations can be found in *Defender*, Feb. 14, 1914, April 15, 1916 (Gold Dust twins), and July 22, 1916; and Grossman, *Land of Hope*, 146. Booker T. Washington was still preaching the message of hygiene in 1915, and annual National Negro Health Weeks kept proclaiming it through the 1920s. See, for example, *Hygeia* 10 (April 1932): 349.

112. Quotations are from Nancy J. Weiss, *The National Urban League, 1910–1940* (New York: Oxford Univ. Press, 1974), 117, 119; and "I AM GEORGE," *Pullman News* 2 (June 1923): 55. See also *Defender*, May 25, 1918; and Chicago Commission on Race Relations, *The Negro in Chicago*, 301–3.

113. Quoted in Weiss, *National Urban League*, 121; and Braunstein and Joselit, *Getting Comfortable in New York*, 25. See also Selma Berrol, "When Uptown Met Downtown: Julia Richman's Work in the Jewish Community of New York, 1880–1912," *American Jewish History* 70 (Sept. 1980): 35–51.

114. Starr, *Social Transformation of American Medicine*, 197.

CHAPTER 5. PERSUADING THE MASSES

1. Quoted in *Fortune* 22 (Nov. 1940): 116.

2. Ruth Miller Elson, *Guardians of Tradition: American Schoolbooks of the Nineteenth Century* (Lincoln: Univ. of Nebraska Press, 1964), 313; the last quotation is from John Daniels, *America via the Neighborhood* (New York: Harper & Brothers, 1920), 249–50, as quoted in David B. Tyack, *The One Best System: A History of American Urban Education* (Cambridge: Harvard Univ. Press, 1974), 241. On immigrant mothers, see Helen Varick Boswell, "Promoting Americanization," *Annals of the American Academy of Political and Social Science* 64 (March 1916): 205 (quote).

3. David Tyack and Elisabeth Hansot, *Managers of Virtue: Public School Leadership in America, 1820–1980* (New York: Basic Books, 1982), 110–12, 190–91; and Wayne E. Fuller, *The Old Country School: The Story of Rural Education in the Middle West* (Chicago: Univ. of Chicago Press, 1982), 159–61.

4. Graham Taylor, *Religion in Social Action* (New York: Dodd, Mead, 1913), 151 (quote). See also Mary Kingsbury Simkhovitch, "The Enlarged Function of the Public School," in National Conference of Charities and Correction, *Proceedings* (n.p., 1904), 476, 485; and Morris Isaiah Berger, *The Settlement, the Immigrant and the Public School: A Study of the Influence of the Settlement Movement and the New Migration upon Public Education: 1890–1924* [1956] (New York: Arno Press, 1980), 36–37, 82–83.

5. Julia Richman is quoted in Berger, *The Settlement, the Immigrant and the Public School*, 92; and Jane Addams, *Twenty Years at Hull-House: With Autobiographical Notes* (Urbana: Univ. of Illinois Press, 1990), 148.

6. Quotations are from Neil M. Cowan and Ruth Schwartz Cowan, *Our Parents' Lives: The Americanization of Eastern European Jews* (New York: Basic Books, 1989), 99; and "Helps in Homemaking," *Commons* 5 (Jan. 1, 1900): 10. See also Sarah B. Cooper, "Free Kindergartens: Practical Results of Ten Years Work [in and around San Francisco]," in National Conference of Charities and Correction, *Proceedings* (n.p., 1889), 191; S. E. Weber, "The Kindergarten as an Americanizer," *Educational Review* 59 (March 1920): 210; Lawrence A. Cremin, *American Education: The Metropolitan Experience, 1876–1980* (New York: Harper & Row, 1988), 299–300; and Maxine Seller, "The Education of Immigrant Children in Buffalo, New York, 1890–1916," *New York History* 57 (April 1976): 191.

7. See Selma Berrol, "Immigrant Children at School, 1880–1940: A Child's Eye View," in Elliott West and Paula Petrik, *Small Worlds: Children & Adolescents in America, 1850–1950* (Lawrence: Univ. Press of Kansas, 1992), 57; and Kate Simon, "Birthing," in Pat C. Hoy II, Esther H. Schor, and Robert DiYanni, eds., *Women's Voices: Visions and Perspectives* (New York: McGraw-Hill, 1990), 619 (quotes). I thank Charlene Avallone for telling me about this incident. See also Edward M. Hartwell, "School Hygiene—What It Is and Why We Need It," *Proceedings and Addresses of the National Education Association Meeting* (n.p., 1898), 501, 503.

8. Cowan and Cowan, *Our Parents' Lives*, 100–101 (quotes); and Mabelle S. Welsh, "Campaigning against Pediculosis," *Public Health Nursing* 16 (Aug. 1924): 388. See also Lina Rogers Struthers, "The School Nurse and Her Work," in Louis W. Rapeer, ed., *Essentials of Educational Hygiene* [1915] (New York: Charles Scribner's Sons, 1919), 206–8.

9. Margaret E. Greenwood and Eleanor M. Fonda, "Clara Cleans Her Teeth," *Hygeia* 2 (March 1924): 192 (quote). The most prevalent contagious diseases were diphtheria, scarlet fever, measles, small pox, chicken pox, whooping cough, and mumps. See Severance Burrage and Henry Turner Bailey, *School Sanitation and Decoration: A Practical Study of Health and Beauty in Their Relations to the Public Schools* (Boston: D. C. Heath, 1899), 137. On dental problems, see Luther Halsey Gulick and Leonard P. Ayres, *Medical Inspection of Schools* (New York: Survey Associates, 1913), 114–21; and William H. Allen, *Civics and Health* (Boston: Ginn, 1909), 95.

10. Robertson Davies, *What's Bred in the Bone* (New York: Viking, 1985), 347 (quote); Arthur De Voe, "The Care of the Teeth," *Cosmopolitan* 29 (Oct. 1900): 653 (quote); and Thomas Fleming, "Visions of My Father," *American Heritage* 42 (July/Aug. 1991): 90. See also Anzia Yezierska, *Bread Givers* [1925] (New York: Persea Books, 1975), 28–29; W. G. Ebersole, "The Place of Mouth Hygiene in the Public Health Movement," *American Journal of Public Health* 5 (May 1915): 387–88; and Allen, *Civics and Health*, 93, 96.

11. John Duffy, "School Buildings and the Health of American School Children in the Nineteenth Century," in Charles E. Rosenberg, ed., *Healing and History: Essays for George Rosen* (New York: Science History Publications, 1979), 161–78, especially 166–70. See also Chicago Commission on Race Relations, *The Negro in Chicago: A Study of Race Relations and a Race Riot* (Chicago: Univ. of Chicago Press, 1922), 243. According to this study, black and white teachers alike realized that migrant children from the South presented special problems of adjustment to city life, especially when both parents were working (pp. 241 and 301). See also James R. Grossman, *Land of Hope: Chicago, Black Southerners, and the Great Migration* (Chicago: Univ. of Chicago Press, 1989), chap. 9, esp. 247–50 and 257–58.

12. Duffy, "School Buildings," 173–74; Leo H. Pleins, "Sanitation of the Modern School Building," *Modern School Houses: Being a Series of Authoritative Articles on Planning, Sanitation, Heating and Ventilation* (New York: Swetland, 1910), 31–34; and Harriet S. Farwell, *Lucy Louisa Flower, 1837–1920: Her Contribution to Education and Child Welfare in Chicago* (Chicago: Privately printed, 1924); along with "How Would You Uplift the Masses" and "Cleanliness," which are clippings in the Lucy Flower Scrapbooks (Nos. 3 and 4), Lucy Flower Papers, Chicago Historical Society. I thank Lana Ruegamer for sending me copies of these clippings. See also Marilyn Thornton Williams, *Washing "The Great Unwashed": Public Baths in Urban America, 1840–1920* (Columbus: Ohio State Univ. Press, 1991), 85; and Florence Kelley, "Hull House," *New England Magazine* 18 (July 1898): 554–55.

13. Robert D. Cross, "Origins of the Catholic Parochial Schools in America," in F. Michael Perko, S.J., ed., *Enlightening the Next Generation: Catholics and Their Schools 1830–1980* (New York: Garland, 1988), 321–22 (quote); Timothy Walch, "Catholic School Books and American Values: The Nineteenth Century Experience," in Perko, ed., *Enlightening the Next Generation*, 268, 269, 273; and Hasia R. Diner, *Erin's Daughters in America: Irish Immigrant Women in the Nineteenth Century* (Baltimore: Johns Hopkins Univ. Press, 1983), 130–31 (quotes). On cold bathrooms, see Kathleen Guillaume, "Poem of Childhood," in Amber Coverdale Sumrall and Patrice Vecchione, *Catholic Girls* (New York: Penguin Books, 1992), 65.

14. Fuller, *The Old Country School*, 76, 77.

15. Ibid., 198; and Susan Carol Peterson and Courtney Ann Vaughn-Roberson,

Women with Vision: The Presentation Sisters of South Dakota, 1880–1985 (Urbana: Univ. of Illinois Press, 1988), 91.

16. Wayne E. Fuller, "Country Schoolteaching on the Sod-House Frontier," *Arizona and the West* 17 (Summer 1975): 122; Lisa Catherine Heffernan, "The One-Room School: Descriptions of Everyday Education in North Callaway County, Missouri, 1910–1940," *Gateway Heritage* 11 (Winter 1990–91): 27; and Mabel Carney, *Country Life and the Country School: A Study of the Agencies of Rural Progress and of the Social Relationship of the School to the Country Community* (Chicago: Row, Peterson, 1912), 197–98.

17. These quotations are taken from copies of articles by C.-E.A. Winslow located in his papers at Yale Univ. The first one on education can be found in "Euthenics," *Reference Handbook of the Medical Sciences* (post 1911), p. 162, Box 81, Folder 87; the second on germs is from "Organizing a State Campaign of Public Health Education," *American Journal of Public Health* (1916), p. 805, Box 119, Folder 112. On the prominent role played by schools in health campaigns during the 1920s and 1930s, see Elizabeth Fee and Barbara Rosenkrantz, "Professional Education for Public Health in the United States," in Elizabeth Fee and Roy M. Acheson, *A History of Education in Public Health: Health That Mocks the Doctors' Rules* (New York: Oxford Univ. Press, 1991), 234.

18. Richard K. Means, *Historical Perspectives on School Health* (Auburn, Ala.: Auburn University, 1975), 52; Philip J. Pauly, "The Development of High School Biology: New York City, 1900–1925," *Isis* 82 (Dec. 1991): 663 (quote), 676–77; and U.S. Bureau of the Census, *Historical Statistics of the United States, from Colonial Times to 1970* (2 vols.; Washington: Government Printing Office, 1975), I: 377.

19. Tyack, *The One Best System*, 231–33, 236 (quote); and David John Hogan, *Class and Reform: School and Society in Chicago, 1880–1930* (Philadelphia: Univ. of Pennsylvania Press, 1985), 133 (quote). See also Lawrence Augustus Averill, "School Hygiene and Training for Citizenship," *American Journal of Social Hygiene* 3 (June 1919): 37–52.

20. The description of schoolhouses is quoted in William A. Link, "Privies, Progressivism, and Public Schools: Health Reform and Education in the Rural South, 1909–1920," *Journal of Southern History* 54 (Nov. 1988): 627; and National Association of Supervisors and Consultants Interim History Writing Committee, *The Jeanes Story: A Chapter in the History of American Education 1908–1968* (Jackson, Miss.: Southern Education Foundation, 1979), 10. The Southern Education Board (1901) and the General Education Board (1902) were organized to improve public education but had concentrated primarily on white schools until 1907, when Anna T. Jeanes made her contribution. William A. Link, *A Hard Country and a Lonely Place: Schooling, Society, and Reform in Rural Virginia, 1870–1920* (Chapel Hill: Univ. of North Carolina Press, 1986), 83. In the end, the Julius Rosenwald Fund (1914) and its school building program "came to symbolize the crusade for black common schools in the rural South" during the 1920s and 1930s. James D. Anderson, *The Education of Blacks in the South, 1860–1935* (Chapel Hill: Univ. of North Carolina, 1988), 152–53. Because of these kinds of initiatives, the proportion of African-American children enrolled in schools doubled between 1900 and 1930, from 31 to 60 percent; enrollment of whites in the same period rose from 54 to 71 percent. See *Historical Statistics of the United States*, I: 370 (series 435 and 434).

21. John Duffy, *The Sanitarians: A History of American Public Health* (Urbana: Univ. of Illinois Press, 1990), 226; and David Nasaw, *Schooled to Order: A Social*

History of Public Schooling in the United States (New York: Oxford Univ. Press, 1979), 140–41.

22. Lance G. E. Jones, *The Jeanes Teacher in the United States 1908–1933: An Account of Twenty-five Years' Experience in the Supervision of Negro Rural Schools* (Chapel Hill: Univ. of North Carolina Press, 1937), 28; and Link, *A Hard Country and a Lonely Place*, 185.

23. "Virginia Randolph's First Report as Jeanes Teacher," in Jones, *The Jeanes Teacher*, 127–32 (quotes); and Link, *A Hard Country and a Lonely Place*, 186–88.

24. Jones, *The Jeanes Teacher*, 108–9. By 1920 there were 272 Jeanes teachers in the South, and most had been educated at Hampton, Tuskegee, or another industrial or normal school. See Link, *A Hard Country and a Lonely Place*, 186.

25. For quotations, see James H. Cassedy, "The 'Germ of Laziness' in the South, 1900–1915: Charles Wardell Stiles and the Progressive Paradox," *Bulletin of the History of Medicine* 45 (March/April 1971): 159, 167. On hookworm: the larvae get into surface soil from animal and human defecation. When children or adults walk barefooted through the soil, the larvae penetrate the soft skin between the toes, enter the blood stream, then reach the digestive tract. There the worms attach themselves to the intestinal wall and feed on blood, causing anemia (hence listlessness and "laziness") and susceptibility to other diseases. Treatment was "a dose of thymol followed by an Epsom salts chaser (on an empty stomach)," which would "jolt the worms loose from the intestinal wall and then forcibly expel them from the system." See John Ettling, *The Germ of Laziness: Rockefeller Philanthropy and Public Health in the New South* (Cambridge: Harvard Univ. Press, 1981), 5.

26. Ettling, *The Germ of Laziness*, 109–10.

27. Ibid., 146–48.

28. J. Fraser Orr, "Special Report on the Stevens Family of Pike County, Ala.," 1911, Alabama, Folder 51, Papers of the Rockefeller Sanitary Commission Collection, Rockefeller Archive Center (Pocantico Hills, N.Y.). Two years later, Orr wrote to W. W. Dismore in the state health office in Montgomery and described the opening of a dispensary in Jasper, Alabama, as "a sanitary revival." Orr to Dismore, Sept. 9, 1913, Alabama, Folder 52, Rockefeller Sanitary Commission Collection. See also "The Days of Galilee: The Dispensary as Revival," in Ettling, *The Germ of Laziness*, 152–77.

29. Quotations appear in B. E. Washburn, "Report of the Hookworm Campaign in Alamance County, North Carolina: August 8 to September 20, 1913," North Carolina, Folder 100, Rockefeller Sanitary Commission Collection; and William A. Link, " 'The Harvest Is Ripe, but the Laborers Are Few': The Hookworm Crusade in North Carolina, 1909–1915," *North Carolina Historical Review* 67 (Jan. 1990): 6.

30. James L. Leloudis II, "School Reform in the New South: The Woman's Association for the Betterment of Public School Houses in North Carolina, 1902–1919," *Journal of American History* 69 (March 1983): 886–909, esp. 899. See also Link, " 'The Harvest Is Ripe, but the Laborers Are Few,' " 8–9, 15.

31. The two quotations are quoted in Ettling, *The Germ of Laziness*, 195 and 215. The first is from Charles V. Chapin, public health official of Providence, R.I.; the second is a response to a 1939 Rockefeller Foundation questionnaire. See also Duffy, *The Sanitarians*, 229; Ettling, *The Germ of Laziness*, 220; and Link, " 'The Harvest Is Ripe, but the Laborers Are Few,' " 19–20.

32. William A. Link, "Privies, Progressivism, and Public Schools," 635–42.

33. Naomi Rogers, "Germs with Legs: Flies, Disease, and the New Public

Health," *Bulletin of the History of Medicine* 63 (Winter 1989): 599–617. "Dealers in deaths" is from a Charleston County, South Carolina "Healthogram," April 7, 1921, Pamphlet File, Box 1, Folder 4, Rockefeller Sanitary Commission Collection; in the same box and folder is the Winston-Salem health department leaflet, "This Is the Time to Swat the Fly," 1921. See also Martha Bensley Bruère and Robert Bruère, "The Revolt of the Farmer's Wife," *Harper's Bazar* 47 (Feb. 1913): 68 (quote).

34. Quoted in Rogers, "Germs with Legs," 611. See also, "'Cleanliness Is Next to Flylessness,'" *American City* 4 (May 1911): 242. On the 1916 polio epidemic, see Naomi Rogers, *Dirt and Disease: Polio before FDR* (New Brunswick: Rutgers Univ. Press, 1992), 57–71. And on "swat the fly" campaigns in Kansas, see Samuel J. Crumbine, *Frontier Doctor: The Autobiography of a Pioneer on the Frontier of Public Health* (Philadelphia: Dorrance, 1948), 156–64; and Thomas Neville Bonner, *The Kansas Doctor: A Century of Pioneering* (Lawrence: Univ. of Kansas Press, 1959), 123–24, 135–38. A Kansas state board of health "Swat the Fly" pamphlet can be found in Pamphlet File, Box 1, Folder 4, Rockefeller Sanitary Commission Collection.

35. Ken Chowder, "How TB Survived Its Own Death to Confront Us Again," *Smithsonian* 23 (Nov. 1992): 188, 191. In 1943 microbiologists discovered streptomycin, which proved an effective antibiotic (especially when combined with two later discoveries) against the tubercle baccillus. I thank Margaret Mac Curtain for sending me a copy of this article.

36. Duffy, *Sanitarians*, 196 (quote); and Michael E. Teller, *The Tuberculosis Movement: A Public Health Campaign in the Progressive Era* (Westport, Conn.: Greenwood Press, 1988), 57–64, 109–10.

37. Means, *Historical Perspectives on School Health*, 29–33; Teller, *The Tuberculosis Movement*, 118; and the National Association for the Study and Prevention of Tuberculosis, "Record of Health Chores: Based on the Rules of Modern Health Crusaders," 1918, Pamphlet File, Box 2, Folder 25, Rockefeller Sanitary Commission Collection. See also *The Health and Happiness League of the Metropolitan Life Insurance Company* (New York: Metropolitan Life Insurance Company, c. 1911). A copy can be found in the Metropolitan Life Insurance Company Archives, New York City. Metropolitan Life published and distributed numerous other public health brochures and pamphlets to children and their families; some examples are: *The Metropolitan Mother Goose*; *The Magic Health Book*; *ABC* ("B" is for bathing, "T" is for teeth, etc.); and *Care of the Teeth*. Others were aimed at young people and adults, especially mothers. The "Tower Health Talks" addressed such subjects as "Bathing," "The Flying Enemy," and "Disarming Germs."

38. Naomi Rogers, "Vegetables on Parade: Child Health Education in the 1920s," 3–4 (unpublished; used with author's permission); "sanitary conscience" from Charles-Edward Amory Winslow, *The Laws of Health and How to Teach Them* (New York: Charles E. Merrill, 1926), 169; and, finally, a public health official, quoted in Means, *Historical Perspectives on School Health*, 12. On draftee rejections and later school health programs, see also Leslie W. Irwin, James H. Humphrey, and Warren R. Johnson, *Methods and Materials in School Health Education* (St. Louis: C. V. Mosby, 1956), 18–19.

39. On the Child Health Organization and Jean's activities, I have benefited from Means, *Historical Perspectives on School Health*, 33–38 (quote), 46, 51, 137–38.

40. "Minutes of the Executive Committee of the Child Health Organization," Sept. 30, 1919, Box 60, Winslow Papers; "Miss Jean Honored by Bates College," *Mother and Child* 5 (July 1924): 327; and Rogers, "Vegetables on Parade," 12 (quote).

41. Grace T. Hallock to C.-E.A. Winslow, "Healthland Flyer," n.d., Box 60, Winslow Papers. See also Grace T. Hallock, "The Child Health Railroad," *Mother and Child* 3 (July 1922): 298–300; and Mary L. Hicks, "Healthland—All Aboard," ibid., 4 (Jan. 1923): 12–15.

42. Rogers, "Vegetables on Parade," 13–14; Grace T. Hallock and C.-E.A. Winslow, *The Land of Health: How Children May Become Citizens of the Land of Health by Learning and Obeying Its Laws* (New York: Charles E. Merrill, 1922), 3–4; and "Urges Lindbergh Bathtub," *New York Times,* June 24, 1927.

43. Quotations are in J. George Becht, "The Public School and the New American Spirit," *School and Society* 3 (April 12, 1916): 615; and Frances A. Kellor, "Americanization by Industry," *Immigrants in America Review* 2 (April 1916): 25. On the key role of women in the Americanization crusade *and* its ironic idealization of the traditional images of women, see John F. McClymer, "Gender and the 'American Way of Life': Women in the Americanization Movement," *Journal of American Ethnic History* 10 (Spring 1991): 3–20.

44. John F. McClymer, "The Americanization Movement and the Education of the Foreign-Born Adult, 1914–25," in Bernard J. Weiss, ed., *American Education and the European Immigrant: 1840–1940* (Urbana: Univ. of Illinois Press, 1982), 103. For quotations, see also John M. Siddall, "Something Worth Tackling: Peter Roberts" (reprinted from *American Magazine,* July 1910), in YMCA Papers Dealing with Immigrants, Folder 35, Miscellaneous Publications Material, Immigration History Research Center (Univ. of Minnesota).

45. Peter Roberts, *The New Immigration: A Study of the Industrial and Social Life of Southeastern Europeans in America* (New York: Macmillan, 1914), 134 (quote); and Mary F. Sharpe, *Plain Facts for Future Citizens* (New York: American Book Company, 1914), 8. Also Sara R. O'Brien, *English for Foreigners* (New York: Houghton Mifflin, 1909), 16, 23, 24–25, 51, 52, 76; and Frederick Houghton, *First Lessons in English for Foreigners in Evening Schools* (New York: American Book Company, 1911), 69. See too Tyack, *The One Best System,* 235–36; McClymer, "The Americanization Movement and the Education of the Foreign-Born Adult, 1914–25," 104–5, 109; and H. H. Wheaton, "Survey of Adult Immigrant Education," *Immigrants in America Review* 1 (June 1915): 51–53.

46. The quotation appears in Philip Roth, "The Man in the Middle," *New York Times,* Oct. 10, 1992. See also James Weinstein, *The Corporate Ideal in the Liberal State: 1900–1918* (Boston: Beacon Press, 1968), 18–19; Gregory Mason, "An Americanization Factory: An Account of What the Public Schools of Rochester Are Doing to Make Americans of Foreigners," *Outlook* 112 (Feb. 23, 1916): 439, 448; and James R. Barrett, "Americanization from the Bottom Up: Immigration and the Remaking of the Working Class, 1880–1930," *Journal of American History* 79 (Dec. 1992): 1003–4. Barrett notes that "learning also went on at work outside the structured programs"; for instance, new immigrants often learned from "older, more experienced, sometimes politicized workers, who conveyed different notions of what was right or wrong in the workshop and in the United States as a society."

47. The quotation is from Martha May, "The Historical Problem of the Family

Wage: The Ford Motor Company and the Five Dollar Day," *Feminist Studies* 8 (Summer 1982): 414. See also Gerd Korman, *Industrialization, Immigrants, and Americanizers: The View from Milwaukee, 1886–1921* (Madison: State Historical Society of Wisconsin, 1967), 143–47. Details of an ideal factory Americanization program, mentioning Ford's, are in Frances K. Wetmore, "Industrial or Factory Classes," in John J. Mahoney, ed., *Training Teachers for Americanization: A Course of Study for Normal Schools and Teachers' Institutes* (Dept. of the Interior, Bureau of Education, Bulletin No. 12; Washington: Government Printing Office, 1920), 43–48.

48. Olivier Zunz, *Making America Corporate, 1870–1920* (Chicago: Univ. of Chicago Press, 1990), 134; and James MacGregor Burns, *The Workshop of Democracy* (New York: Alfred A. Knopf, 1985), 481. The quotation appears in Stephen Meyer, "Adapting the Immigrant to the Line: Americanization in the Ford Factory, 1914–1921," *Journal of Social History* 14 (Fall 1980): 71.

49. Gregory Mason, " 'Americans First': How the People of Detroit Are Making Americans of the Foreigners in Their City," *Outlook* 114 (Sept. 27, 1916): 193–201. Ford's paternalism, as we know, eventually failed. For a discussion of the reasons why, see Meyer, "Adapting the Immigrant to the Line," 78–79.

50. "Americanization Day," *Kohler of Kohler News* 1 (April 1917): 4 (quote). See also Susan Mahnke, "Kohler of Kohler of Kohler," *Wisconsin Trails* (Spring 1979), 36–37; and "The Early Years," in *Bold Craftsmen* (Kohler: Kohler Company, 1973), 4. I am grateful to Gail and Jim Leonard for introducing me to Kohler, and to Peter J. Fetterer, manager of Media and Civic Services at Kohler, who assisted me during my research trip.

51. Mahnke, "Kohler," 37–38; and "The Early Years," in *Bold Craftsmen*, 5. For the quotation, see "Dedication of the American Club, Sunday, June 23, 1918," *Kohler of Kohler News* 2 (July 1918): 3.

52. "The American Club," ibid. 1 (June 1917): 14–17; and "Dedication of the American Club," 4, 6–12; "The American Club," ibid. 8 (Dec. 1924): 3–6.

53. "Dental Department," ibid. 1 (Feb. 1917): 14; and "Promoting Health and Safety in the Kohler Co. Organization," ibid. 13 (April 1929): 3–5. See also Alice Hamilton, *Exploring the Dangerous Trades: The Autobiography of Alice Hamilton* (Boston: Little, Brown, 1943), 142–43 (quotes).

54. "Kohler Winter Classes," *Kohler of Kohler News* 3 (Sept. 1919): 6–7; and ibid. 9 (Oct. 1925): 5.

55. "Teeth Tell Tales," ibid. 5 (July 1921): 16 (quote). See also, for example, "Health and Safety," ibid. 1 (Nov. 1916): 9; "Tuberculosis," ibid. 1 (Aug. 1917): 10–11; "Preserve Your Health," ibid. 5 (Nov. 1920): 12; and "Rules for Health," ibid. 5 (Dec. 1920): 16.

56. "Kohler, Beacon City," ibid. 1 (July 1917): 12–13; "Dedication Addresses [of Nature Theatre]," ibid. 3 (Oct. 1919): 13; "Americanization Day," ibid. 4 (April 1920): 3; and "Americanization Day at Kohler, Wednesday, April 7," ibid. 10 (May 1926): 3–5.

57. Walter H. Uphoff, *Kohler on Strike* (Boston: Beacon Press, 1966), 9–14.

58. Korman, *Industrialization, Immigrants, and Americanizers*, 164; Meyer, "Adapting the Immigrant to the Line," 78; Uphoff, *Kohler on Strike*, 10; and "The Shrine of Cleanliness," *Kohler of Kohler News* 7 (March 1923): 13 (quote).

59. Stephen Fox, *The Mirror Makers: A History of American Advertising and Its Creators* (New York: Vintage, 1985), 101 (quote); "Telling the World About

Kohler Products," *Kohler of Kohler News* 9 (Jan. 1925): 9; and two ads in 1925 newsletters: "Early reflections are happy ones when the bathroom is a room of magic cleanliness" (July) and "The fun of being clean!" (Sept.). See also two ads in 1927 *Kohler of Kohler News*, vol. 11: "First aid to health, first aid to happiness—such is the bathroom with Kohler fixtures" (June) and "There is also the game of 'Steal-the-Bathroom'" (Sept.).

60. "'Take-a-Bath Week' Starts," *New York Times*, July 10, 1927 (quote); Vincent Vinikas, *Soft Soap, Hard Sell: American Hygiene in an Age of Advertisement* (Ames: Univ. of Iowa Press, 1992), 55; and Lois Banner, *American Beauty* (Chicago: Univ. of Chicago Press, 1983), 271.

61. Vinikas, *Soft Soap*, 82–83. See also *One Hundred Years of Public Works Equipment: An Illustrated History* (Chicago: Public Works Historical Society, 1986), 24–25.

62. "For Cleanliness Education: Organization of Cleanliness Institute Announced at Dinner in New York," and "Half Million Dollars Pledged for Cleanliness Education," *Cleanliness Journal* 1 (July 1927): 3 and 4.

63. Roscoe C. Edlund, *The Business of Cleanliness* [pamphlet] (New York: Cleanliness Institute, 1930), 5. A copy is in the archives of the Soap and Detergent Association in New York City. I thank Mildred Gallik for assisting me during a research trip. See also Roland Marchand, *Advertising the American Dream: Making Way for Modernity, 1920–1940* (Berkeley: Univ. of California Press, 1985), 218. For examples of the Sapolio ads, see the back covers of *Ladies' Home Journal*, Oct. 1896 and July 1899. See also Susan Strasser, *Satisfaction Guaranteed: The Making of the American Mass Market* (New York: Pantheon, 1989), 134; Laurie Freeman, "The House That Ivory Built," *Advertising Age*, Aug. 20, 1987, pp. 12 and 168; and Vinikas, *Soft Soap*, 86.

64. "Shake Hands *Often* with Soap" appears on a Cleanliness Institute poster in the archives of the Soap and Detergent Association. The other quotations are from Roscoe C. Edlund, "Lave and Learn: Study Made by Cleanliness Institute Reveals That Hands of America's 25,000,000 School Children Are Not Washed as Often as Health and Decency Demand," *Cleanliness Journal* 4 (April 1931): 3–5; and Jean Broadhurst, "You Can Lead Him to Water: But You Should Not Expect the Child to Take to Cleanliness Instinctively," ibid. 2 (Oct. 1928): 5. See also L. L. Lumsden, "The Soul of Sanitation: Common Sense Application of Cleanliness Principles to Everyday Life Goes Far to Forestall Spread of Communicable Disease," ibid. 3 (Feb. 1930): 3; School Service, *Outline for Cleanliness Teaching in Three Sections* (New York: Cleanliness Institute, 1929); Vinikas, *Soft Soap*, 87–88, 90; and "Two Hundred Books on Cleanliness Listed in Bibliography," *Cleanliness Journal* 1 (Dec. 1927): 8.

65. Herman N. Bundesen, "Cleanliness First," *Cleanliness Journal* 1 (Feb. 1928): 3 (quote); and Edlund, *The Business of Cleanliness*, 11–12.

66. One author, for instance, said, "Self-respect based on personal cleanliness is one of the essentials of success." Eunice Brown, "Soap as a Cleanser of the Body," *Cleanliness Journal* 1 (July 1926): 4. Many other articles reinforced that message. Samples from other issues of the *Cleanliness Journal* include: "Help Wanted: Employment Managers Tell Why It Pays to Clean Up before Applying for a Job," 3 (Oct. 1929); "What People Expect" and "Cleanliness an Essential in Family Budget: Well Worth the Cost," 3 (Feb. 1930); "Good Form and Good Health Demand

Cleanliness as a Safeguard" and "At a Time When Jobs Are Scarce It Is Doubly Necessary to Keep Up a Clean Front," 4 (Feb. 1931); and "A Clean Shirt Helps Jimmie to Get His Job," 4 (June 1931).

67. Warren I. Susman, "'Personality' and the Making of Twentieth-Century Culture," in Susman, ed., *Culture as History: The Transformation of American Society in the Twentieth Century* [1973] (New York: Pantheon, 1984), 273–78. See also Walter D. Scott, "Habits that Help," *Everybody's Magazine* 25 (Sept. 1911): 415–16; Paula S. Fass, *The Damned and the Beautiful: American Youth in the 1920s* (paper ed., New York: Oxford Univ. Press, 1979), 230, 243; Marchand, *Advertising and the American Dream*, 209; and Robert S. Lynd and Helen Merrell Lynd, *Middletown: A Study in American Culture* [1929] (New York: Harcourt Brace Jovanovich, 1957), 219–20.

68. Quotations appear in Marchand, *Advertising the American Dream*, 210, 211; "Don't Fool Yourself: A Tip for Office Workers," *Ladies' Home Journal*, Sept. 1927, p. 57; and "Don't Fool Yourself: Rings Aren't Binding," ibid., 55. On the "discovery" of halitosis, see Fox, *The Mirror Makers*, 97–98; and on the halitosis campaign as an early example of advertising hype see Stuart Chase, "Putting Halitosis on the Map," *Survey* 41 (Nov. 1, 1928): 127–29, 183–85.

69. On the prosperity of the 1920s, see William E. Leuchtenburg, *The Perils of Prosperity, 1914–32* (Chicago: Univ. of Chicago Press, 1958), 9 (quote); and Vinikas, *Soft Soap*, 23. On the ad men, who were young and largely from "small-town Protestant America," see Thomas J. Schlereth, *Victorian America: Transformations in Everyday Life, 1876–1915* (New York: Harper Collins, 1991), 157; and Marchand, *Advertising the American Dream*, 70 (quote). On the behaviorist psychology and mass advertising's explosion in the 1920s, see David E. Shi, "Advertising as Literary Imagination during the Jazz Age," *Journal of American Culture* 2 (Summer 1979): 167. The final quote is from L. B. Jones, "Advertising Men as the 'Cheer Leaders' of the Nation," *Printers' Ink* 102 (Feb. 7, 1918): 62.

70. Quotations can be found in "Tell Me What To Do! Coupon Clippers Ask for Help in Cleanliness Problems," *Cleanliness Journal* 4 (Nov. 1930): 9; and *Coupon Returns: One Advertiser's Experience* (New York: Newell-Emmett Company, 1932), 7–11, 62.

71. "'What's Wrong with Me, Mother?,'" *Good Housekeeping*, April 1932, p. 105; "Hygienic Freedom: Such as Women Never Knew Before," *Ladies' Home Journal*, July 1927, p. 82; and "The Safe Solution of Women's Greatest Hygienic Problem," ibid., Nov. 1927, p. 79. "Sanitary napkins," which appeared on the market in 1921, were invented during World War I; but women's magazines did not begin advertising them until the late 1920s. Women had previously used "rags," "linens," or "diapers" that they washed and reused each month. Janice Delaney, Mary Jane Lupton, and Emily Toth, *The Curse: A Cultural History of Menstruation* (New York: E. P. Dutton, 1976), 108–9; and Fox, *The Mirror Makers*, 99. Kotex's chief selling points were disposability and protection from social embarrassment. Jane Celia Busch, "The Throwaway Ethic in America" (Ph.D. dissertation, Univ. of Pennsylvania, 1983), 102–4.

72. Daniel Pope, *The Making of Modern Advertising* (New York: Basic Books, 1983), 247; T. J. Jackson Lears, "From Salvation to Self-Realization: Advertising and the Therapeutic Roots of the Consumer Culture, 1880–1930," in Richard Wightman Fox and T. J. Jackson Lears, eds., *The Culture of Consumption: Critical Essays in*

American History, 1880–1980 (New York: Pantheon, 1983), 27; and Marchand, *Advertising the American Dream*, 54–58, 65.

73. "Teaching Mrs. Rizzuto American Ideas," *Survey* 65 (June 1, 1930): 251 (quote). See also "The Zitis Are Summering on the Fire-Escape," ibid. 68 (July 1, 1932): 317; "Moving the Orozcos Next Door to Godliness," ibid. 62 (May 1, 1929): 215; and "Little Graziella Wants a Gold Star," ibid. 68 (Nov. 15, 1932): 659.

74. For quotations, see A. B. Messer, "What the Foreigner Means to America," *Judicious Advertising* 19 (March 1921): 63, 64; and T. Coleman Du Pont, "The Inter-Racial Council—What It Is and Hopes to Do," *Advertising and Selling* 29 (July 5, 1919): 2. "Interracial" here meant relations among native-born and immigrants, not between whites and African-Americans.

75. Marchand, *Advertising the American Dream*, 64; "Po Kilku Tancach Zwykle Jej *Unikano*," *Kuryer Polski*, June 23, 1926; "Why Is Maizie So Popular?," Chicago *Defender*, Aug. 11, 1923; and "Yes, Sir . . . She's My Baby . . . Now!," ibid., July 3, 1926. I am especially grateful to Michal Rozbicki for translating several Polish ads. Between 1910 and 1914 the Yiddish press acquired numerous national advertisers, including Ivory soap. See Andrew R. Heinze, *Adapting to Abundance: Jewish Immigrants, Mass Consumption, and the Search for American Identity* (New York: Columbia Univ. Press, 1990), 159–60.

76. Copies of the Cleanliness Institute posters can be found in the archives of the Soap and Detergent Association. See also "Behind His Back: What Are People Saying . . . About You?," *Saturday Evening Post*, May 14, 1941, p. 104.

77. Quotations are from "New Self-Sharpening Ronson Razor," *Saturday Evening Post*, May 14, 1932, p. 83; and "Get Orders or Give Orders with a Face That's Fit," ibid., June 4, 1932, p. 85. See also Marchand, *Advertising the American Dream*, 188–89; Schlereth, *Victorian America*, 165; and "Women Men Despise," *Ladies' Home Journal*, July 1935, p. 38. For information on Gillette razors, the first disposable ones, see Strasser, *Satisfaction Guaranteed*, 97–101.

78. Quotations are from "The General Manager Says OK to the Face That's Fit," *Saturday Evening Post*, May 7, 1932, p. 109; and "Why Do We Advertise Men's Underwear in a Woman's Magazine?," *Ladies' Home Journal*, May 1925, p. 114.

79. Vinikas, *Soft Soap*, 14–16; and Marchand, *Advertising the American Dream*, 149.

80. "Mr. Countway Takes the Job," *Fortune* 22 (Nov. 1940): 94–100, 114, 116.

81. Paul F. Lazarsfeld, *Radio and the Printed Page: An Introduction to the Study of Radio and Its Role in the Communication of Ideas* (New York: Duell, Sloan and Pearce, 1940), 255 (quote); "The Culture of Democracy," *Fortune*, Feb. 1940, p. 83; "The Fortune Quarterly Survey: VIII," ibid., Jan. 1938, p. 88; Marchand, *Advertising the American Dream*, 110, 306; and Hugh Beville, "A Research-Suggested Approach to Commercials," in Charles Hull Wolfe, ed., *Modern Radio Advertising* (New York: Funk & Wagnalls and Printer's Ink, 1953), 483 (quote).

82. Studs Terkel, *Hard Times: An Oral History of the Great Depression* [1970] (New York: Avon Books, 1978), 80; and Melvin Patrick Ely, *The Adventures of Amos 'n' Andy: A Social History of an American Phenomenon* (New York: Free Press, 1991), 58, 118 (quote)–19, 245.

83. "Cleanliness Is Broadcast in Series of Talks over Nation-wide Network," *Cleanliness Journal* 3 (July 1930): 11; and "Houseworking Your Way to Good Looks: Five Radio Talks Prepared by the Cleanliness Institute," copy in archives of Soap and

Detergent Association. When the Cleanliness Institute shut down in Dec. 1932, its 48 staff members were dismissed and their exodus completed by Jan. 15, 1933. W. W. Peter to "Editor," *American Journal of Public Health* 23 (Jan. 1933): 53.

84. Quotations are from Barbara Ehrenreich and Deirdre English, *For Her Own Good: 150 Years of the Experts' Advice to Women* (New York: Anchor Books, 1979), 173; and interview with Victor Giustino, Allstate Insurance Claims Representative, Jan. 5, 1980, "Italians in Chicago" Oral History Project, Chicago Historical Society.

85. *Hygeia* 20 (May 1942): 331 (editorial).

CHAPTER 6. WHITER THAN WHITE—AND A GLIMMER OF GREEN

1. P.B., "An American Paradox," *The Twentieth Century* [British publication] 1561 (May 1952): 394.

2. William E. Leuchtenburg, *A Troubled Feast: American Society since 1945* (rev. ed., Boston: Little, Brown, 1979), 37 (quote), 39, 63; and James Gilbert, *Another Chance: Postwar America, 1945–1985* [1981] (Chicago: Dorsey Press, 1986), 58–59.

3. Witold Rybczynski, *Home: A Short History of an Idea* (New York: Viking, 1986), 219–24. The "cleanest clean" quotation is from a Tide ad in *Ladies' Home Journal*, Jan. 1956, front matter.

4. Daniel E. Sutherland, "Modernizing Domestic Service," in Jessica H. Foy and Thomas J. Schlereth, eds., *American Home Life, 1880–1930: A Social History of Spaces and Services* (Knoxville: Univ. of Texas Press, 1992), 243–45; and Ruth Schwartz Cowan, *More Work for Mother: The Ironies of Household Technology from the Open Hearth to the Microwave* (New York: Basic Books, 1983), 155–58; 173–74. The quotation is from a Eureka ad in *Ladies' Home Journal*, Nov. 1927, p. 129.

5. Elizabeth Ross Haynes, "Negroes in Domestic Service in the United States," *Journal of Negro History* 8 (Oct. 1923): 429–32; Susan Tucker, *Telling Memories among Southern Women: Domestic Workers and Their Employers in the Segregated South* (Baton Rouge: Louisiana State Univ. Press, 1988), 76–77; Phyllis Palmer, *Domesticity and Dirt, 1920–1945* (Philadelphia: Temple Univ. Press, 1989), 67–69; Mario T. Garcia, "The Chicana in American History: The Mexican Women of El Paso, 1880–1920—A Case Study," *Pacific Historical Review* 49 (May 1980): 325–26; and Amerika Nadeshiko, "Japanese Immigrant Women in the United States, 1900–1924," ibid., 349.

6. Cowan, *More Work for Mother*, 160–72 (quote on p. 166).

7. Ibid., 189–91. See also Ruth Schwartz Cowan, "Coal Stoves and Clean Sinks: Housework between 1890 and 1930," in Foy and Schlereth, eds., *American Home Life*, 222–23; and Miriam Cohen, *Workshop to Office: Two Generations of Italian Women in New York City, 1900–1950* (Ithaca: Cornell Univ. Press, 1992), 189.

8. Ellen H. Richards, "Housekeeping in the Twentieth Century," *American Kitchen Magazine* 12 (March 1900): 205; Campbell, *Household Economics*, 196; and Ellen H. Richards, *The Cost of Cleanness* (New York: John Wiley & Sons, 1908), frontispiece.

9. Helen Campbell, "Household Art and the Microbe," *House Beautiful* 6 (Oct. 1899): 218–21. Linoleum, enamel, and tile became the preferred materials for kitchens and bathrooms; and the color white was considered best, since it would show dirt immediately. See Jonquil K. Seager, " 'Father's Chair': Domestic Reform and Housing Change in the Progressive Era" (Ph.D. dissertation, Clark Univ., 1988), 152–53. See also the following ads from which the quotations are taken: Creolin-Pearson disinfectant in *Ladies' Home Journal*, Jan. 1902, back of cover; Standard Floor dressing in *Survey*, Sept. 3, 1910, n.p.; Dutch Cleanser in *Ladies' Home Journal*, Jan. 1912, p. 60; Lysol disinfectant in *Good Housekeeping*, Jan. 1923, p. 137; and Bon Ami cleanser in *Parents' Magazine*, Feb. 1933, p. 51.

10. A quotation from Ellen H. Richards in Caroline L. Hunt, *The Life of Ellen H. Richards* (Washington, D.C.: American Home Economics Association, 1958), 159; Barbara Ehrenreich and Deirdre English, *For Her Own Good: 150 Years of the Experts' Advice to Women* (Garden City, N.Y.: Anchor Books, 1978), 128–31; and Charlotte Perkins Gilman, *Women and Economics: A Study of the Economic Relation between Men and Women as a Factor in Social Evolution* [1898] (New York: Harper & Row, 1966), 257.

11. Maxine L. Margolis, *Mothers and Such: Views of American Women and Why They Changed* (Berkeley: Univ. of California Press, 1984), 139; and Laura Shapiro, *Perfection Salad: Women and Cooking at the Turn of the Century* (New York: Henry Holt, 1986), 8 (quote), 185–86. The 1920 Girl Scout manual admonished girls to become adept at "domestic science," but in the 1950s they learned that "the greatest career is homemaking." Cleanliness was always one of the explicit values in the Girl Scout creed. Elizabeth Israels Perry, "From Achievement to Happiness: Girl Scouting in Middle Tennessee, 1910s–1960s," *Journal of Women's History* 5 (Fall 1993): 79, 84, 90.

12. Carolyn Goldstein, "From Service to Sales: The Rise and Fall of Home Economics in Light and Power, 1920–1940" (unpublished paper presented at the annual meeting of Society for the History of Technology, Washington, D.C., October 1993). I thank Ms. Goldstein for sending me a copy of her paper and permitting me to quote from it.

13. Caroline Shillaber, "Christine McGaffey Frederick," in Barbara Sicherman and Carol Hurd Green, eds., *Notable American Women: The Modern Period* (Cambridge: Harvard Univ. Press, 1980), 249–50; and Christine Frederick, *Selling Mrs. Consumer* (New York: The Business Bourse, 1929), 168.

14. Frederick, *Selling Mrs. Consumer*, 171; Christine Frederick, *The New Housekeeping: Efficiency Studies in Home Management* (Garden City, N.Y.: Doubleday, 1913), 70; and Christine Frederick, *The Ignoramus Book of Housekeeping* (New York: Sears Publishing, 1932), 4.

15. Frederick, *Selling Mrs. Consumer*, 3, 22, 40, 62, and 76.

16. Ibid., 47, 59, 171; and Ruth Schwartz Cowan, "Two Washes in the Morning and a Bridge Party at Night: The American Housewife between the Wars," *Women's Studies* 3 (1976): 150–51. See also the following ads: General Electric dishwasher, N. W. Ayer Advertising Agency Collection, Box 245 (National Museum of American History, Smithsonian Institution, Washington, D.C.); Rinso soap in *Ladies' Home Journal*, July 1935, front matter; and Sani-Flush scouring powder, Ayer Collection, Box 425. Advertisers tried to create new demands and often modeled themselves after the successful Lambert Pharmaceutical Company. The story of Listerine's vic-

tory over "halitosis" is well-known; it is also well told in Roland Marchand, *Advertising the American Dream: Making Way for Modernity, 1920–1940* (Berkeley: Univ. of California Press, 1985), 18–20.

17. Christine Frederick, *Household Engineering: Scientific Management in the Home* (Chicago: American School of Home Economics, 1919), 146; Jacqueline Jones, *Labor of Love, Labor of Sorrow: Black Women, Work, and the Family from Slavery to the Present* (New York: Vintage, 1986), 165; and Heather Biola, "The Black Washerwoman in Southern Tradition," *Tennessee Folklore Society Bulletin* 45 (1979): 20. The Automatic Electric Washer ad appears in Victoria Leto, "'Washing, Seems It's All We Do': Washing Technology and Women's Communication," in Cheris Kramarae, ed., *Technology and Women's Voices: Keeping in Touch* (New York: Routledge & Kegan Paul, 1988), 168. The final quotation is from Arwen Palmer Mohun, "Women, Work, and Technology: The Steam Laundry Industry in the United States and Great Britain, 1880–1920" (Ph.D. dissertation, Case Western Reserve Univ., 1992), 300.

18. Cowan, "Two Washes in the Morning," 147–49; Annegret S. Ogden, *The Great American Housewife: From Helpmate to Wage Earner, 1776–1986* (Westport, Conn.: Greenwood Press, 1986), 141–50; and Frederick, *Ignoramus Book of Housekeeping*, 174.

19. Janet Anne Hutchison, "American Housing, Gender, and the Better Homes Movement, 1922–1935" (Ph.D. dissertation, Univ. of Delaware, 1989), 18–34; Margaret Marsh, *Suburban Lives* (New Brunswick: Rutgers Univ. Press, 1990), 132–33; and "Color in Industry," *Fortune*, Feb. 1930, p. 92 (quote).

20. General Federation of Women's Clubs, "Home Equipment Survey, 1925–1926," Program Records, RG 7, Mary K. Sherman Collection, Box 1, Folder 23 (General Federation of Women's Clubs Archives, Washington, D.C.); Robert S. Lynd and Helen Merrell Lynd, *Middletown: A Study in Modern American Culture* [1929] (New York: Harcourt Brace Jovanovich, 1957), 98; Harold L. Platt, *The Electric City: Energy and the Growth of the Chicago Area, 1880–1930* (Chicago: Univ. of Chicago Press, 1991), 235; and Marilyn Thornton Williams, *Washing "The Great Unwashed": Public Baths in Urban America, 1840–1920* (Columbus: Ohio State Univ. Press, 1991), 137.

21. Eleanor Arnold, ed., *Party Lines, Pumps and Privies: Memories of Hoosier Homemakers* (Indianapolis: Indiana Extension Homemakers Association, 1984), 42–43, 47.

22. Deborah Fink, *Agrarian Women: Wives and Mothers in Rural Nebraska, 1880–1940* (Chapel Hill: Univ. of North Carolina, 1992), 43, 67–68; and LuAnn Jones, "'The Task That Is Ours': White North Carolina Farm Women and Agrarian Reform, 1886–1914," in *Institute News* [of the North Carolina Division of Archives and History] 4 (March 1985), 3 (quote).

23. Arnold, ed., *Party Lines, Pumps and Privies*, 92–94; 101–2.

24. Deborah Fink, *Open Country Iowa: Rural Women, Tradition and Change* (Albany: State Univ. of New York Press, 1986), 53; Arnold, ed., *Party Lines, Pumps and Privies*, 94–96.

25. Arnold, ed., *Party Lines, Pumps and Privies*, 82 (quote).

26. Robert A. Caro, *The Path to Power: The Years of Lyndon Johnson* (New York: Vintage, 1983), 508–9.

27. Arnold, ed., *Party Lines, Pumps and Privies*, 70–71; and Caro, *Path to Power*, 508–9 (quote).

28. Arnold, ed., *Party Lines, Pumps and Privies*, 72–73, 78–79 (quotes).

29. Quotations are from Jones, "'The Task That Is Ours,'" 5; and Mrs. Alfred Abbuhl, Greene, New York, to C. J. Galpin, Economist, Rural Life Studies, U.S. Department of Agriculture, June 2 and 10, 1921, Records of Bureau of Agricultural Economics, RG 83, General Correspondence, 1919–34, Box 12, Folder "Farm Women" (National Archives, Washington, D.C.)

30. Quotations are from Abbuhl to Galpin, June 2, 1921; and Christine Frederick, "What the New Housekeeping Means to the Farm Home" (Feb. 22, 1916), 86, copy in Christine Isobel MacGaffey Frederick Papers (Schlesinger Library, Radcliffe College, Cambridge, Mass.). See also Katherine Jellison, "Women and Technology on the Great Plains, 1910–40," *Great Plains Quarterly* 8 (Summer 1988): 146–47; and Marquis Childs, *The Farmer Takes a Hand: The Electric Power Revolution in Rural America* (Garden City, N.Y.: Doubleday, 1952), 170, 239.

31. Florence E. Ward, "The Farm Woman's Problems," *Journal of Home Economics* 12 (Oct. 1920): 442, 446–47; Arnold, ed., *Party Lines, Pumps and Privies*, 44–46, 47; and D. Clayton Brown, *Electricity for Rural America: The Fight for REA* (Westport, Conn.: Greenwood Press, 1980), xiii.

32. Dorothy Schwieder and Deborah Fink, "Plains Women: Rural Life in the 1930s," *Great Plains Quarterly* 8 (Spring 1988): 82–84. The quotations can be found in Katherine Kay Jellison, "Entitled to Power: Farm Women and Technology, 1913–1963" (Ph.D. dissertation, Univ. of Iowa, 1991), 160, 168.

33. Jones, "'The Task That Is Ours,'" 4–5 (quote).

34. George D. Aiken, "Foreword," in Childs, *The Farmer Takes a Hand*, 13; and David E. Nye, *Electrifying America: Social Meanings of a New Technology, 1880–1940* (Cambridge: MIT Press, 1990), 294–95.

35. Nye, *Electrifying America*, 299–301; and Brown, *Electricity for Rural America*, x.

36. Jellison, "Entitled to Power," 206–7; Platt, *The Electric City*, 265–66; and Caro, *Path to Power*, 524–25.

37. Ronald R. Kline, "Less Work for the Farm Woman? Rural Electrification and Household Work in the United States" (unpublished paper presented at the annual meeting of the Society for the History of Technology, Washington, D.C., Oct. 1993). According to Kline, studies done at the time showed that "farm women with more technology often worked more hours in what was then called 'homemaking'" (p. 4). I thank Mr. Kline for sending me a copy of his paper and permitting me to quote from it.

38. Childs, *The Farmer Takes a Hand*, 117–18.

39. Louisan Mamer to John W. Asher, Nov. 13, 1950, Records of the Rural Electrification Administration, RG 221, Correspondence 1946–53, Box 3 (Federal Records Center, Suitland, Maryland). See also Louisan Mamer, "Electricity Pays Its Way in the Rural Home," copy found in Records of the Rural Electrification Administration, RG 221, Correspondence 1946–53, Box 3, from which the quotations are taken.

40. The first quotation can be found in both Nye, *Electrifying America*, 304, and Platt, *The Electric City*, 262. The other two are in Jellison, "Entitled to Power," 208, and "Editorial: Not Words, But Deeds," *Farmer's Wife Magazine* 41 (May 1938): 42. See also "Another Year," ibid. 42 (Jan. 1939): 26.

41. "Not Words, But Deeds," 42 (quote). See also Frederick, "What the New Housekeeping Means to the Farm Woman," 89; Jellison, "Entitled to Power," 234–35; Rural Electrification Administration, *Farm Plumbing* (Washington, D.C.:

Government Printing Office, c. 1949–50), 7–13. A copy can be found in Rural Electrification Administration Records, RG 221, "Applications and Loans Division, 1946–53," Box 5.

42. Nye, *Electrifying America*, 144 (quote); Jellison, "Entitled to Power," 235; Childs, *Farmer Takes a Hand*, 144–45; and Arnold, ed., *Party Lines, Pumps and Privies*, 64–65.

43. U.S. Bureau of the Census, *Historical Statistics of the United States, Colonial Times to 1970* (2 vols.; Washington: Government Printing Office, 1975), II: 829–30. Quotations can be found in Fink, *Open Country Iowa*, 2, 105; and Alice Walker, "Beyond the Peacock: The Reconstruction of Flannery O'Connor," *In Search of Our Mothers' Gardens* (New York: Harcourt Brace Jovanovich, 1983), 44–45.

44. This is, of course, the central argument of Cowan's *More Work for Mother* and Susan Strasser's *Never Done: A History of American Housework* (New York: Pantheon, 1982). Their main focus is on urban women, but their thesis generally holds true for farm women too. Higher standards of cleanliness often resulted in more housework (especially consuming); many farm women also undertook new purchasing tasks, particularly in recent times. See Katherine Jensen, "Mother Calls Herself a Housewife, But She Buys Bulls," in Jan Zimmerman, ed., *The Technological Woman: Interfacing with Tomorrow* (New York: Praeger, 1983), 140–42. Quotations are from Arnold, ed., *Party Lines, Pumps and Privies*, 49; and Clara H. Zillessen, "When Housework Is Not Drudgery," *Ladies' Home Journal*, Jan. 1937, p. 127.

45. "The Fortune Survey: XXVII, The People of the U.S.A.—A Self-Portrait," *Fortune* 21 (Feb. 1940): 20; and U.S. Bureau of the Census, *Historical Statistics of the United States*, I: 139. It should be remembered that the "new middle class" depended very much on the wife/mother's second income. See William H. Chafe, "World War II as a Pivotal Experience for American Women," in Maria Diedrich and Dorothy Fischer-Hornung, eds., *Women and War: The Changing Status of American Women from the 1930s to the 1950s* (New York: Berg, 1990), 32.

46. D'Ann Campbell, *Women at War with America: Private Lives in a Patriotic Era* (Cambridge: Harvard Univ. Press, 1984), 72; Alice Kessler-Harris, *Out to Work: A History of Wage-Earning Women in the United States* (New York: Oxford Univ. Press, 1982), 275–76; and David Halberstam, *The Fifties* (New York: Villard Books, 1993), 588.

47. Kessler-Harris, *Out to Work*, 276; Jones, *Labor of Love, Labor of Sorrow*, 237; Campbell, *Women at War with America*, 76–77, 85, 119, 125 (quote).

48. Campbell, *Women at War with America*, 133; Susan M. Hartmann, *The Home Front and Beyond: American Women in the 1940s* (Boston: Twayne, 1982), 78–79; and Kessler-Harris, *Out to Work*, 274, 278 (quote).

49. Campbell, *Women at War with America*, 169, 173; and Kenneth T. Jackson, *Crabgrass Frontier: The Suburbanization of the United States* (New York: Oxford Univ. Press, 1985), 232.

50. Campbell, *Women at War with America*, 169–72, 174.

51. Carl N. Degler, *At Odds: Women and the Family in America from the Revolution to the Present* (New York: Oxford Univ. Press, 1980), 421; Campbell, *Women at War with America*, 128; Hartmann, *The Home Front and Beyond*, 87; and Jones, *Labor of Love, Labor of Sorrow*, 238–40 (quote).

52. National Life Insurance Company ad in *Life*, Oct. 1, 1945, p. 125 (quote); and Halberstam, *The Fifties*, 132–33.

53. Hartmann, *The Home Front and Beyond*, 163 (quote); Walter Nugent, *Structures of American Social History* (Bloomington: Indiana Univ. Press, 1981), 127; Steven Mintz and Susan Kellogg, *Domestic Revolutions: A Social History of American Family Life* (New York: Free Press, 1988), 178–79; and Brett Harvey, *The Fifties: A Women's Oral History* (New York: HarperCollins, 1993), xv (quote), 70.

54. Richard S. Blaisdell, "More Women Are Working," *Journal of Home Economics* 50 (April 1958): 261–65. See also Kessler-Harris, *Out to Work*, 286–87; Stephanie Coontz, *The Way We Never Were: American Families and the Nostalgia Trap* (New York: Basic Books, 1992), 158–60; and Tamara K. Hareven, "Introduction: The Historical Study of the Life Course," in *Transitions: The Family and Life Course in Historical Perspective* (New York: Academic Press, 1978), 37 (quote).

55. Mintz and Kellogg, *Domestic Revolutions*, 180–82; Hartmann, *The Home Front and Beyond*, 163–64; Halberstam, *The Fifties*, 589–90; Mary Beth Haralovich, "Sit-coms and Suburbs: Positioning the 1950s Homemaker," in Lynn Spigel and Denise Mann, eds., *Private Screenings: Television and the Female Consumer* (Minneapolis: Univ. of Minneapolis Press, 1992), 114; and Elaine Tyler May, *Homeward Bound: American Families in the Cold War Era* (New York: Basic Books, 1988), 141–42. On the postwar return to domesticity and "the problem that has no name," see Betty Friedan, *The Feminine Mystique* [1963] (New York: Laurel, 1984), esp. 15–32.

56. A "Cleaner Clean" (in the section head) appears in a Prell shampoo ad; see photograph in "Advertising," *New York Times*, Jan. 28, 1993. See also Mintz and Kellogg, *Domestic Revolutions*, 182; and Kohler ads (quote), Ayer Collection, Box 305 (National Museum of American History Archives, Smithsonian Institution, Washington, D.C.).

57. "The Great Housing Shortage," *Life*, Dec. 24, 1945, p. 27 (quote); Herbert J. Gans, *The Levittowners: Ways of Life and Politics in a New Suburban Community* (New York: Pantheon, 1967), 284–86; and Jackson, *Crabgrass Frontier*, 233.

58. W. D. Wetherell, *The Man Who Loved Levittown* (New York: Avon, 1985), 3.

59. Jackson, *Crabgrass Frontier*, 234–35; Halberstam, *The Fifties*, 135 (quote); and Barbara M. Kelly, *Expanding the American Dream: Building and Rebuilding Levittown* (Albany: State Univ. of New York Press, 1993), 44 (quote).

60. Quotations can be found in Kelly, *Expanding the American Dream*, 44; and in Harvey, *The Fifties: A Women's Oral History*, 113–14. See also Jackson, *Crabgrass Frontier*, 236–37.

61. Gilbert, *Another Chance*, 105–7; Alexander O. Boulton, "The Buy of the Century," *American Heritage* 44 (July-Aug. 1993): 65; and Jackson, *Crabgrass Frontier*, 238–41 (quote).

62. For a detailed discussion of how owners of Levittown houses changed them, see Kelly, *Expanding the American Dream*, 119–47. See also M. Susan Bland, "Henrietta the Homemaker, and 'Rosie the Riveter': Images of Women in Advertising in *Maclean*'s Magazine, 1939–50," *Atlantis* 8 (Spring 1983): 67–70; Maytag and Schick ads (quotes), *Life*, Oct. 1 and Nov. 19, 1945, pp. 125 and 46 respectively.

63. Clifford E. Clark, Jr., "Ranch-House Suburbia: Ideals and Realities," in Lary May, ed., *Recasting America: Culture and Politics in the Age of Cold War* (Chicago: Univ. of Chicago Press, 1989), 181; "Dream House," *Life*, May 6, 1946, p. 86; and Alice McDermott, *That Night* (New York: Harper & Row, 1987), 97.

64. Kelly, *Expanding the American Dream*, 96–97; Clark, "Ranch-House Subur-

bia," 179; "Dream House," 84 (quote); Margolis, *Mothers and Such*, 166; and General Electric dishwasher ad, *Life*, May 27, 1946, p. 5 (quote).

65. Friedan, *Feminine Mystique*, 233–57, esp. 241. "Shows how much you care" appears in an All dishwasher-soap ad in *Ladies' Home Journal*, March 1956, p. 171.

66. See Marshall McLuhan, "How Not to Offend," *The Mechanical Bride: Folklore of Industrial Man* (New York: Vanguard, 1951), 60–62. The quotations are from a number of ads: Sani-Flush scouring powder, Ayer Collection, Box 425; Air-wick, *Life*, Jan. 6, 1950, p. 4; Dutch Cleanser, ibid., May 3, 1954, p. 84; and Arm & Hammer baking soda (for "a sweet refrigerator"), *Ladies' Home Journal*, July 1951, p. 117.

67. "Billions of Dollars for Prettiness," *Life*, Dec. 24, 1956, p. 121. The material on the kitchen garbage disposer is taken, with permission, from Suellen Hoy, "The Garbage Disposer, the Public Health, and the Good Life," *Technology and Culture* 26 (Oct. 1985): 758–84.

68. Quotations appear in a variety of ads: Kotex, *Life*, Jan. 9, 1950, p. 50; Tampax, ibid., Aug. 3, 1959, p. 80; and Veto deodorant, ibid., May 6, 1957, p. 203. See also Jane Celia Busch, "The Throwaway Ethic in America" (Ph.D. dissertation, Univ. of Pennsylvania, 1983), 100–104; and Harvey, *The Fifties: A Women's Oral History*, xv. Women generally did not remove hair from legs or underarms before World War I. Only when fashions changed—first with the appearance of evening gowns, then sheer stockings—did women begin to shave. Ads, for the most part, stressed fashion rather than hygiene; occasionally, though, they mentioned mild perspiration odors that underarm growth somehow harbored. See Christine Hope, "Caucasian Female Body Hair and American Culture," *Journal of American Culture* 5 (Spring 1982): 93–99, esp. 97.

69. According to the National Advertising Review Board (1971), women on television were often "depicted as obsessed with cleanliness, as being embarrassed or feeling inadequate or guilty because of various forms of household dirt." Quoted in United States Commission on Civil Rights, *Window Dressing on the Set: Women and Minorities in Television* (Washington, D.C.: Government Printing Office, 1977), 13. See also another series of ads: Dial, *Life*, July 6, 1957, p. 39; Gleem, *Life*, May 13, 1957; Tide, *Ladies' Home Journal*, March 1951, n.p.

70. Gilbert, *Another Chance*, 27; John Duffy, *The Sanitarians: A History of American Public Health* (Urbana: Univ. of Illinois Press, 1990), 280–83; and Stanley Lebergott, *Pursuing Happiness: American Consumers in the Twentieth Century* (Princeton, N.J.: Princeton Univ. Press, 1993), 98–101.

71. Beth L. Bailey, *From Front Porch to Back Seat: Courtship in Twentieth-Century America* (Baltimore: Johns Hopkins Univ. Press, 1988), 10; Harvey, *The Fifties: A Women's Oral History*, xvii; Sidonie Matsner Gruenberg, "Will They Ever Be Neat and Clean?," *Parents' Magazine* 34 (Nov. 1959): 145–46; "Have *you* got what it takes to be popular?," *Seventeen*, Nov. 1955, p. 158; "Dial soap keeps complexions clearer by keeping skin cleaner!," ibid., Feb. 1952, p. 24; Wini Breines, *Young, White, and Miserable: Growing Up Female in the Fifties* (Boston: Beacon Press, 1992), 95; Mintz and Kellogg, *Domestic Revolutions*, 181; and Joseph F. Kett, *Rites of Passage: Adolescence in America, 1790 to the Present* (New York: Basic Books, 1977), 265 (quote).

72. Listerine ad, *Life*, June 7, 1954, p. 155; Bailey, *From Front Porch to Back Seat*, 71–73; "Getting and Spending the Teen-Age Allowance," *Life*, May 13, 1957,

p. 150; Breines, *Young, White, and Miserable*, 95; and Dial ad, *Life*, June 16, 1950, p. 9.

73. On the 1952 poll, see Bailey, *From Front Porch to Back Seat*, 11. See also Daniel J. Boorstin, "Welcome to the Consumption Community," *Fortune* 76 (Sept. 1, 1967): 132–38; and Paul Fussell, *Class: A Guide through the American Status System* [1983] (New York: Simon & Schuster, 1992), 39.

74. Lebergott, *Pursuing Happiness*, 101–2; "Cleanliness: The Germ's Last Stand?," *Newsweek*, Nov. 24, 1958, p. 99; and Michael Harrington, *The Other America: Poverty in the United States* (New York: Macmillan, 1962).

75. Edna Ferber is quoted in the *New York Times*, Dec. 6, 1954. William C. Stolk, chairman of the newly created Keep America Beautiful, called Americans' habit of littering "a national disgrace." See ibid., Oct. 14, 1954.

76. Samuel P. Hays, *Beauty, Health, and Permanence: Environmental Politics in the United States, 1955–1985* (Cambridge: Cambridge Univ. Press, 1987), 22–26; and Suellen Hoy and Michael C. Robinson, *Recovering the Past: A Handbook of Community Recycling Programs, 1890–1945* (Chicago: Public Works Historical Society, 1979), 1–5.

77. John B. Rae, *The American Automobile: A Brief History* (Chicago: Univ. of Chicago Press, 1965), 176; and Virginia Scharff, *Taking the Wheel: Women and the Coming of the Motor Age* (New York: Free Press, 1991), 137-38, 150.

78. Martin V. Melosi, *Garbage in the Cities: Refuse, Reform, and the Environment, 1880–1980* (College Station: Texas A&M Univ. Press, 1981), 210–11; and Busch, "The Throwaway Ethic in America," esp. 124–27.

79. Harrison Salisbury, "City Wages Constant Battle to Keep Streets Litter Free," *New York Times*, Dec. 6, 1954.

80. "Minutes of Organization Meeting of 'Keep Our Roadsides Clean Council,'" Oct. 15, 1953; "Minutes of Second Organization Meeting of 'Keep Our Roadsides Clean Council,'" Nov. 13, 1953; and "Minutes of Third Organization Meeting of Keep America Beautiful, Inc.," Dec. 17, 1953 (Archives, Keep America Beautiful, Inc., Stamford, Conn.). I am grateful to Roger Powers who responded to my questions and gave me copies of these minutes.

81. Ibid., Dec. 17, 1953; and "Minutes of First Meeting of Advisory Council to the Board of Directors of Keep America Beautiful, Inc.," May 26, 1954.

82. Philip Shabecoff, *A Fierce Green Fire: The American Environmental Movement* (New York: Hill and Wang, 1993), 90 (quote), 111–20; and "Minutes of Meeting of Advisory Council to the Board of Directors of Keep America Beautiful, Inc." (quote), Nov. 19, 1954.

83. Melosi, *Garbage in the Cities*, 213–14; "A Clean Sweep in Georgia," *Time*, May 19, 1980, p. 51; APWA Research Foundation, *Cost/Benefit Analysis of Selected Clean Community System Cities* (Chicago: American Public Works Association, 1982), 1–10; and Keep America Beautiful, Inc., "The Ten-Year Assessment of the Behavioral Foundations of the Keep America Beautiful System," pamphlet, Dec. 1986, pp. 5–10.

84. Timothy Miller, *The Hippies and American Values* (Knoxville: Univ. of Tennessee Press, 1991), 109, 111–12; 116–18; and "Youth: The Hippies," *Time*, July 7, 1967, pp. 18–22.

85. The quotations can be found in Todd Gitlin, *The Sixties: Years of Hope, Days of Rage* (New York: Bantam, 1987), 215, 217.

86. Ibid., 216; and Edward P. Morgan, *The 60s Experience: Hard Lessons about Modern America* (Philadelphia: Temple Univ. Press, 1991), 232, 241.

87. John Steele Gordon, "The American Environment," *American Heritage* 44 (Oct. 1993): 45 (quote); Rachel Carson, *Silent Spring* (Boston: Houghton Mifflin, 1962), 3 (quote); and Shabecoff, *A Fierce Green Fire*, 107–9.

88. On women sanitarians and conservationists, see Suellen Hoy, " 'Municipal Housekeeping': The Role of Women in Improving Urban Sanitation Practices, 1880–1917," in Martin V. Melosi, ed., *Pollution and Reform in American Cities, 1870–1930* (Austin: Univ. of Texas Press, 1980), 173–98; and Carolyn Merchant, "Women of the Progressive Conservation Movement: 1900–1916," *Environmental Review* 8 (Spring 1984): 57–85. See also Paul Brooks, "Rachel Carson," in Barbara Sicherman and Carol Hurd Green, eds., *Notable American Women: The Modern Period* (Cambridge: Belknap Press of Harvard Univ. Press, 1980), 139 and 140 (quotes); and Lewis L. Gould, *Lady Bird Johnson and the Environment* (Lawrence: Univ. of Kansas Press, 1988), 1–6.

89. Gould, *Lady Bird Johnson*, 228 (quote), 243–45 (quote on p. 244); and Hays, *Beauty, Health, and Permanence*, 53.

90. Morgan, *The 60s Experience*, 242 (quote); and Shabecoff, *A Fierce Green Fire*, 129–41.

91. Gordon, "American Environment," 47–51. See also Shabecoff, *A Fierce Green Fire*, 142–48; Dena Kleiman, "Recycling Household Trash: A Chore Becomes a Cause," *New York Times*, July 26, 1989; John Schall, "Recycling, Minus the Myths," ibid., Aug. 22, 1992; Joseph Berger, "New York City Fights Road Squalor," ibid., April 28, 1990; "The (Dirty) Sidewalks of New York," ibid., May 17, 1991; and Matthew Wald, "Guarding Environment: A World of Challenges—Earth Day at 20," ibid., April 22, 1990.

POSTSCRIPT

1. Molly O'Neill, "Drop the Mop, Bless the Mess: The Decline of Housekeeping," *New York Times*, April 11, 1993; Carolyn Swartz, "Hers: All That Glitters Is the Tub," *New York Times Magazine*, Nov. 5, 1989 (quote). See also Barbara Ehrenreich, "Housekeeping Is Obsolescent," *Time*, Oct. 25, 1993, p. 92; Lynne Cascio, "Cleanliness Is Next to . . . Insanity," *Air Destinations* 2 (April 1989): 25–26; and Carroll Stoner, "Dollhouses," in Laurie Abraham, Mary Beth Danielson, Nancy Eberle, Laura Green, Janice Rosenberg, and Carroll Stoner, eds., *Reinventing Home: Six Working Women Look at Their Home Lives* (New York: Plume of Penguin Books, 1991), 27–28.

2. Ruth Sidel, *On Her Own: Growing Up in the Shadow of the American Dream* (New York: Viking, 1990), 169–92, esp. pp. 170, 179, 182, 186. See also Susan Chira, "New Realities Fight Old Images of Mother," and Tamar Lewin, "Rise in Single Parenthood is Reshaping U.S.," *New York Times*, Oct. 4 and 5, 1992. Both were part of a series on "The Good Mother."

3. Marian Burros, "Even Women at Top Still Have Floors to Do," *New York Times*, May 31, 1993; Rebecca Piirto, "New Women's Revolution," *American Demographics* 13 (April 1991): 6 (quote); Arlie Hochschild with Anne Machung, *The Second Shift* (New York: Avon, 1989), 6–9 (quote, p. 8). See also Heidi I. Hartmann,

"The Family as the Locus of Gender, Class, and Political Struggle: The Example of Housework," *Signs* 6 (Spring 1981): 386–94.

4. "The Superwoman's Syndrome," *McCall's*, July 1986, p. 93. Quotations are from: Lisa Belkin, "In Busy Lives, Housework Is No Longer a Top Priority," *New York Times*, April 11, 1985; Steven D. Stark, "Housekeeping Today: A Lick and a Promise," ibid., Aug. 20, 1987; and Douglas Martin, "For Many Fathers, Roles Are Shifting," ibid., June 20, 1993. See also Ruth Schwartz Cowan, *More Work for Mother: The Ironies of Household Technology from the Open Hearth to the Microwave* (New York: Basic Books, 1983), 217–19.

5. Phyllis Palmer, *Domesticity and Dirt: Housewives and Domestic Servants in the United States, 1920–1945* (Philadelphia: Temple Univ. Press, 1989), 156–60; and Michael Kelly, "Household Hiring Is Trickier with New Broom in Capital," *New York Times*, Feb. 12, 1993.

6. Michael J. McDermott, "The Boom Continues in Cleaning Franchises," *The Franchise Handbook* (Fall 1992), 21–24; Deborah Blumenthal, "Coping with Spring Cleaning," *New York Times*, March 18, 1989; James Barron, "Spring Cleaning Is Giving Way to Age of Dirt," ibid., April 19, 1990; Lynie Arden, "Profitable Maids All in a Row," *Income Opportunities* (Sept. 1992), 87; and "Maid Services Mop Up," *Executive Female* (March/April 1992), 26. I am grateful to Paul M. Wiljanen in Ann Arbor, Michigan, for sending me information on Molly Maid.

7. Dolores Hayden, *The Grand Domestic Revolution: A History of Feminist Designs for American Homes, Neighborhoods, and Cities* (Cambridge, Mass.: MIT Press, 1981), esp. pp. 299–305. See also Cowan, *More Work for Mother*, 149–50; and Juliet B. Schor, *The Overworked American: The Unexpected Decline of Leisure* (New York: Basic Books, 1992), 99–103.

8. For a full understanding of how housewives lost their self-esteem, see Glenna Matthews, *"Just a Housewife": The Rise and Fall of Domesticity in America* (New York: Oxford Univ. Press, 1987). See also Women's Liberation Movement, "Help Wanted: Female, 99.6 Hours a Week," *Ladies' Home Journal*, Aug. 1970, p. 67; and Abraham et al., eds., *Reinventing Home*, 3–4 (quote). Thanks to the women's movement, income-earning opportunities expanded for some women during this period, and many others, despite their low-salaried jobs, found new sources of support and self-esteem in feminism. See, for example, Vivian Gornick, "Who Says We Haven't Made a Revolution? A Feminist Takes Stock," *New York Times Magazine*, April 15, 1990, pp. 52–53. The final quotation appears in "This Task Above All," *New York Times*, Aug. 20, 1987.

INDEX